MANUAL OF TRAUMA MANAGEMENT IN THE DOG AND CAT

MANUAL OF TRAUMA MANAGEMENT IN THE DOG AND CAT

EDITORS

KENNETH J. DROBATZ, DVM, MSCE, DACVIM, DACVECC

Professor, Section of Critical Care
School of Veterinary Medicine
University of Pennsylvania
Philadelphia, PA 19104

MATTHEW W. BEAL, DVM, DACVECC

Associate Professor; Emergency and Critical Care Medicine
Director of Interventional Radiology Services
College of Veterinary Medicine
Michigan State University
East Lansing, MI 48824-1314

REBECCA S. SYRING, DVM, DACVECC

Staff Veterinarian, Section of Critical Care
School of Veterinary Medicine
University of Pennsylvania
Philadelphia, PA 19104

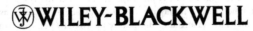

WILEY-BLACKWELL

A John Wiley & Sons, Ltd., Publication

Wiley-Blackwell is an imprint of John Wiley & Sons, formed by the merger of Wiley's global Scientific, Technical and Medical business with Blackwell Publishing.

Registered office: John Wiley & Sons Ltd, The Atrium, Southern Gate, Chichester, West Sussex, PO19 8SQ, UK

Editorial offices: 2121 State Avenue, Ames, Iowa 50014-8300, USA
9600 Garsington Road, Oxford, OX4 2DQ, UK

For details of our global editorial offices, for customer services and for information about how to apply for permission to reuse the copyright material in this book please see our website at www.wiley.com/wiley-blackwell.

Library of Congress Cataloging-in-Publication Data

Manual of trauma management of the dog and cat/editors: Kenneth J. Drobatz, Matthew W. Beal, and Rebecca S. Syring.
   p. ; cm.
   Includes bibliographical references.
   ISBN 978-0-470-95831-5 (pbk. : alk. paper)
   1. Veterinary traumatology–Handbooks, manuals, etc.   2. Dogs–Wounds and injuries–Handbooks, manuals, etc.   3. Cats–Wounds and injuries–Handbooks, manuals, etc.   I. Drobatz, Kenneth J.   II. Beal, Matthew W.   III. Syring, Rebecca S.
   [DNLM: 1. Wounds and Injuries–veterinary–Outlines.   2. Cats–Outlines.   3. Dogs–Outlines.   4. Wounds and Injuries–therapy–Outlines. SF 914.3]
   SF914.3.M36 2011
   636.089'71–dc22

                                                                            2010039464

A catalogue record for this book is available from the British Library.

This book is published in the following electronic formats: eBook 9780470959299; ePub 9780470959305

Set in 9.5/11.5pt Berkeley by Aptara® Inc., New Delhi, India

Disclaimer

1   2011

I would like to dedicate this book to my mother and father, who taught me to have a strong work ethic, to be kind to others, and to have a strong loyalty and love for friends and family. Their level of generosity and caring is certainly a goal to strive for but one that will likely be too high for me to ever achieve.

Ken Drobatz

To my mentors Ken Drobatz, Dez Hughes, Cindy Otto, and Lesley King, for their wisdom, enthusiasm, guidance, and encouragement.

To my colleagues in the ECCM Service at MSU both past and present for making it fun to come to work each day.

To the veterinary nurses and technicians for their caring and expertise. We couldn't do our job without you.

And to my family for their love and support.

Matt Beal

To the doctors and veterinary nurses who I have worked with over the years, who have provided me immeasurable mentorship and assistance.

To my family, who has provided me with endless support through these endeavors.

Rebecca Syring

CONTENTS

PREFACE

Trauma is one of the most common problems that dogs and cats encounter. Traumatic injuries range in severity from the simple breaking of a toenail to massive, life-threatening blunt or penetrating injuries involving multiple organ systems. Emergency veterinarians and criticalists are truly specialists in trauma. Traditionally, trauma has always fallen into the surgeon's arena since they induce tissue trauma on a daily basis through their surgical manipulations. As the field of traumatology has evolved, there is greater understanding of the systemic physiologic affects of massive trauma that may contribute as much, if not more, to the clinical consequences experienced by the animal than just the inciting incident. As this greater understanding of trauma developed, so in parallel did the development of the specialty of Emergency and Critical Care Medicine. These parallel developments resulted in veterinary Emergency and Critical Care specialists taking a major interest in the treatment of trauma patients. The field has developed rapidly, yet we are only beginning to understand the full ramifications of trauma and what it can do. As specialists in this area, we find the full understanding of this field of medicine daunting despite our clear focus on it. Yet, emergency and critical care specialists are not the only veterinarians to see these patients. General practitioners see traumatized patients on a daily basis. General practitioners are truly the veterinarians who "work in the trenches" and have the best global understanding of all conditions affecting the health of animals. The requirement for global understanding is very challenging, and hence, it is impossible to have an intimate understanding of every condition—trauma being one of them. With this realization, we have developed a manual that applies a practical approach to traumatized patients. We have produced it in a logical and easily accessible organization that provides rapid but adequately detailed information about the general approach to the trauma patient as well information on specific traumatic injuries. Our goal was to make this manual something that the practicing veterinarian can use on the clinic floor to assist in the quick assessment and treatment of these very diverse and challenging patients. We have asked our chapter authors to make their portions clinically useful and as practical as possible, and yet provide an understanding of the underlying principles of what is being written. To this end, we have organized this book into an outline format that provides the essential facts that are necessary to understand and implement the principles in the clinical approach to trauma patients. The initial chapters provide a background in the global assessment of the traumatized patients followed by chapters dealing with very specific types of traumas. It is our hope that the practitioner will find this not an "Ivory Tower Manual" but one that will be used in the "trenches", one that will get dirty and worn out due to its frequent use on the clinic floor.

ACKNOWLEDGMENTS

The editors would like to acknowledge all of our contributors for their diligent and persistent effort in making this book a reality. Additionally, we are most grateful to Lianna Drobatz for her assistance in some of the medical illustrations and Dr. Garret Pachtinger for his help on formatting many of the images. A book is only as good as its contributors and this final product reflects the high standards of our fine collaborators.

Manual of Trauma Management in the Dog and Cat

CONTRIBUTOR LIST

Matthew W. Beal, DVM, DACVECC
Associate Professor, Emergency and Critical Care
  Medicine
Director of Interventional Radiology Services
College of Veterinary Medicine
Michigan State University
East Lansing, Michigan

Benjamin M. Brainard, VMD, DACVA, DACVECC
Assistant Professor, Critical Care
Department of Small Animal Medicine and Surgery
University of Georgia
Athens, Georgia

Andrew J. Brown, MA, VetMB, DACVECC, MRCVS
VetsNow Referral Hospital
123-145 North Street
Glasgow
G3 7DA
SCOTLAND

Dana L. Clarke, VMD, DACVECC
Lecturer in Emergency and Critical Care
Fellow in Interventional Radiology
Department of Small Animal Clinical Sciences
University of Pennsylvania
Philadelphia, Pennsylvania

Merilee F. Costello, DVM, DACVECC
Staff Criticalist
Boston Road Animal Hospital
Springfield, MA

William T. Culp, VMD, DACVS
Assistant Professor, Small Animal Surgery
Department of Surgical and Radiological Sciences
School of Veterinary Medicine
University of California
Davis, California

Kenneth J. Drobatz, DVM, MSCE, DACVIM, DACVECC
Professor, Section of Critical Care
School of Veterinary Medicine
University of Pennsylvania
Philadelphia, Pennsylvania

Daniel J. Fletcher, PhD, DVM, DACVECC
Assistant Professor of Emergency and Critical Care
Cornell University College of Veterinary Medicine
Ithaca, New York

David E. Holt, BVSc, DACVS
Professor of Surgery
Department of Clinical Studies
School of Veterinary Medicine
University of Pennsylvania
Philadelphia, Pennsylvania

John R. Lewis, VMD, FAVD, DAVDC
Assistant Professor of Dentistry and Oral Surgery
Department of Clinical Studies
School of Veterinary Medicine
University of Pennsylvania
Philadelphia, Pennsylvania

Deborah C. Mandell, VMD, DACVECC
Staff Criticalist, Emergency Service
Adjunct Assistant Professor
Department of Clinical Studies
School of Veterinary Medicine
University of Pennsylvania
Philadelphia, Pennsylvania

Lauren R. May, VMD, DACVS
Staff Surgeon
Department of Surgery
Veterinary Specialists of Rochester
Rochester, New York

Philipp D. Mayhew, BVM&S, MRCVS, DACVS
Assistant Professor, Small Animal Surgery
Department of Surgical and Radiological Sciences
School of Veterinary Medicine
University of California–Davis
Davis, California

Charles S. McBrien Jr., DVM, MS
Northeast Veterinary Referral Hospital
Plains, PA

Stephen J. Mehler, DVM, DACVS
Staff Surgeon
Department of Surgery
Veterinary Specialists of Rochester
Rochester, New York

Alexander M. Reiter, Dipl. Tzt., Dr. med. vet., DAVDC, DEVDC
Associate Professor of Dentistry and Oral Surgery
Department of Clinical Studies
School of Veterinary Medicine
University of Pennsylvania
Philadelphia, Pennsylvania

Jessica M. Snyder, DVM, DACVIM (Neurology)
Staff Neurologist
Department of Neurology
VCA Veterinary Specialty Center of Seattle
Lynnwood, Washington

Lindsey Beth Culp Snyder, DVM, MS, DACVA
Clinical Assistant Professor, Anesthesia and Pain
  Management
Department of Surgical Sciences
University of Wisconsin—Madison
Madison, Wisconsin

Rebecca S. Syring, DVM, DACVECC
Staff Criticalist, Section of Critical Care
School of Veterinary Medicine
University of Pennsylvania
Philadelphia, Pennsylvania

GLOBAL APPROACH TO THE TRAUMA PATIENT

Kenneth J. Drobatz

1. GLOBAL APPROACH TO THE TRAUMA PATIENT

a. Trauma is defined as a "wound or injury" and may occur secondary to motor vehicle accidents, fall from heights, animal interactions, human-animal interactions, etc. Severity may range from mild to fatal. Trauma may affect only one organ system or multiple organ systems, either directly or indirectly. Therefore, a global and thorough approach is required to improve survival and decrease morbidity in trauma patients.

b. Initial assessment of the trauma patient occurs quickly but can theoretically be broken down into two major phases; primary survey and secondary survey:

    i. Primary survey is the assessment of the respiratory and cardiovascular systems, followed by assessment of the central nervous system and urinary tract system.

    ii. Secondary survey is assessment of all other systems once the animal's most immediately life-threatening problems, identified during the primary survey, are dealt with.

c. The primary goal in attending to a critically injured trauma patient is to optimize oxygen delivery to the tissues. In fact, during the initial approach and resuscitation of these patients, all procedures are oriented toward this goal. Oxygen delivery is dependent upon cardiac output,

hemoglobin concentration, and oxygen saturation of hemoglobin. It is important to optimize these variables at all times.

2. BRIEF PATHOPHYSIOLOGY

a. Traumatic shock results in a maldistribution of blood flow because of increased circulating catecholamines, hypovolemia, and increased vasoactive hormones.

b. Persistent microcirculatory perfusion failure may lead to sludging of blood and increased cellular and platelet aggregation.

c. Endothelial injury due to trauma may result in release of inflammatory mediators and stimulation of coagulation.

d. Damaged cellular membranes, due to poor perfusion or direct trauma, result in release of phospholipids. The enzymes phospholipase, cyclooxygenase, and lipoxygenase produce thromboxane and leukotrienes:

    i. Thromboxane causes vasoconstriction, further compromising tissue perfusion and stimulating platelet aggregation.

    ii. Leukotrienes and activation of the complement cascade propagates the inflammatory response with mobilization and activation of neutrophils.

    iii. Neutrophil release of lysosomal enzymes and toxic oxygen metabolites cause further cellular damage, leading to edema with subsequent

Manual of Trauma Management in the Dog and Cat, First Edition. Edited by Kenneth J. Drobatz, Matthew W. Beal and Rebecca S. Syring.

increase of oxygen diffusion distance to the cells from the capillaries.

    iv. Optimizing tissue oxygen delivery will minimize the perpetuation of these inflammation-producing cascades.

3. ASSESSING AND MAINTAINING OXYGEN SATURATION OF HEMOGLOBIN—THE RESPIRATORY SYSTEM

    a. At presentation, supplemental oxygen should be provided to the severely affected trauma patient until assessment of an arterial blood gas or measurement of hemoglobin saturation confirms that oxygen supplementation is not required:

        i. Clinical signs of respiratory compromise include increased respiratory rate or effort, flail chest, pale or cyanotic mucous membranes, increased heart rate, increased upper airway sounds, or altered lower airway sounds (increased or decreased airways sounds). If these signs are present, oxygen supplementation is essential.

    b. Physical assessment of the respiratory system (Figure 1.1):

        i. Look:

            1. Signs of respiratory compromise include increased respiratory rate and effort, restlessness, extended head and neck, abducted elbows, and paradoxic movement of the chest and abdominal walls (normally should move in and out together but with paradoxical movement they move in opposite directions).

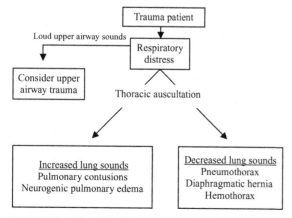

FIGURE 1.1 Algorithm for assessment of the patient with respiratory distress following trauma.

            2. Remember: animals in severe respiratory distress do not have to have all of these signs (especially cats), *but* if they do have all of these signs they have severe respiratory compromise.

        ii. Listen:

            1. Loud upper airway sounds heard without the stethoscope indicate upper airway compromise (from the carina forward).

            2. Traumatic causes of upper airway problems include cervical tracheal crush injury (bite wounds are most common), pharyngeal injury (swelling/bleeding), and tracheal avulsion (see Chapter 6: Trauma-Associated Thoracic Injury):

                a. Note that nasal airway injuries and frontal sinus injuries can result in bleeding into the nasal passages, causing upper airway sounds. Despite this problem, most animals do not suffer respiratory compromise from these injuries.

            3. Decreased air sounds on auscultation:

                a. Indicates pleural space disease.

                b. Traumatic causes of pleural space disease:

                    i. Pneumothorax (most common)

                    ii. Diaphragmatic hernia

                    iii. Severe hemothorax (least common)

                c. Thoracocentesis:

                    i. If the patient is in respiratory distress and you cannot hear the lung sounds well, then thoracocentesis is warranted.

            4. Increased lung sounds on auscultation (not the upper airway sounds referred to earlier):

                a. Indicate lower airway/pulmonary parenchymal injury:

                  i. Pulmonary contusions:

                    1. Therapy for pulmonary contusions is largely supportive with caution on overzealous fluid therapy.

            5. Open chest wound/"sucking" chest wound:

                a. Open wounds connecting to the pleural space should be immediately covered with a sterile bandage, which will create a seal, and thoracocentesis should then be performed to remove the residual air.

b. If respiratory distress persists, intubation and positive pressure ventilation should be provided until the wounds can be surgically repaired.

6. Flail chest:

a. Recognized by paradoxic movement of the chest wall. The flail segment moves in on inspiration and is a result of a "floating" segment of the chest wall because consecutive ribs are broken in more than one place.

b. Primary physiologic consequences are pain and underlying lung damage and pleural space injury in most instances.

4. ASSESSING CARDIAC OUTPUT/TISSUE PERFUSION

a. Initial assessment of adequate cardiac output and circulating volume includes mucous membrane color, capillary refill time, pulse rate, and quality:

i. Abnormalities indicating poor tissue perfusion

1. Pale or gray mucous membranes
2. Prolonged capillary refill time (>1–2 seconds)
3. Weak and rapid pulses

b. Measurement of arterial blood pressure directly or indirectly by Doppler or oscillometric techniques should be performed when possible:

i. A Doppler systolic blood pressure of <80 is suggestive of decreased tissue perfusion.

ii. A mean arterial pressure of <60 mm Hg is suggestive of decreased tissue perfusion.

iii. It should be kept in mind that blood pressure may be normal or even high and peripheral tissue perfusion could still be inadequate for the body's requirements.

c. More objective evaluation is obtained by pulmonary artery catheter placement and actual measurement of cardiac output, oxygen delivery, and oxygen consumption; although this is uncommonly done in veterinary emergency medicine and carries its own complications.

d. The most common cause of poor tissue perfusion in the trauma patient is hypovolemia from blood loss:

i. Most common areas for hemorrhage causing hypovolemia are in order of frequency; the peritoneal space, retroperitoneal space, thigh musculature, pleural space, external, or a combination of spaces (e.g., retroperitoneal and peritoneal spaces).

e. The less common causes of poor tissue perfusion are cardiac arrhythmias, tension pneumothorax, diaphragmatic hernia, peritoneopericardial diaphragmatic hernia, and cardiac tamponade due to hemopericardium from traumatic atrial rupture.

f. Therapy of poor tissue perfusion:

i. Thoracocentesis if a tension pneumothorax is present (this is extremely rare).

ii. Intravenous fluids/colloids/blood products/hemoglobin substitutes:

1. Caution with fluids when pulmonary contusions are present.

5. ASSESSMENT OF THE NEUROLOGIC SYSTEM

a. It is important to assess brain function at presentation to obtain a baseline for potential dynamic changes that may occur.

b. Conclusions regarding brain and neurologic function (brain and spinal cord) should be withheld until perfusion is adequate and function is reassessed:

i. Profound neurologic changes may be found with poor tissue perfusion and corrected once tissue perfusion is improved.

c. Assessment of brain function:

i. Mentation:

1. Grades of mentation:

a. Excited/agitated

b. Normal

c. Depressed

d. Obtunded (markedly decreased level of consciousness, but arousable with auditory or tactile stimulation)

e. Stupor (unconscious but responds to noxious stimuli)

f. Coma (unconscious and does not respond to noxious stimuli)

2. Cranial nerve assessment:

a. Assessment of facial sensation, jaw tone (be careful with jaw fractures), eye position and movement, papillary light responses, menace reflex, eye blink, and gag reflex.

3. Evidence of potential brain injury:
   a. Obvious head trauma (skull fractures, bleeding from ear, jaw fractures, scleral, or ocular hemorrhage, etc.)
   b. Altered mentation
   c. Altered cranial nerve function
4. General principles of treating brain injury:
   a. Primary injury (direct trauma to tissues)—no specific treatment for this.
   b. Secondary injury (swelling, inflammation, reperfusion injury, increased intracranial pressure):
       i. Maintain good perfusion/blood pressure (MAP at least 80 mm Hg, systolic at least 90 mm Hg).
       ii. Maintain good oxygenation via oxygen supplementation, ventilation, etc. ($PaO_2 > 80$ mm Hg, $SpO_2 > 95\%$).
       iii. Hyperosmotics:
           1. Mannitol
           2. Hypertonic saline/colloid combination to treat decreased blood pressure and poor tissue perfusion
       iv. Elevate head 30° from horizontal if increased intracranial pressure is suspected.
d. Assessing spinal cord function:
    i. Ensure that tissue perfusion is adequate.
    ii. Palpate full length of the spine and pelvis.
    iii. Note the voluntary movement of all legs.
    iv. Assess the ability to stand/ambulate.
    v. Check anal tone and anal reflex.
    vi. Check proprioception of limbs.
    vii. Assess limb reflexes.
    viii. Evidence of spinal cord injury:
        1. Spinal or sacral fractures/displacement
        2. Spinal pain
        3. Changes in limb function or sensation.
        4. Change in tail tone, bladder, or anal sphincter function
    ix. General principles of treating spinal cord injury:
        1. Stabilization of fractures/luxations
        2. Decompression surgery (e.g., hemilaminectomy for ruptured intervertebral disk)
        3. Corticosteroids (controversial)
        4. Time

6. **ASSESSING THE RENAL SYSTEM**
   a. Physical assessment of the urinary tract is limited to palpation of the urinary bladder and kidneys.
   b. Urinary tract injury seems to occur more commonly with pelvic fractures.
   c. BUN and serum creatinine may not have substantial increases until several hours after urinary tract rupture or injury.
   d. Hematuria indicates urinary tract injury.
   e. Manifestations of renal damage may not be immediately evident at presentation and may not be detected until several hours later, after continuous monitoring.
   f. Potential trauma-induced urinary tract injuries:
       i. Kidney contusions, rupture, or avulsion
       ii. Renal pelvis disruption
       iii. Urethral disruption
       iv. Urinary bladder rupture
       v. Urethral trauma/rupture
   g. General therapy for urinary tract trauma:
       i. IV fluid diuresis
       ii. Stabilization of cardiovascular manifestations of urinary tract injury (hyperkalemia)
       iii. Surgical repair and/or urinary diversion of injuries if necessary

7. **SECONDARY SURVEY**
   a. Full physical examination.
   b. Particular attention should be paid to the following:
       i. Musculoskeletal system:
           1. Observe limb function of all four legs.
           2. Observe ambulation.
           3. Complete palpation of appendicular and axial skeleton including rectal examination, palpation of skull, and manipulation of jaw.
       ii. Peripheral nervous system:
           1. Full evaluation of peripheral nerves.
       iii. Examine the animal from the tip of the nose to the tip of the tail.

8. **MONITORING**
   a. Monitoring of all the above systems should be done for at least 24–48 hours for animals that have had significant trauma.

b. Generally, if significant injury has occurred, clinical signs will usually develop within 24–48 hours of the traumatic incident:

    i. Biliary tract rupture can sometimes result in clinical signs several days after the trauma.

    ii. Patients with diaphragmatic hernias may not develop respiratory distress for months to years.

c. The intensity of the monitoring should be proportional to the degree of compromise of the patient.

TRIAGE AND PRIMARY SURVEY

Matthew W. Beal

1. INTRODUCTION

a. Success in the management of small animal emergency patients or dynamic critically ill patients will largely be based on the ability of the veterinary health care team to rapidly identify and manage immediately life-threatening problems.

b. The following pages will focus on facility readiness, triage and major body systems assessment, and the primary survey of the traumatized dog or cat.

2. FACILITY READINESS

a. Infrastructure:

i. Preparedness for small animals presented with potentially life-threatening problems should not just be reserved for emergency hospitals and large referral centers. Through a minimal amount of staff training in the art of triage (see the following), attention to physical examination findings, delegation of responsibilities to the team, and minimal financial outlay for necessary equipment, any veterinary facility can be equipped to handle immediate stabilization of life-threatening problems.

ii. There is no substitute for practice or "mock" emergencies for honing the skills of the team.

b. Initial contact:

i. Emergency management begins at the front desk / receptionist, whether a client is calling on the phone regarding a crisis with a pet, or walking through the front door with an ill or injured pet. Of critical importance to client satisfaction is that the reception personnel display a "can-do" attitude.

ii. Emergencies are not scheduled for appointments. When the client brings a patient through the door, an *immediate* series of events should be triggered beginning with a call to the doctor(s), technicians, or veterinary assistants so that a triage and major body systems assessment can be performed (see the following).

c. Equipment:

i. If, based on triage, the pet is judged to have potentially life-threatening problems, it is immediately moved to the treatment area.

ii. The treatment area should provide ready access for oxygen supplementation and ideally monitoring equipment including an ECG, Doppler blood pressure monitor, and pulse-oximeter. A defibrillator is desirable.

iii. Crash cart versus crash box:

1. A fully stocked "crash cart" is not likely to be practical for the small private practice; however, a large tackle box that is ONLY used for emergencies is an appropriate substitute.

2. The crash box should be restocked after every usage and a seal placed over the latch to document this. The crash box should be opened weekly to check drug expiration dates and to ensure adequate stock of required supplies. These tasks can easily

Manual of Trauma Management in the Dog and Cat, First Edition. Edited by Kenneth J. Drobatz, Matthew W. Beal and Rebecca S. Syring.
© 2011 John Wiley & Sons, Inc. Published 2011 by John Wiley & Sons, Inc.

TABLE 2.1
CRASH CART AND CRASH BOX SUPPLIES. SHADED AREAS DENOTE CRITICAL SUPPLIES

Equipment	Purpose
Laryngoscope + small and large blades	Facilitate difficult intubation
Cuffed endotracheal tubes of sizes 2, 3, 4, 5, 6, 7, 8, 9, 10, 12, 14	Endotracheal intubation of dogs and cats of all sizes
Cuff syringe	Endotracheal tube cuff inflation
Roll gauze	Secure endotracheal tube
Ambu-bag (to be connected to O_2 source)	Positive pressure ventilation with 100% O_2
Epinephrine	CPCR
Atropine	CPCR and bradyarrhythmias
Naloxone 0.4 mg/mL	Reversal of opiates
Calcium gluconate (10%)	Antagonize conduction disturbances associated with hyperkalemia
Reversal agents for any anesthetics commonly utilized (e.g., atipamezole, flumazenil)	Reversal of anesthetics
Small surgical pack (scalpel, mayo scissors, hemostats (3), drape, and tissue forceps)	Emergency thoracotomy, venous cutdown and occlusion of arterial hemorrhage
Sterile gloves	Maintain sterile technique
Scalpel blades (10, 11)	Surgical procedures
Drug dosing scale (based on body weight) for all drugs in box	Quick dose reference
IV catheters (24 g, 22 g, 20 g, 18 g, 16 g, 14g)	Intravenous access for drug and fluid therapy
IV fluid set	Intravenous fluid delivery
Red rubber catheter	Intratracheal drug delivery for CPCR
Syringes and needles of various sizes	Drug delivery
250 mL 0.9% Saline	Flush solution for drug delivery
Butterfly needles (19 g, 21 g)	Feline thoracocentesis
IV extension tubing	Canine thoracocentesis
3-way stopcock	Canine and feline thoracocentesis
22 g and 20 g spinal needles	Intraosseous access in puppies and kittens

be delegated to a technician or veterinary assistant.

3. A crash box should contain the equipment listed in Table 2.1. This equipment will allow the practitioner to maintain an open airway, institute rescue breathing, and carry out all aspects of cardiopulmonary-cerebral resuscitation (CPCR). In addition, the necessary supplies for venous or intraosseous access, the reversal of sedatives and anesthetics, management of pleural space diseases, emergency tracheostomy, control of arterial or severe venous hemorrhage are included.

3. TRIAGE
    a. Definition and philosophy:
      i. Triage is defined as "the process of prioritizing sick or injured people for treatment according to the seriousness of the condition or injury" (Encarta 2001).
      ii. Triage of small animal patients presented for emergent problems or those that appear to be acutely changing during the course of hospitalization will serve the dual purpose of allowing the clinician to prioritize one patient over another, but will also identify life-threatening problems and the need for immediate intervention.

iii. Triage should be performed by trained personnel immediately upon the arrival of a new patient to the hospital.

iv. Triage is performed to rapidly assess patient stability and identify immediately life-threatening problems. Triage should take no more than 30–60 seconds.

v. Triage does not include obtaining a full medical history or performing a complete physical examination.

vi. The end result of triage is a decision as to whether the patient requires one of the following:

1. Immediate care for stabilization of major body systems abnormalities.

2. Immediate further evaluation to better assess patient stability.

3. Evaluation, but not immediately. In this scenario, the patient will be placed in the queue for evaluation based on the seriousness of the perceived problem.

vii. In the authors' practice, a history of trauma always triggers triage for immediate stabilization or the need for further assessment. Trauma patients are physiologically dynamic and their clinical condition can change rapidly.

b. Triage history:

i. Presenting Complaint (PC) is simply the reason for presentation.

ii. Last Normal (LN) refers to when the patient was last normal. In the trauma setting, this will include the date and time of the trauma.

iii. Full medical historical examination is critical, but will be performed at a later time once the primary survey is complete and initial stabilization is underway.

c. Triage technique:

i. The "physical examination" aspects of triage are focused on assessment of the ABCs and on cursory evaluation of the major body systems.

ii. ABCs:

1. A: Does the patient have a patent airway?

2. B: Is the patient breathing?

3. C: Does the patient have spontaneous circulation?

4. A "no" answer to any of these questions will prompt immediate movement of the patient to the treatment area for the initiation of CPCR and further assessment.

iii. Major Body Systems (MBS) assessment focuses on the cardiovascular, respiratory, and central nervous system:

1. Cardiovascular system:

a. The status of the cardiovascular system can be assessed in less than 20 seconds through examination of the following:

i. Mucous membrane color

ii. Capillary refill time (CRT)

iii. Pulse rate

iv. Pulse quality

b. Mucous membrane color:

i. Normal mucous membrane color is pink. However, the patient with compensated hypovolemia may still demonstrate pink mucous membranes.

ii. Pale mucous membranes result from anemia or peripheral vasoconstriction induced by hypovolemia, pain, hypothermia, or stress:

1. The patient with euvolemic anemia may present with pale mucous membranes. An example of this situation is a trauma patient that had acute blood loss, but was stabilized with appropriate intravenous fluid therapy prior to presentation.

2. Identification of pale mucous membranes on triage examination should trigger movement to the treatment area for further evaluation and therapy.

iii. Icteric mucous membranes result from hemolysis, primary hepatic disease, or posthepatic cholestatic disease. Icterus may be seen in the traumatized patient with longstanding (days) biliary disruption.

iv. Brown mucous membranes result from the presence of methemoglobinemia. In the small animal patient, this is most common with acetaminophen ingestion in cats and is uncommon in the trauma patient, unless an owner administered this medication for pain control prior to seeking veterinary care.

v. Cyanotic mucous membranes are present when at least 5 g/dL of hemoglobin is not saturated with oxygen. In a dog or cat with a normal hematocrit, the pulse oximeter will read less than 66% when cyanosis is present. It is critical to recognize that severe hypoxemia may be present even without the presence of cyanosis. For example, a dog with severe pneumothorax and pulmonary contusion that has an SpO_2 of 75% will not be cyanotic. Cyanosis implies *severe* and immediately life-threatening compromise to the respiratory system. Identification of cyanotic mucous membranes on triage examination should trigger movement to the treatment area for oxygen support and further evaluation.

vi. Red mucous membranes are most often associated with vasodilation (vasodilator therapy, sepsis, and hyperthermia). Vasodilatative processes are uncommon in the acute trauma patient. However, a traumatized patient that is presenting hours to days after the inciting injury (Example: massive dog bite injury) may manifest with acute sepsis and peripheral vasodilation. Identification of red mucous membranes should trigger movement to the treatment area for additional evaluation.

c. CRT:

i. CRT is assessed by applying transient gentle pressure to the mucous membrane and evaluating the time for color to "flow" back to the mucous membrane.

ii. CRT should be considered a very crude indicator of cardiac output.

iii. Normal CRT is approximately 1.5 seconds in dogs and cats examined at veterinary hospitals.

iv. CRT may be prolonged in low cardiac output states (hypovolemia due to blood loss) and may be more rapid in high cardiac output states (stress and / or pain not accompanied by severe hypovolemia). A CRT greater than or equal to two seconds in the trauma patient should prompt immediate movement to the treatment area for further assessment.

d. Pulse rate:

i. The pulse rate provides an excellent assessment of the overall status of the cardiovascular system.

ii. Normal pulse rate in the dog is 60–120 bpm.

iii. Normal pulse rate in the cat is 170–220 bpm.

iv. Animals with a normal pulse rate most likely do not have significant compromise to the cardiovascular system.

v. Tachycardia in the traumatized patient may be associated with hypovolemia, pain, stress, anxiety, or excitement. Hypoxemia may also be associated with tachycardia. Tachycardia should prompt movement to the treatment area for assessment for evidence of hypovolemia, hypoxemia, and the management of pain.

vi. Bradycardia is relatively uncommon in the traumatized patient:

1. The patient that has sustained head trauma may demonstrate overt or relative bradycardia due to increased intracranial pressure.

2. The patient that has uroperitoneum may demonstrate overt or relative bradycardia associated with hyperkalemia.

3. Blunt cardiac injury is a very rare cause of bradycardia.

4. Bradycardia should prompt movement of the patient to the treatment area for further assessment.

e. Pulse quality can provide valuable information about the status of the cardiovascular system in the traumatized dog or cat:

i.   The femoral pulse should be assessed in the dog and cat and the dorsal pedal pulse can often be assessed in the dog. The dorsal pedal (dorsal metatarsal) pulse is best palpated just below the hock between the 2nd and 3rd metatarsals.

ii.   Palpation of a pulse pressure is the difference between systolic and diastolic pressure and despite a trend toward blood pressure, is not a very accurate assessment of it. The pulse pressure is influenced by vasomotor tone, stroke volume, and diastolic runoff. In the traumatized patient, decreased stroke volume due to hypovolemia (decreased preload) is the most common cause of poor pulse quality:

1.   Inability to feel the pulse at the dorsal metatarsal region in the dog could imply compromise to the cardiovascular system and should signal the need for further investigation.

2.   Inability to palpate the pulse of a dog or cat at the femoral artery implies life threatening cardiovascular compromise and should be a trigger for immediate movement to the treatment area.

iii.   Pulse quality is very subjective and is something that many individuals have developed a variety of different adjectives to describe:

1.   Pulse quality should be assessed as normal, weaker than normal, or stronger than normal.

2.   In the traumatized patient, weaker than normal pulses may occur in response to conditions including but not limited to hypovolemia. Weaker than normal pulse quality should trigger movement to the treatment area for further evaluation.

3.   In the traumatized patient, stronger-than-normal pulses may occur with euvolemia coupled with sympathetic stimulation due to pain or stress. In addition, peripheral vasodilation and increased cardiac output as seen in patients with sepsis or acute inflammatory conditions may also manifest with stronger-than-normal pulses. Stronger than normal pulse quality should trigger movement to the treatment area for further evaluation.

f.   Abnormalities in the aforementioned criteria (mucous membrane color, CRT, pulse rate, and pulse quality) that trigger movement to the treatment area and immediate further patient assessment are quite strict (and thus highly sensitive) and designed to identify as many patients with potentially life-threatening problems as possible. The downside of such strict criteria is that many patients that do not have life-threatening problems will be subjected to time-consuming further assessment.

g.   Upon movement to the treatment area due to suspicion of cardiovascular compromise, further assessment of the cardiovascular system should focus on the primary survey (see the following) and a full physical examination (secondary survey), blood pressure measurement, and ECG assessment. Oxygen therapy should be delivered to all animals with suspected cardiovascular compromise to help maximize blood oxygen content and thus oxygen delivery to the tissues. Volume expansion is necessary in the hypovolemic patient.

2.   Respiratory system:

a.   The status of the respiratory system can be determined in less than 20 seconds through assessment of the following:

i.   Respiratory rate

ii.   Respiratory effort

b.   A commonly overlooked technique for assessing the respiratory system is simply to "take a step back" and observe the patient (hands off) for 10 seconds (respiratory rate can be taken at this time as well).

c. Respiratory rate:

i. Assessment of the respiratory rate provides an excellent assessment of the overall status of the respiratory system.

ii. Normal respiratory rate for dogs and cats presented in an emergency setting is approximately 20–30 breaths per minute.

iii. As a general rule, a normal respiratory rate makes severe compromise to the respiratory system unlikely.

iv. Tachypnea in the traumatized patient may occur due to compromise to any portion of the respiratory tract from the upper airway to the lungs, pleural space, diaphragm, and chest wall. Pain, stress, anxiety, shock, or a combination thereof may also result in tachypnea. Tachypnea should trigger immediate movement to the treatment area for further assessment of the respiratory system.

d. Respiratory effort:

i. Assessment of respiratory effort may help illustrate the presence of respiratory distress while helping localize the site of the injury(ies) to the respiratory system.

ii. Most patients with respiratory compromise will position themselves sternally. Often, the neck is extended and the elbows are abducted. Observation of this posture should trigger immediate movement to the treatment area for further evaluation and oxygen therapy.

iii. Open-mouth breathing in the cat is seen with respiratory compromise and occasionally with extreme stress. Open-mouth breathing in the cat should trigger immediate movement to the treatment area for further evaluation and oxygen therapy. Open-mouth breathing (panting) in the dog may indicate respiratory compromise or a normal response to pain, stress, excitement, or hyperthermia.

iv. A restricted breathing pattern characterized by frequent short breaths of small tidal volume is common in animals with pleural space disease after trauma (pneumothorax, pleural effusion, and diaphragmatic hernia). A restricted breathing pattern should trigger movement to the treatment area for further evaluation and oxygen therapy.

v. Stridorous breathing may be observed in upper airway obstruction:

1. Inspiratory stridor generally implies dynamic obstruction of the extrathoracic airway.

2. Inspiratory stridor and expiratory stridor generally imply fixed obstruction of the extrathoracic airway.

3. Airway obstruction is not common in the trauma patient but may result from hemorrhage into and around the respiratory system, crushing injury to the larynx and trachea associated with dog bite wounds, tracheal avulsion, head trauma, and other injuries.

4. Airway obstruction is a life-threatening problem necessitating further evaluation, provision of oxygen, and efforts to provide a patent airway.

vi. Paradoxical abdominal movement (PAM) is a subtle finding that may be observed during triage:

1. Normally, during inspiration, the chest wall and abdomen move outward in a synchronous fashion.

2. Normally, during expiration, as the chest wall recoils, the abdomen also moves synchronously inward.

3. During inspiration, animals with PAM will demonstrate outward movement of the thoracic wall and inward movement of the abdomen.

4. In the traumatized patient, PAM implies diaphragmatic disease or dysfunction most

often associated with diaphragmatic hernia. Less frequently, airway obstruction or severe decreases in pulmonary compliance associated with massive pulmonary contusion may also cause PAM in the traumatized patient. PAM should trigger movement to the treatment area for further evaluation and oxygen therapy.

vii. A moist cough or hemoptysis may be observed in animals with severe pulmonary contusion. Cough or hemoptysis in the trauma patient should trigger movement to the treatment area for further evaluation and oxygen therapy.

viii. Upon movement to the treatment area due to suspicion of respiratory compromise, further assessment of the respiratory system should focus on a full physical examination, pulse-oximetry or arterial blood gas analysis, and initial treatment including oxygen administration. Emergency procedures including thoracocentesis may be necessary if pneumothorax or hemothorax is suspected.

3. Central nervous system:

a. A simple assessment of the patient's level of consciousness and the historical question of whether or not the patient was able to walk are appropriate for the triage assessment of the central nervous system.

b. Altered levels of consciousness include obtunded, stuporous, and comatose (see Chapter 7: Traumatic Brain Injury). Hyperexcitable states might also be noted. Any alteration in level of consciousness should prompt movement to the treatment area for further assessment and treatment.

c. The attending clinician should keep in mind that severe cardiovascular compromise may impair delivery of oxygen to the brain and may manifest as an obtunded to a stuporous level of consciousness.

d. Any dog or cat that has sustained trauma, that does not have a history of normal ambulation after trauma, should be treated as if a spinal injury is present. Immobilization should be accomplished immediately.

e. Upon movement to the treatment area due to suspicion of CNS compromise, further assessment should focus on a full physical and neurologic examinations, modified Glasgow coma scoring, and provision of oxygen support and volume expansion measures (if indicated).

4. **PRIMARY SURVEY**

a. Definition and philosophy:

i. The primary survey is considered by the author to be an extension of triage. Whereas the goal of triage is to rapidly evaluate the major body systems to screen for potentially life-threatening problems, the goal of the primary survey is to perform a more in-depth assessment of those major body systems.

ii. In contrast to triage, which is performed by any trained personnel, the attending veterinarian performs the primary survey.

b. Primary survey technique:

i. As previously mentioned, the primary survey should be considered an extension of the triage. All parameters examined on initial triage will be reassessed during the primary survey. In addition, a more in-depth evaluation of the major body systems will be performed.

ii. In human medicine, the primary survey is often approached utilizing the **ABCD** principle. This principle can be appropriately applied in veterinary medicine as well:

1. **A**irway: The veterinarian should assess for the presence of a patent airway. If the airway is not patent or cannot be maintained by the patient, intubation should be performed and positive pressure ventilation instituted at 10–15 breaths per minute utilizing 100% oxygen. Caution should be exercised during intubation of the traumatized patient to minimize movement of the cervical spine and thus prevent exacerbation of injury secondary to spinal trauma.

2. **B**reathing: The veterinarian should assess for the presence of breathing and a

full examination of the respiratory system should be performed:

    a. Respiratory rate (see 3.c.iii.2.)

    b. Respiratory effort (see 3.c.iii.2.)

    c. Palpation and visual inspection of the neck and chest should be performed. Abnormalities to be noted include, but are not limited to, bruising, full thickness skin wounds, subcutaneous emphysema, subcutaneous fluid accumulation, displacement of a rib/ribs, sternal irregularities, and paradoxical movement of a floating thoracic segment (flail chest).

    d. Auscultation of the chest should be performed to evaluate for pulmonary parenchymal or pleural space injuries:

        i. Pleural space injuries (pneumothorax, hemothorax, chylothorax, and diaphragmatic hernia) cause decreased lung sounds.

        ii. Pulmonary parenchymal injuries (pulmonary contusion) generally are associated with increased lung sounds.

        iii. For a complete summary of assessment of the respiratory system in the traumatized patient; see Chapter 6: Trauma-Associated Thoracic Injury.

    e. Initial diagnostic testing for further evaluation of respiratory system injuries based on primary survey results may include the following:

        i. Thoracocentesis: Thoracocentesis is both diagnostic and therapeutic for both pneumothorax and pleural fluid accumulations after trauma.

        ii. Indicators of oxygenation: Determination of oxygen saturation (SpO_2) or arterial blood gas analysis will help dictate the need for oxygen support. Oxygen should be administered to all patients with increased respiratory rate and effort and/or SpO_2 <94%. Hypoxemia in the traumatized dog or cat signifies injury to the respiratory system.

        iii. Thoracic radiographs may be performed after cardiovascular and respiratory system stabilization is underway. Thoracic radiographs will allow for confirmation of injuries suspected based on primary survey of the respiratory system.

    f. Initial therapy for respiratory system injuries based on primary survey results may include the following:

        i. Oxygen support is uniformly administered to all patients who have sustained trauma that has any evidence of injury associated with the respiratory (or cardiovascular) systems:

        1. High (100%) concentrations of oxygen delivered over short periods of time (<24 hours) will not cause harm.

        2. Importantly, the balance between maximizing oxygen support while minimizing stress must be found.

        3. A variety of methods are available for oxygen support that vary in terms of stress of use, cost, inspired oxygen concentration that can be achieved, and contact with the patient. These methods are:

        a. Nasal insufflation:

        i. Achieved by placement of a soft red rubber catheter or other cannula into the nose. Before placement, 2–5 drops of lidocaine should be placed in the nostril(s) every 5 minutes for three doses. 5F is appropriate for use in cats and very small dogs. 8F is appropriate in dogs of most sizes. A measurement is taken from the medial canthus of the eye to the external nares. (Figure 2.1) 1 cm is added to this distance and the cannula is marked. The well-lubricated cannula is then advanced in a ventral and medial direction to the predetermined mark. The cannula

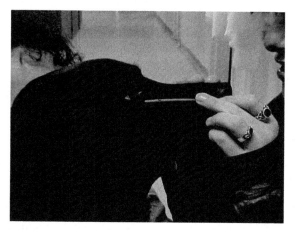

FIGURE 2.1 Nasal insufflation. A measurement is taken from the medial canthus of the eye to the external nares. 1 cm is added to this distance and the cannula is marked. After local anesthetic administration, the cannula will be advanced to this mark and sutured in place.

is then secured in place just adjacent to the alar fold of the nose (adjacent to the nasal planum). The author prefers to suture using a finger trap pattern.

ii. Moderate to high FiO_2 is achieved with this method. $FiO_2 = 0.5$ (50%) may be achieved in normal dogs with oxygen flow rates of 50–100 mL/Kg/min through 8Fr red rubber catheters (Dunphy et al 2002).

iii. Method is inexpensive.

iv. Moderately stressful to place.

v. Excellent for longer term oxygen support in dogs.

vi. Should be utilized in conjunction with a humidification system to minimize airway irritation/damage.

b. Oxygen cage:

i. Easy to achieve high FiO_2.

ii. Minimizes stress.

iii. Expensive to purchase and to fill the environment and to refill it when the doors are opened to assess the patient.

iv. Separation of patient and veterinary health care team is detrimental to ongoing assessment and monitoring.

v. Excellent method for use in cats.

vi. Should be utilized in conjunction with a humidification system to minimize airway irritation/damage.

c. Flow-by oxygen:

i. Achieved by simply placing a hose for the delivery of oxygen in front of the face of the patient.

ii. Low FiO_2 achieved.

iii. Minimizes stress.

iv. Good for early delivery of oxygen when access to the patient for vascular access and other stabilizing therapeutics is needed.

v. Inexpensive.

d. Mask oxygen:

i. Achieved by simply placing a mask over the nose/face of the patient.

ii. Can achieve high FiO_2.

iii. Mild to moderately stressful.

iv. Good for early delivery of oxygen when access to the patient for vascular access and other stabilizing therapeutics is needed.

v. Inexpensive.

e. Vented baggie or E-collar with plastic wrap:

i. Achieved by placing a large, clear, well-vented bag over the head +/− body of the patient in a "tent" fashion. Alternatively, clear, plastic wrap may be placed over the front of an Elizabethan collar leaving approximately a 2–3 cm vent at the top. Oxygen is then insufflated into the vented environment.

   ii. Can achieve high FiO_2.

   iii. Cats tolerate vented baggie method well (short term).

   iv. Inexpensive.

   v. Disadvantages include the potential for hyperthermia and condensation if inappropriately vented.

  f. Endotracheal intubation:

   i. Allows for the delivery of 100% oxygen ($FiO_2 = 1.0$) as well as positive pressure ventilation.

   ii. Allows for control of airway in upper airway obstruction.

   iii. Minimizes stress because the patient is anesthetized.

   iv. Inexpensive.

   v. Disadvantages include the need for general anesthesia and intensive monitoring of the anesthetized patient.

  ii. Thoracocentesis may be rapidly performed if pneumothorax or pleural effusion is suspected; see Chapter 6: Trauma-Associated Thoracic Injury.

3. Circulation: The veterinarian should assess for the presence of spontaneous circulation and a full evaluation of the cardiovascular system including evaluation for evidence of hemorrhage should be performed. Hypovolemia secondary to hemorrhage is very common in the trauma patient:

  a. Mucous membranes (see 3.c.iii.1)

  b. CRT (see 3.c.iii.1)

  c. Pulse rate (see 3.c.iii.1)

  d. Pulse character (see 3.c.iii.1)

  e. Evaluate for hemorrhage:

   i. Five sites for large volume blood loss after trauma:

    1. Peritoneal space

    2. Retroperitoneal space

    3. Pleural space

    4. Externally

    5. Around proximal long-bone fractures (primarily femur)

  f. Auscultation of the heart should be performed to evaluate for the presence of the following:

   i. Arrhythmia:

    1. Arrhythmias are relatively uncommon in the acutely traumatized patient and more commonly manifest 12–48 hours after the traumatic event. Arrhythmias associated with trauma may result from any of the following:

     a. Hypoxemia

     b. Myocardial contusion

     c. Ischemia-reperfusion injury

    2. Underlying cardiac disease such as dilated cardiomyopathy may result in arrhythmias that are detected incidentally during primary survey of the trauma patient. The presence of underlying cardiac disease may influence initial fluid therapy decisions toward a more conservative resuscitation protocol.

   ii. Heart murmur:

    1. Underlying cardiac disease may result in the presence of a heart murmur detected on primary survey.

    2. Presence of a heart murmur may influence initial fluid therapy decisions toward a more conservative resuscitation protocol.

   iii. Decreased heart sounds:

    1. Decreased heart sounds may be noted on initial auscultation of the heart during the primary survey.

    2. Pleural space diseases (pneumothorax, pleural effusion, and diaphragmatic hernia) and pericardial effusion may result in decreased heart sounds due to the presence of fluid surrounding the heart.

3. Hypovolemia may also result in decreased heart sounds.

g. Assessment of the jugular vein should be performed:

i. The jugular furrow is clipped free of hair for evaluation.

ii. The jugular vein may be difficult to palpate and may not distend rapidly when transiently occluded in hypovolemic states. The jugular vein should not be transiently occluded in the patient with head trauma.

iii. Jugular venous distention may be noted in animals with pericardial effusion, massive hemorrhage into the mediastinum, or massive air accumulations in the mediastinum.

h. Initial diagnostic testing for further evaluation of cardiovascular system injury based on primary survey results are directed primarily toward the identification of sources of hemorrhage:

i. Focused assessment with sonography for trauma, or the FAST scan, of the abdomen to evaluate for peritoneal and retroperitoneal hemorrhage (see Chapter 3: Shock in the Trauma Patient, Figure 3.5).

ii. Rapid ultrasonographic evaluation of the pleural and pericardial spaces for evidence of hemorrhage.

iii. Trauma series of radiographs once patient stability has been achieved. The trauma series of radiographs helps identify spinal injuries as well as major cavitary injury and pelvic injury while minimizing the necessity for initial manipulations. Four radiographic views are acquired:

1. Lateral neck

2. Lateral thorax

3. Lateral abdomen

4. Lateral pelvis

iv. Bloodwork should include the following:

1. Packed cell volume/ Total protein by refractometry (PCV/TS):

a. A normal to increased PCV may be noted in conjunction with decreased TS in dogs with acute hemorrhage.

b. PCV/TS is not a good reflection of intravascular volume. An animal can acutely bleed to death and still have a normal PCV/TS.

2. Blood glucose:

a. Hyperglycemia is common in dogs and very common in cats that have sustained trauma.

b. Persistent hyperglycemia in the face of appropriate resuscitation may indicate underlying diabetes mellitus. A urinalysis should be acquired.

3. Lactate:

a. Lactate is a byproduct of anaerobic glycolysis (metabolism).

b. Lactate is a global indicator of adequacy of oxygen delivery to the tissues or oxygen utilization by the tissues.

c. Normal lactate is <2.5 mmol/L.

d. An elevated lactate in a traumatized patient indicates inadequate oxygen delivery to the tissues. Efforts to optimize cardiac output and blood oxygen content (Hgb and SpO_2) should be undertaken.

e. An elevated lactate should be monitored in concert with resuscitation. Efforts should be made to rapidly normalize lactate.

f. Persistent hyperlactatemia (hours) indicating an ongoing deficiency in oxygen delivery to the tissues may carry a guarded prognosis.

4. Venous blood gas + electrolytes + BUN/CREA:

a. Metabolic acidosis is common in dogs and cats

that have sustained trauma and is most often lactic acidosis:

    i. Metabolic acidosis is characterized by acidemia in association with a decreased bicarbonate (HCO_3^-) concentration.

    ii. Metabolic acidosis occurs with hyperlactatemia. Lactate is produced from hypoxic tissues in concert with hydrogen ion (H^+).

  b. Metabolic acidosis also may occur in animals with urinary tract disruption due to failure to excrete hydrogen ion.

5. Blood type:

  a. Determination of DEA 1.1 status is useful in directing whole blood or packed red blood cell transfusions to traumatized patients:

    i. DEA 1.1(+) dogs may receive DEA 1.1(+) or DEA 1.1(−) blood.

    ii. DEA 1.1(−) dogs may only received DEA 1.1(−) blood to avoid sensitization to DEA 1.1.

  b. Blood typing is not critical for initial whole blood or packed red blood cell transfusion in dogs because they lack significant naturally occurring antibodies to other blood types. Cats absolutely require blood typing prior to any blood transfusion therapy.

  c. Blood typing is critical to prevent DEA 1.1 incompatibility if the recipient has been transfused in the past.

i. Initial therapy for cardiovascular system injury based on primary survey results may include the following:

    i. Oxygen support is uniformly administered to all patients that have sustained trauma that have any evidence of injury associated with the respiratory (or cardiovascular) systems; see 4.b.ii.2.f.i.

    ii. Acquisition of vascular access and resuscitation from hypovolemic states (see Chapter 3: Shock in the Trauma Patient).

4. Disability (neurologic evaluation). The veterinarian should assess for any evidence of CNS injury. A limited neurologic examination should be performed that does not involve significant patient manipulation. Once it is clear that there is no spinal injury, a more complete neurologic examination may be performed:

  a. Level of consciousness (see 3.c.iii.3).

  b. Evaluation of the head for evidence of trauma including but not limited to ocular trauma, mandibular fractures, maxillofacial injuries, dental trauma, injuries to the hard palate, blood in the ears, and abrasions.

  c. Determination of the modified Glasgow coma score (MGCS). See Chapter 7: Traumatic Brain Injury. Determination of the MGCS will help provide objective information as to the severity of CNS injury. Repeated evaluation of the MGCS will allow for more objective determination of patient improvement or deterioration.

  d. Evaluate for the presence of deep pain perception in all four limbs.

  e. Evaluate for the presence voluntary motor function in all four limbs.

  f. Evaluate spinal segmental reflexes in all four limbs.

  g. Initial diagnostic testing for further evaluation of CNS system injury based on primary survey results are directed primarily toward the identification of spinal fracture or luxation.

    i. Trauma series (see 4.b.ii.h.iii).

c. Full medical history:

  i. While the primary survey is being performed, a team member trained in history taking should be dispatched to collect any relevant acute or chronic medical history including the circumstances surrounding the traumatic event that occurred.

ii. Critical pieces of historical information that may impact how a traumatized dog or cat is managed will include the following:

1. Time/date of the traumatic event.

2. Progression of signs since the traumatic event occurred.

3. Whether the dog or cat has displayed any specific systemic signs of illness since the traumatic event. These systemic manifestations of illness might include, but are not limited to increased respiratory rate or effort, coughing, presence of blood loss, vomiting, loss of consciousness, seizure activity, urination or defecation, and inability to ambulate.

4. Current medications.

5. Allergies to foods or medications.

6. Previous history of blood or blood product transfusion.

5. SECONDARY SURVEY

a. The secondary survey includes a complete physical examination and is focused on the identification of all trauma-associated injuries.

b. Aspects of the secondary survey will be discussed in individual chapters devoted to the various body systems.

BIBLIOGRAPHY

Encarta® World English Dictionary [North American Edition] © & (P) 2001 Microsoft Corporation. All rights reserved.

Dunphy ED, Mann FA, Dodam JR, *et al.* Comparison of unilateral versus bilateral nasal catheters for oxygen administration in dogs. *J Vet Emerg Crit Care* 2002; 12: 245–251.

SHOCK IN THE TRAUMA PATIENT

Rebecca S. Syring

1. **PATHOPHYSIOLOGY OF SHOCK**
   a. One of the most vital functions of the circulation is to maintain tissue oxygen delivery at a level that meets the tissue's metabolic requirement for oxygen:
   i. When tissue oxygen delivery and the tissue's metabolic requirement for oxygen are in balance, aerobic metabolism can be sustained:
   1. In this scenario, 1 mole of glucose can be oxidized to yield 36 moles of ATP.
   2. Aerobic metabolism is an efficient way to maintain ATP production and, therefore, cell membrane pump function and cellular integrity.
   b. Shock occurs when tissue oxygen delivery is insufficient to meet the metabolic requirement for oxygen delivery at the tissue level (Figure 3.1):
   i. Aerobic metabolism can no longer be sustained when this occurs.
   ii. In this scenario, anaerobic metabolism ensues, with 1 mole of glucose yielding *only* 2 moles of ATP, which are rapidly consumed.
   iii. Anaerobic metabolism is an inefficient means of ATP production and leads to generation of a lactic acidosis.
   iv. Left uncorrected, a tissue oxygen debt develops, cells and organs become hypoxemic, and cellular and/or end-organ damage occurs, which can ultimately result in cell death and organ failure.

   c. Compensatory responses to shock:
   i. When tissue oxygen delivery is decreased, the body initially mounts a compensatory response in order to maintain tissue oxygen delivery at an acceptable level to maintain aerobic metabolism.
   ii. Cardiac output is increased by increasing heart rate and cardiac contractility. Venoconstriction occurs to shunt pooled blood into the effective circulating volume and vasoconstriction occurs to shunt blood to vital organs such as the brain, heart, and kidneys. Neurohormonal activation of the renin–angiotensin–aldosterone system occurs to conserve electrolytes and water to restore circulating volume.
   iii. At the capillary level, the oxygen extraction ratio to tissues increases. Normally, a standard proportion of the oxygen delivered from the arterial side is extracted at the capillary/tissue level, leaving approximately 35–40 mm Hg of oxygen (or an oxygen saturation >70%) on the venous side. When the oxygen extraction ratio increases, this results in a decreased venous oxygen saturation. Measurement of mixed or central venous oxygen saturations in blood samples, obtained from catheters located in the pulmonary artery or just proximal to the right atrium, respectively, can provide some information about global oxygen delivery, where

Manual of Trauma Management in the Dog and Cat, First Edition. Edited by Kenneth J. Drobatz, Matthew W. Beal and Rebecca S. Syring.
© 2011 John Wiley & Sons, Inc. Published 2011 by John Wiley & Sons, Inc.

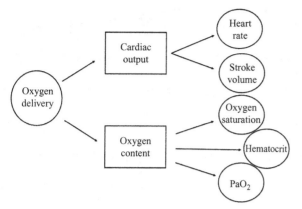

FIGURE 3.1   This diagram depicts the important components of oxygen delivery.

optimal mixed/central venous saturations exceed 70%.

iv.   Eventually, these compensatory responses fail to maintain oxygen delivery. This results in tissue hypoxia, acidosis, and cellular injury, which ultimately can lead to organ dysfunction or failure.

2. PHYSICAL EXAMINATION OF THE CARDIO-VASCULAR SYSTEM

a. Auscultation of the heart:

i.   Heart rate and rhythm should be evaluated on initial assessment of the traumatized patient prior to fluid therapy. The presence of tachycardia or an irregular rhythm may warrant further therapeutics (i.e., fluid resuscitation, analgesics) or diagnostics (i.e., electrocardiogram, thoracic radiographs following stabilization):

1.   The normal heart rate for a dog varies according to its size. For large or giant breeds of dog, a heart rate ranging from 60 to 100 beats/min should be considered normal. For small to medium breeds of dog, a heart rate ranging from 100 to 140 beats/min should be considered normal. Heart rates in excess of 100 beats/min in large dogs and 140 beats/min in small dogs warrant further investigation.

2.   The normal heart rate for a cat in the hospital is usually 160–220 beats/min. Heart rates higher and lower than this range warrant further investigation. Bradycardia (<160 beats/min) is particularly common in critically ill cats and should

not be ignored. Two of the most common causes of bradycardia in the traumatized cat include hyperkalemia and hypothermia.

ii.   The heart should be carefully auscultated for the presence of a murmur or gallop. While murmurs or gallops are not likely to occur as a result of traumatic injury unless severe anemia has developed, the detection of a murmur or gallop provides information about the possibility of underlying cardiac disease and the likelihood that the animal will tolerate intravenous fluid therapy:

1.   When a murmur or gallop is noted in a traumatized patient, thoracic radiographs may be useful to discern if the murmur is innocent or related to underlying cardiac pathology (chamber enlargement detected on radiographs).

2.   Many animals with heart murmurs can tolerate fairly aggressive intravenous fluid therapy when hypovolemia is present. In this scenario, the patient should be closely monitored during resuscitation for any increase in respiratory rate or effort. In addition, a central venous catheter can be used to guide fluid resuscitation when a concern for fluid overloading is present (see Chapter 4: Monitoring of the Trauma Patient).

iii.   The ability to hear the heart adequately should be assessed. Inability to adequately auscultate the heart may indicate severe hypovolemia, pericardial effusion or pleural space disease.

b. Assessment of peripheral pulses:

i.   Palpation of peripheral pulses should be performed routinely in all traumatized patients. Pulse palpation can give information about heart rate, regularity of heart rhythm, and perfusion status.

ii.   Pulse quality:

1.   Peripheral pulse quality, over the dorsal metatarsal/pedal region, should be assessed on triage of the traumatized dog. In cats, distal pulses can be difficult to palpate even in good health; therefore palpation of the femoral pulse is sufficient. Warm extremities and good peripheral pulse quality indicate good peripheral tissue perfusion. When the limbs are cooler to the touch than

the body's core and/or the peripheral pulse quality is diminished to unappreciable levels, this indicates either excessive peripheral vasoconstriction or reduced cardiac output, resulting in impaired tissue perfusion.

2. It is important to realize that pulse quality and blood pressure do not necessarily equate. For instance, an animal may profoundly vasoconstrict the peripheral vascular beds to maintain systemic blood pressure; however, in this instance blood pressure is maintained at the cost of tissue perfusion.

3. Pulse quality is determined by the pulse pressure, which is the difference between the systolic and diastolic pressures. This difference can be altered by changes in stroke volume, vasomotor tone, and diastolic runoff of blood.

c. Assessment of mucous membranes:

i. Mucous membranes should be assessed for color and capillary refill time. In a normal animal, the mucous membranes should be pink and moist with a capillary refill time of 1–2 seconds.

ii. Pale mucous membranes can be caused by either peripheral vasoconstriction or anemia. The capillary refill time is often prolonged beyond 2 seconds with peripheral vasoconstriction, or, in anemic patients with, concurrent hypovolemia.

iii. Cyanosis is an insensitive marker of hypoxemia! When present, one can assume the animal is severely hypoxic; however, the absence of cyanosis does not correspond to the absence of hypoxemia. In animals with normal hemoglobin concentrations, cyanosis will not be detectable until the PO_2 is below 40 mm Hg, corresponding to a pulse oximeter reading of approximately 66%.

3. REASONS FOR CIRCULATORY COMPROMISE AND SHOCK IN THE TRAUMATIZED PATIENT

a. Hypovolemic shock:

i. Acute blood loss:

1. The blood volume in dogs is approximately 90 mL/kg, while in cats it is approximately 66 mL/kg.

2. Clinical signs of acute hemorrhage are subtle until approximately 30% of blood volume is shed. This is equivalent to an acute blood loss of 30 mL/kg in a dog and 22 mL/kg in cat:

a. Mild hemorrhage (15–30%): The presence of tachycardia may be the only clinical sign present in the early stages of hemorrhagic shock. Tissue perfusion is maintained in this early stage of hemorrhage; therefore, mucous membrane color, capillary refill time, and pulse quality will still be assessed as normal.

b. Moderate hemorrhage (30–40%): Impaired peripheral tissue perfusion develops at this point. Pale mucous membranes, delayed capillary refill time, weak peripheral pulses, and cold extremities may be noted at this stage. Blood pressure may still be maintained despite impaired tissue perfusion. Urine output will decrease once 30–40% of blood volume is lost.

c. Severe/life-threatening hemorrhage (>40%): Marked signs of circulatory collapse are present. At this point, not only is tissue perfusion impaired but attempts to maintain blood pressure fail and marked hypotension results.

3. Areas where a significant amount of blood can be lost following trauma that results in cardiovascular compromise:

a. External hemorrhage—external hemorrhage from open wounds is often an obvious and easily identifiable cause of hypovolemia.

b. Abdominal cavity—the abdominal cavity is probably the most common site for significant blood loss in the traumatized patient. Hemorrhage into the abdomen often results from hepatic or splenic fractures following blunt trauma, or from direct vascular or parenchymal organ damage in penetrating trauma:

i. Many animals with clinically significant abdominal hemorrhage will NOT have an obvious fluid wave on abdominal palpation.

ii. Rarely, the presence of a hemorrhagic ring around the umbilicus, known as the Cullen's sign, may be seen in animals with

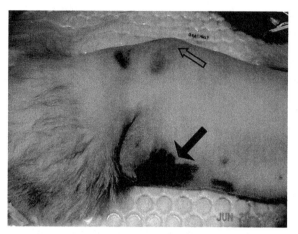

FIGURE 3.2 This dog sustained both blunt and penetrating trauma after being picked up, shaken, and being bitten. Note the large area of hemorrhage around the umbilicus (closed arrow). Peri-umbilical hemorrhage, referred to as the Cullen's sign, suggests intra-abdominal hemorrhage. This dog had an avulsed right kidney which was herniated through the body wall (note the swelling in the dorsal flank region and bruising (open arrow)) and several liver fractures resulting in a significant hemoabdomen. Photograph courtesy of Dr. Susan Volk.

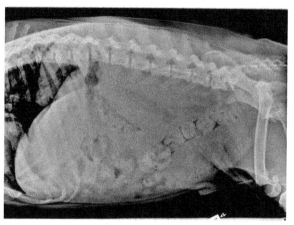

FIGURE 3.3 Lateral abdominal radiograph of a dog that sustained blunt vehicular trauma. On this radiograph, you cannot appreciate the silhouette of the kidneys, there is a wispy appearance in the retroperitoneal space, and the colon is markedly ventrally deviated. These radiographic findings are highly suggestive of retroperitoneal effusion, which may be caused by either blood or urine secondary to trauma.

significant intraperitoneal hemorrhage (Figure 3.2).

c. Retroperitoneal space—the retroperitoneal space is a relatively common site for a significant amount of blood loss in the traumatized animal:

i. Clinically, it is difficult to discern retroperitoneal hemorrhage only through physical examination. Some animals will exhibit pain or discomfort on paraspinal or renal palpation.

ii. Rarely, bruising may be present in the region of the inguinal ring(s), indicating the presence of retroperitoneal hemorrhage.

iii. Retroperitoneal hemorrhage should be suspected in the traumatized patient who is cardiovascularly unstable when external, abdominal, and long-bone fracture-associated hemorrhage have been ruled-out.

iv. Radiographically, there will be loss of retroperitoneal detail obscuring the ability to visualize the kidneys, the presence of a "wispy" pattern in the retroperitoneal space, and possibly ventral deviation of the colon on a lateral radiograph (Figure 3.3).

d. Muscles and fascia surrounding long bone and pelvic fractures (Figure 3.4):

i. This is most commonly seen with femoral and humeral fractures, but is also seen with pelvic fractures.

ii. Clinically, the affected limb or peri-pelvic region will be visibly swollen or may be noted to enlarge during fluid resuscitation.

e. Pleural space and mediastinum:

i. Clinically, this is an uncommon site for significant hemorrhage following trauma in veterinary medicine, though it does occur on occasion. Significant thoracic bleeding may develop with such rapidity that these animals never make it to a veterinarian before the animal arrests. Most hemothoraces are of a small volume and clinically insignificant.

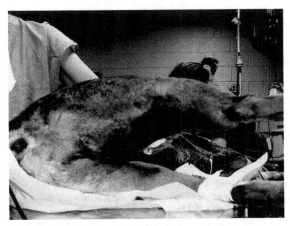

FIGURE 3.4 This dog sustained a mid-shaft femoral fracture of the right hindlimb after being hit by a car. He demonstrated cardiovascular instability on initial presentation to the hospital and bloodwork was consistent with acute blood loss. It was determined that the source of blood loss was into the thigh musculature from the medullary cavity of the broken femur. Note the marked increase in size of the right thigh compared to the left and the bruising on the medial aspect of the limb.

       ii. Penetrating trauma (i.e. gunshot wounds, impalements, stabbing) is more likely to result in significant intra-thoracic hemorrhage than blunt trauma.
       f. While hemorrhage can occur into the lungs (pulmonary contusions) and brain/spinal cord, the amount of blood lost into those regions would be insufficient to cause cardiovascular compromise.
  ii. Third-spacing of fluids:
    1. Third-spacing is seen most often in traumatized patients with chemical peritonitis, such as occurs with urinary bladder rupture or bile peritonitis.
    2. The irritant (urine, bile) within the peritoneal cavity induces an inflammatory response that causes vascular leak, which can result in hypovolemia.
    3. In addition to vascular leak, this inflammatory response often results in a vasodilatory state (see the following).
  iii. Decreased intake of fluids:
    1. Animals who have sustained trauma resulting in an altered state of consciousness (i.e., head trauma) or an altered ability to access free water will eventually become dehydrated and potentially hypovolemic (when dehydration is marked, i.e., 10–15%) unless parenteral fluid therapy is provided.
    2. This would likely take days beyond the traumatic incident to become evident, unless other confounding factors, such as blood loss, third-spacing, or mannitol administration, are concurrently present.
  b. Cardiogenic shock:
    i. Direct myocardial trauma:
      1. Cardiac trauma can occur secondary to blunt or penetrating trauma.
      2. Mechanisms of cardiac injury include acceleration-deceleration forces which result in compression of heart, rapid transfer of kinetic injury from direct trauma to the thorax, direct cardiac trauma (more often as a result of penetrating trauma) or rapid increases in intrathoracic and/or intraabdominal pressure leading to increased venous return and overdistention of the ventricle, causing bruising or rupture.
      3. These injuries result in variable degrees of cardiac petechiation, gross or microscopic contusions, hematomas, and/or lacerations. Ultimately, these injuries can cause focal or global impairment in myocardial function.
      4. Impaired myocardial function leads to a decreased stroke volume and compensatory tachycardia, which likely increases myocardial workload and oxygen demand.
      5. Ultimately, myocardial ischemia and necrosis result, leading to arrhythmia generation.
      6. Atrial rupture/tearing is uncommon, but has been reported in dogs following trauma. The resulting hemorrhagic pericardial effusion can lead to shock. This is not because of the volume of blood lost; instead, it is because the pericardial effusion reduces venous return (preload) to the heart and therefore reduces cardiac output.
    ii. Indirect myocardial injury:
      1. Generalized or localized tissue hypoxia and injury result in ischemia-reperfusion injury, liberation of reactive oxygen species,

and up-regulation of inflammatory media-tors, such as tumor necrosis factor-α (TNF-α) that can induce both cardiac dysrhyth-mias and reversible myocardial depression.

iii. Pericardial effusion:

1. Atrial rupture/tearing is uncommon, but has been reported in dogs following blunt and penetrating thoracic trauma.

2. The resulting hemorrhagic pericardial effusion can lead to shock.

3. This is not because of the volume of blood lost; instead, it is because the peri-cardial effusion reduces venous return (preload) to the heart and therefore reduces cardiac output.

iv. Thoracic tamponade:

1. Definition: Decreased cardiac output as a result of impaired venous return to the heart as a result of increased intrathoracic pressure.

2. Causes:

a. Tension pneumothorax (see Chapter 6: Trauma-Associated Thoracic Injury)

b. Diaphragmatic hernia (see Chapter 6: Trauma-Associated Thoracic Injury)

3. Improvement in cardiac output can be achieved by thoracocentesis, when pneu-mothorax is present, or by removal of the abdominal contents from the thorax, when a diaphragmatic hernia is present:

a. When the stomach has herniated into the thoracic cavity, it can become distended with gas and result in a vicious cycle of respiratory distress, which causes more gas to accumulate in the stomach secondary to aerophagia. Attempts to decompress the stomach via orogastric intubation or by transtho-racic gastrocentesis can improve both hemodynamic stability and signs of res-piratory distress.

c. Vasodilatory shock:

i. Vasodilatory shock refers most commonly to inflammatory disease states that are charac-terized by a lack of arterial vascular tone and maldistribution of blood flow, often resulting initially in a high cardiac output normotensive state, but later progresses to a hypotensive state often coupled with impaired myocardial func-tion.

ii. The systemic inflammatory response syn-drome (SIRS) is a term used to characterize those patients that have, or are at a risk of developing, an overwhelming inflammatory process that may have started locally within the body but has resulted in a diffuse inflammatory state throughout the body:

1. Patients who meet the SIRS criteria (see Section 4: Clinical Signs) are at risk for vasodilatory shock.

2. SIRS can be caused by systemic infection (sepsis) or a sterile inflammatory process:

a. Sepsis refers to a patient who meets the SIRS criteria AND an infectious agent (bacterial, viral, protozoal, or fungal) has been identified. Of these, bacterial infec-tions are most likely following trauma:

i. Bacterial peritonitis may occur in the traumatized animal secondary to penetrating abdominal injury, perfo-rating bowel trauma, or rarely from rupture of an infected gall bladder or urinary bladder.

ii. Overwhelming bacterial infec-tions may occur secondary to bite wounds, degloving wounds, other cutaneous injuries, or even as a result of improper bandage management.

b. Sterile inflammation:

i. Chemical peritonitis—rupture of the urinary bladder or gall bladder releases urine or bile, respectively, which can induce an intense inflam-matory response in the peritoneal cav-ity. Most cases of chemical peritonitis are sterile.

ii. Traumatic pancreatitis can occur as a result of blunt force trauma to the abdomen or as a result of decreased pancreatic perfusion following injury.

iii. Massive tissue trauma as a result of blunt or penetrating trauma can induce a marked inflammatory response. This could be secondary to crushing injury, shearing injury to the skeleton when being dragged along the ground, or even following bite wounds when bacterial contami-nation has been controlled.

iv. Prolonged hypoperfusion as a result of hypovolemia following trauma can ultimately induce inflammation, leading to a vasodilatory state following resuscitation.

4. CLINICAL SIGNS OF CARDIOVASCULAR COMPROMISE

  a. Hypovolemic shock:

  i. Pale mucous membranes: pallor to the mucous membranes is a normal compensatory response to hypovolemia as a result of vasoconstriction of the peripheral vasculature and shunting of blood to vital organs.

  ii. Prolonged capillary refill time (>1.5 seconds): The capillary refill becomes prolonged as a result of decreased blood flow through nonvital tissues as a result of vasoconstriction and decreased stroke volume.

  iii. Weak to absent peripheral pulse quality: Peripheral pulse quality is often diminished as a result of peripheral vasoconstriction and shunting of blood to vital organs. Cool to cold extremities are often noted in these animals. *Note*: Pulse quality does not necessarily correspond to blood pressure as it possible to maintain an acceptable blood pressure via peripheral vasoconstriction despite poor distal limb perfusion.

  iv. Tachycardia: Since cardiac output is equal to Heart Rate × Stroke Volume, a compensatory increase in heart rate will help to maintain cardiac output when stroke volume is reduced as a result of hypovolemia.

  v. Tachypnea: Tachypnea develops during hypovolemic shock as a result of the lactic acidosis that occurs with poor tissue perfusion—the animal will hyperventilate in order to compensate for the metabolic acidosis. In addition, tachypnea may be a response to improved oxygen content and therefore tissue oxygen delivery. Finally, tachypnea in the traumatized patient may also result from injury to the chest wall, pleural space, lungs, or stress/pain/fear.

  vi. Decreased mentation: When perfusion becomes impaired, decreased oxygen delivery to the brain can result in decreased mentation. Mentation should always be reassessed following resuscitation.

  vii. Decreased urine output: Urine output decreases as a normal compensatory response to hypovolemia in order to retain fluid and expand intravascular volume. These animals should have concentrated urine in the face of hypovolemia so long as adequate renal function is present. With severe and prolonged hypovolemia, decreased urine output may occur as a result of decreased renal blood flow and secondary acute tubular injury.

  b. Cardiogenic shock:

  i. Cardiogenic shock is uncommon in the traumatized patient.

  ii. All of the aforementioned signs of hypovolemic shock can be seen in animals with cardiogenic shock. Cardiogenic shock may be difficult to differentiate from hypovolemic shock based upon physical examination alone. Subjective evaluation of the jugular vein may be helpful to differentiate cardiogenic from hypovolemic shock:

  1. With hypovolemic shock, the jugular vein should be collapsed and difficult to elevate with compression at the thoracic inlet.

  2. With cardiogenic shock, the jugular vein may be distended or may easily fill with compression at the thoracic inlet.

  iii. Animals who exhibit cardiogenic shock secondary to cardiac dysrhythmias may have a discernable irregularity in cardiac rhythm on auscultation, or palpable pulse deficits.

  iv. Animals who exhibit cardiogenic shock secondary to atrial tears and pericardial effusion may have quiet or dull heart sounds on auscultation and either weak peripheral pulses or pulsus paradoxus:

  1. Pulsus paradoxus refers to a cyclical variation in pulse quality associated with the respiratory cycle. On inspiration, the pulse quality is dampened, and on expiration, the pulse quality improves.

  v. Cardiogenic shock secondary to thoracic tamponade, as occurs with tension pneumothorax and herniation of abdominal organs into the chest or pericardium, may be characterized by quiet heart and lungs sounds (unilaterally or bilaterally), a distended or "sprung" thorax, and/or a restrictive respiratory pattern (short, shallow breathing). Animals with diaphragmatic hernia may demonstrate a paradoxical abdominal movement during respiration, wherein the abdomen expands on expiration and collapses during inspiration.

c. Vasodilatory shock:

   i. Suggested criteria to characterize SIRS (must meet two of four criteria to classify as SIRS):

   1. Dogs: Heart rate >160 beats/min, respiratory rate >40 breaths/min, rectal temperature >103.5°F or <100°F, and/or white blood cell count >12,000 or <4000 (Hauptman et al., 1997; Okano et al., 2002).

   2. Cats: Heart rate >225 beats/min or <140 beats/min, respiratory rate >40 breaths/min, rectal temperature >104°F or <100°F, and/or white blood cell count >19,000 or <5000 (Brady et al., 2000).

   3. The aforementioned criteria are subject to much debate in the medical community, including veterinary medicine. These criteria are vague and may not be sensitive or specific enough to accurately identify patients with SIRS. There is much discussion about altering the SIRS inclusion criteria with respect to number of criteria to be fulfilled, and if additional criteria such as additional physical examination findings or biomarkers of inflammation should be included.

   ii. Severe sepsis or SIRS refers to these states with associated hypoperfusion or hypotension (systolic blood pressure <90 mm Hg).

   iii. Septic shock or SIRS with shock refers to the patient with persistent hypotension (systolic < 90 mm Hg) despite adequate fluid resuscitation and continued perfusion abnormalities such as lactic acidosis, oliguria, or mental depression.

   iv. Compensated vasodilatory shock: In this phase the patient is usually hyperdynamic. These patients demonstrate high cardiac output hypotension as a result of mild to moderate vasodilation and the following are noted clinically:

   1. Injected/bright pink-red mucous membranes

   2. Capillary refill times <1 second

   3. Warm extremities

   4. Bounding peripheral pulse quality

   5. Hyperthermia or normothermia

   6. Hyperglycemia may be detected in this phase

   v. Decompensated vasodilatory shock: In this phase the patient becomes hypodynamic. These patients frequently demonstrate reduced cardiac output secondary to concurrent hypovolemic and/or myocardial depression. The following may be noted clinically:

   1. Injected, pink or pale mucous membranes

   2. Capillary refill times >2 seconds

   3. Normal to cold extremity temperature

   4. Reduced peripheral pulse quality

   5. Markedly reduced mentation

   6. Normothermia or hypothermia

   7. Hypoglycemia is often detected in this phase.

5. DIAGNOSTICS TO ASSESS THE CARDIOVAS-CULAR SYSTEM IN SHOCK

a. Bloodwork:

   i. Packed cell volume (PCV)/Total Protein by refractometry (TS):

   1. Immediately following hemorrhage, PCV and TS concentration may be normal. When blood is shed, all components are lost in equal proportion; however, the absolute circulating volume is decreased. Peracutely, no changes can be detected in PCV and TS, even with significant hemorrhage.

   2. In response to a decrease in circulating volume, fluid shifts into the vasculature to expand the circulating blood volume. Therefore, a decrease in TS concentration will be detected prior to a fall in PCV, as PCV can be maintained by splenic contraction and release of high PCV blood into the circulatory system. The presence of a total protein of < 5.5 g/dL following trauma should prompt a search for blood loss.

   3. Eventually, both the PCV and TS will decrease.

   ii. Blood gas analysis:

   1. Venous:

   a. The presence of a high anion-gap metabolic acidosis, in the absence of ketosis or azotemia, often indicates the accumulation of lactate as a result of poor tissue perfusion in the traumatized patient. As perfusion deficits are corrected, this metabolic acidosis should rapidly resolve. For every 1 mmol/L elevation in lactate, the bicarbonate/base excess concentration will decrease by approximately 1 mmol/L.

b. Profound hypoperfusion can markedly elevate PCO_2 concentrations in peripheral venous blood samples, exacerbating the extent of acidosis in the sample:

    i. The elevated PCO_2 should not be confused with hypoventilation. Instead, the increased PCO_2 represents decreased local tissue perfusion and accumulation of CO_2 which is not being picked up by the venous circulation and returned to the lungs for excretion.

    ii. Arterial blood gas sampling will more accurately reflect the patient's ventilatory status in this scenario.

  2. Arterial:

    a. Arterial blood gas sampling should be used to obtain information about ventilation and oxygenation. Calculation of the Alveolar-arterial oxygen gradient will help both identify and quantitate the presence and severity of pulmonary gas exchange abnormalities (see Chapter 4: Monitoring of the Trauma Patient).

 iii. Lactate:

  1. Lactate concentrations can be measured by several commercial blood gas analyzers (Critical Care Xpress, Nova Biomedical, Waltham, MA; iStat, Abbott Point of Care, East Windsor, NJ) or independently with handheld point-of-care analyzers (Accutrend Lactate, Roche, Basel, Switzerland).

  2. Blood samples should be processed within 5 minutes of collection to minimize artificial elevations in lactate concentrations.

  3. Normal lactate concentrations should be less than 2.0 mmol/L in cats and dogs.

  4. Elevations in lactate often correlate to the severity of hypoperfusion and subsequent decrease in oxygen delivery:

    a. Mild hypoperfusion: lactate concentrations between 3 and 5 mmol/L:

      i. Mild increases in lactate may also be noted in animals that struggle during blood sampling or when the vessel has been occluded for a prolonged period of time. This should be considered when elevations in lactate do not match the clinical picture of the patient.

    b. Moderate hypoperfusion: lactate concentrations between 5 and 7 mmol/L:

      i. Shivering and excessive muscle activity can cause moderate elevations in lactate and should be considered when clinical signs of perfusion do not match with the lactate concentration obtained.

    c. Severe hypoperfusion: lactate concentrations above 7 mmol/L.

  5. When elevations in lactate do not correspond to physical examination findings regarding perfusion, the following should be considered: decreased hepatic or renal function (impaired clearance), excessive muscular activity or injury, severe hypoxia (<40 mm Hg), severe anemia (<15%), or impaired tissue oxygen utilization.

  6. Lactate concentrations should decrease as tissue perfusion is improved. Persistence of moderate to severe hyperlactatemia despite resuscitative efforts is a poor prognostic indicator:

    a. The kinetics of lactate clearance will vary depending upon the cause of hyperlactatemia and hepatic function.

    b. If the liver functions normally and perfusion is restored, the half-life of lactate is approximately 60 minutes.

    c. However, with ongoing hypoperfusion and/or impaired hepatic function the half-life of lactate can increase to 16 hours.

    d. Rechecking lactate concentrations within the first 1–2 hours of treatment will provide useful information on response to therapy and prognosis.

 iv. Complete blood count (CBC):

  1. In an emergency setting, the evaluation of a blood smear can provide as much, if not more, information than an automated CBC can. Blood smears should routinely be evaluated when automated CBCs are performed in practice.

2. Red blood cells:

   a. While ongoing monitoring of packed cell volume and total protein concentration is often sufficient to assess for bleeding and response to therapy, the quantitative and qualitative information regarding red blood cells obtained from a CBC can provide additional useful information, such as if an appropriate regenerative response is mounting to anemia.

3. White blood cells:

   a. A stress leukogram may be noted in traumatized patients. The stress leukogram is characterized by a mature neutrophilia (there should not be a left shift, nor should there be evidence of toxic change), lymphopenia, and monocytosis.

   b. A blood smear evaluation should be performed to look for evidence of left shifting or toxic change, which may indicate an inflammatory process that may predispose to vasodilatory shock.

4. Platelets:

   a. Thrombocytopenia is frequently seen in following significant hemorrhage, as a result of platelet consumption. Platelet counts as low as 50,000 cells/uL have been documented shortly after bleeding.

   b. Another reason for thrombocytopenia following trauma is the development of disseminated intravascular coagulation (DIC) as a result of severe trauma or inflammation. Evaluation of complete coagulation (which should include evaluation of clotting times, platelet counts and some combination of fibrinogen, fibrin degradation products, or D-dimers) should be considered in patients at risk for DIC.

v. Serum chemistry profile:

   1. The hepatocellular enzymes, alanine aminotransferase (ALT) and aspartate aminotransferase (AST), are frequently moderately to markedly elevated in the patient traumatized with shock:

   a. ALT is liver specific, but AST may also be elevated with muscular injury.

   b. These liver values increase immediately following direct hepatic injury or in response to impaired hepatic perfusion.

   c. The half-life of ALT is approximately 2–3 days—therefore, a 50% reduction in ALT is expected within 2–3 days of injury so long as there is no ongoing hepatic injury.

   d. AST has a much shorter half-life (<5 hours) and would be expected to subside earlier once injury has ceased.

   e. Elevations in AST without elevated ALT indicate muscle damage/injury.

   2. Creatinine phosphokinase (CPK), also known as creatinine kinase (CK), is also often moderately to markedly elevated in patients following significant trauma, as it is released from traumatized and hypoperfused muscle cells.

   3. Decreased total protein, albumin, and globulin are seen primarily with hemorrhage, but can also be seen with inflammatory disease states causing increased vascular permeability and with severe cutaneous wounds and burns where proteins exude from the surfaces. In the latter two conditions, albumin may decrease more so than globulin, as globulins are larger molecules making them less likely to leak in states of increased vascular permeability. In addition, systemic inflammation may stimulate globulin production.

b. Blood pressure measurements should be obtained upon presentation in all patients following significant trauma, and ongoing monitoring performed during and following the resuscitation period. It is important to note that good blood pressure does not equate to good tissue perfusion. Intense vasoconstriction may be sufficient to maintain blood pressure at the cost of impaired peripheral tissue perfusion. Therefore, blood pressure should be interpreted in light of other physical examination findings and treatment should be based on a combination of these parameters (see Chapter 4: Monitoring of the Trauma Patient).

c. Electrocardiogram (ECG):
   i. A lead-II ECG should be used in the resuscitation phase following trauma. It is valuable for the following reasons:
      1. As a marker for underlying cardiac disease, such as detecting alteration in the magnitude and duration of the ECG complexes as seen with chamber enlargement, or noting atrial fibrillation as seen with diseases resulting in atrial enlargement.
      2. To diagnose and monitor dysrhythmias associated with trauma, such as ventricular tachycardia or ventricular premature contractions. These arrhythmias may occur immediately following trauma, but are often noted within the first 24 hours following a traumatic injury.
   ii. Probably the most effective use of ECG monitoring in the trauma patient is to noninvasively monitor the patient's response to resuscitation efforts or other therapies, by allowing continuous assessment of the animal's heart rate.
d. Focused Assessment with Sonography for Trauma (FAST Ultrasound) (Figure 3.5):
   i. The FAST ultrasound examination is designed as a diagnostic tool to allow veterinarians with minimal ultrasonographic training to rapidly assess for free fluid in the chest and abdomen in traumatized patients:
      1. To be performed within minutes of initial triage following traumatic injuries.
      2. Entire examination should take less than 5 minutes.
      3. Purpose of the examination is to look for the presence or absence of free fluid and not to look for other underlying pathology.
   ii. The patient should be restrained in lateral recumbency for the examination.
   iii. There are four different sites that should be evaluated during the FAST examination:
      1. Ventral midline subxiphoid: this site is evaluated for fluid accumulation between liver lobes and the diaphragm, in the pleural and pericardial spaces.
      2. Flank (both the gravity dependent and gravity independent flank should be evaluated): this site is evaluated for fluid accumulation in the peritoneal space

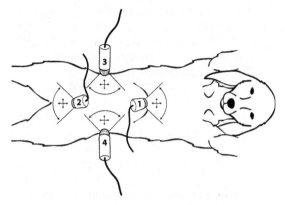

FIGURE 3.5 Focused assessment with sonography for trauma (FAST) can be used to rapidly detect fluid in the abdominal, retroperitoneal, pleural, and pericardial spaces utilizing four ultrasonographic views on the abdomen. The ultrasound transducer should be placed in the subxiphoid region to assess for fluid around liver lobes and in the pleural and pericardial spaces. Placement of the ultrasound transducer in the left and right flanks, assessing both the dependent and independent regions, will assess for fluid around the kidneys and spleen. Lastly, placement of the ultrasound transducer above the pubis will assess for fluid accumulation around the bladder: Reprinted with permission: Boysen SR, Rozanski EA, Tidwell AS, et al. Evaluation of a focused assessment with sonography for trauma protocol to detect free abdominal fluid in dogs involved in motor vehicular accidents. J Am Vet Med Assoc 2004; 225: 1198–1204.

(between bowel loops, spleen, and liver) and retroperitoneal space around the kidney.
      3. Ventral midline prepubic: this site is evaluated for for fluid accumulation around the urinary bladder and pelvis.
      4. Each site should be evaluated with two views: a transverse view and a longitudinal view, which can be obtained by rotating the ultrasound transducer 90°.
   iv. Accuracy: The FAST is a highly sensitive test to determine if free fluid has accumulated in the abdomen and thorax. Its sensitivity is increased even further when a second examination is performed after fluid resuscitation when the initial examination is negative. However, this examination does not specify the reason for effusion. Centesis is required to help determine the cause of fluid accumulation (i.e. hemorrhage, urine, bilious effusion, etc.) (Boysen et al., 2004)

e. Urine output (see Chapter 4: Monitoring of the Trauma Patient):

  i. Urine output in a euvolemic animal with normal renal function should be approximately 0.5–1.0 mL/kg/h. One should always take into account the volume of fluid being administered when considering normal urine output. For instance, if an animal is volume expanded, well hydrated, and has no other losses (i.e. diarrhea, third-spacing) urine output should be only slightly lower than fluid input.

  ii. In the presence of hypovolemia, a decrease in urine output is a normal compensatory response, which serves to conserve water and attempt to correct deficits in circulatory volume:

    1. The presence of highly concentrated urine (urine specific gravity >1.035) suggests volume depletion and the need to administer additional fluids to replace fluid deficits.

  iii. In the presence of hypotension, or inadequate renal perfusion, the urine output will decrease to an oliguric state. Mean arterial blood pressures below 80 mm Hg can affect urine output. This occurs not only because of reduced renal blood flow resulting in decreased glomerular filtration rate, but also secondary to stimulation of a variety of neurohormonal chemicals which act to conserve volume. Restoration of renal perfusion often restores urine output.

  iv. Urine output can be measured noninvasively by free catching all urine and by using absorbent cage pads which can be weighed (1 mL = 1 gram) or by placement of an indwelling urinary catheter and connection to a closed collection system.

f. Thoracic radiographs:

  i. While not recommended as an initial diagnostic in the cardiovascularly unstable trauma patient, thoracic radiographs can provide useful information in these patients:

    1. The cardiac silhouette and size of the caudal vena cava can be assessed for degree of volume expansion (Figure 3.6).

    2. Thoracic radiographs may help in the evaluation of preexisting cardio-respiratory disease.

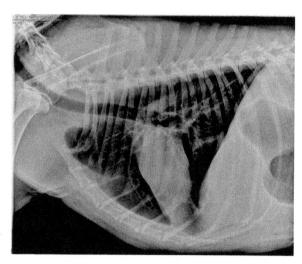

FIGURE 3.6 This lateral thoracic radiograph was taken in a hypovolemic dog who had been hit by a car. Note that the microcardia (the heart spans only 2 rib spaces) and the caudal vena cava is thin as a result of hypovolemia.

    3. Detection of interstitial to alveolar infiltrates may indicate pulmonary contusions secondary to trauma. Pulmonary contusions can result in variable degrees of hypoxemia, which may explain some signs of cardiovascular compromise.

    4. Detection of a pneumothorax or diaphragmatic hernia, which may have gone undiagnosed based upon physical examination, may help to explain ongoing cardiovascular compromise.

  ii. Thoracic radiographs should never be performed until stabilizing therapy has been initiated and the patient can tolerate the stress of restraint. Analgesics should be considered prior to radiographs.

g. Echocardiogram:

  i. In the face of persistent hypoperfusion, or when underlying cardiac disease is of concern, an echocardiogram may be used to assess global cardiac function and how well the patient will tolerate ongoing fluid challenges.

  ii. In the hands of a skilled echocardiographer, more objective assessments of hemodynamic variables in the critically ill patient, such as overall volume status, ventricular filling pressures, stroke volume, and cardiac output, can be obtained.

h. Pulmonary artery catheter:
  i. Cardiac output:
  1. Cardiac output can be directly measured with either the traditional pulmonary artery catheter, or with less invasive transpulmonary cardiac output methodology, both using either thermo- or indicator-dilution techniques. More recently, indirect measures of cardiac output have been developed which allow for less invasive and even continuous monitoring via echocardiographic assessment and pulse contour analysis of the arterial waveform.
  2. In the absence of cardiac output monitoring, one can use either physical examination parameters or central venous pressure (CVP) to assess adequacy of peripheral tissue perfusion and intravascular volume, respectively. These parameters are often used to estimate tissue perfusion and adequacy of vascular filling volume:
    a. If cardiac output is measured or subjectively thought to be decreased: measure CVP or PAOP/PCWP to determine if the low cardiac output is because of decreased cardiac filling volume (hypovolemia) or decreased cardiac contractility:
      i. If CVP is <4 mm Hg (PAOP <6 mm Hg) there is a need for volume resuscitation. Fluids should be administered until the CVP approaches 8–10 mm Hg (PAOP 13–15 mm Hg).
      ii. If CVP is high (>10 mm Hg) (PAOP >15 mm Hg) the patient is volume replete or has underlying myocardial disease resulting in a decrease in cardiac compliance. In this scenario, positive inotropes such as dobutamine or dopamine should be used to augment cardiac output.
  ii. Systemic vascular resistance can be measured with indicator-dilution curves injected through a traditional pulmonary artery catheter or via transpulmonary cardiac output calculations:
    1. Systemic vascular resistance (SVR) is a determinant of blood pressure according to the following equation: $CO \times SVR = Blood\ Pressure$.
    2. Measurement of CO and SVR can be helpful to ascertain the reason for hypotension. If SVR is normal or high, hypotension is caused by decreased cardiac output. If SVR is low, hypotension is caused by decreased vasomotor tone that can be augmented by vasopressors such as dopamine, norepinephrine, epinephrine, or vasopressin.
  iii. Mixed venous oxygen saturation can be obtained from the pulmonary artery sampling port of the pulmonary artery catheter:
    1. Monitoring of mixed venous oxygen saturation can provide information about tissue oxygen delivery. Close monitoring of mixed venous oxygen saturation in severely injured patients may aid in early recognition of shock.
    2. Resuscitation of the patient until mixed venous oxygen saturation exceeds 70% is thought to reflect adequate resuscitation.
    3. Alternatively, monitoring central venous oxygen saturation, which is obtained via a central venous catheter just outside the right atrium, may be a less invasive way to assess adequacy of resuscitation. Similar values (>70%) should be targeted.

6. MECHANISMS TO IMPROVE TISSUE OXYGEN DELIVERY (See Figure 3.1)
  a. Improve oxygen content in circulation:
    i. The goal should be to maintain oxygen saturation of hemoglobin (SaO_2) minimally above 90%, and optimally around 96% or higher.
    ii. Increase the inspired oxygen concentration in the environment until the SaO_2 exceeds 90%:
      1. Note: once hemoglobin is fully saturated, further increases in PaO_2 result in minimal improvements in oxygen delivery. Therefore, supplementing oxygen to obtain a PaO_2 in excess of 97–100 mm Hg will have minimal effect on oxygen delivery and could result in oxygen toxicity.
      2. If the SaO_2 cannot be maintained above 90% despite increased inspired oxygen concentrations no higher than 60%, then intubation and positive pressure ventilation may

be required. Positive pressure ventilation is often used successfully in dogs and cats with massive thoracic trauma resulting in hypoxemia. Positive pressure ventilation, however, will worsen and pneumothorax and thoracostomy tubes attached to continuous suction are likely to be needed.

b. Improve cardiac output:

    i. Intravenous fluids as needed to correct hypovolemia (see the following).

    ii. Positive inotropes, such as dobutamine (3–15 mcg/kg/min), to improve cardiac contractility.

c. Improve hemoglobin concentration in circulation (see Chapter 4: Monitoring of the Trauma Patient):

    i. Acute blood loss and decreases in hematocrit can significantly impair tissue oxygen delivery, from the perspective of reducing both cardiac output and hemoglobin concentrations in circulation.

    ii. If it is difficult to recommend an exact hematocrit/hemoglobin concentration where one should consider blood transfusions:

        1. Experimentally, myocardial ischemia is noted when hemoglobin drops below 5 g/dL (hematocrit 15%) and anaerobic metabolism emerges when hemoglobin drops below 3 g/dL (hematocrit 9%) during euvolemic anemia.

        2. In human medicine, critically ill patients with hemoglobin concentrations below 7 g/dL (hematocrit less than 21%) warrant transfusion. Transfusions are considered when hemoglobin approaches 10 g/dL in critically ill patients.

        3. With acute blood loss, it will take some time for hemoglobin levels to decrease and therefore transfusion may be indicated prior to arriving at a specific low hemoglobin trigger.

        4. With more long-standing anemia, patients develop tolerance for lower hemoglobin concentrations.

7. VASCULAR ACCESS

a. Intravenous:

    i. Catheter choice:

        1. Short, large-bore, over-the-needle catheters (i.e., 12–18 gauge, 1–2 inch) placed in peripheral veins are preferred in the early management of traumatized patients. These catheters are inexpensive, easy to use, and afford the ability to rapidly initiate fluid resuscitation.

        2. Many central venous catheters are longer than peripheral catheters–this is not helpful when attempting to rapidly administer fluids during resuscitation as the rate at which fluids can be administered decreases as the length of the catheter increases.

    ii. Catheter location:

        1. When vascular access is needed in the traumatized patient, the initial catheter should be placed at a site that is easily accessed with minimal stress to the patient and is familiar to the person placing the catheter. Most often, this is a peripheral catheter placed in the cephalic or lateral saphenous vein:

            a. Care should be taken to avoid catheter placement in broken limbs, limbs with significant soft tissue injuries, or limbs with known or suspected vascular disruption proximal to the catheter site.

            b. Alternative sites for peripheral vascular access include the medial saphenous vein (more frequently used in cats), the accessory cephalic vein distal to the carpus, and the auricular veins that run along the ear margins.

        2. Animals with severe cardiovascular compromise may benefit from catheter placement in the jugular vein.

            a. The jugular vein is larger and therefore more likely to be accessible despite marked peripheral vascular collapse.

            b. Jugular venous catheterization will not only facilitate placement of a larger bore catheter, but also allow for more rapid fluid administration a result of the larger circumference of the vessel into which the fluids enter.

            c. Jugular catheterization is often more stressful for the animal than peripheral vessel catheterization. Some animals will have depressed mentation as a result of cardiovascular collapse and therefore will allow this procedure with minimal to no distress. However, if placement of a catheter at this site causes distress, one or two peripheral venous catheters should be placed depending upon the size of the patient and the required fluid volume for resuscitation. Use of systemic analgesics that spare the cardiovascular system should be administered prior to jugular catheterization (see Chapter 5: Analgesia and Anesthesia for the Trauma Patient).

d. Catheterization of the jugular vein may allow for monitoring of central venous pressure if the tip of the catheter extends beyond the thoracic inlet, but this is usually not possible when a short, large-bore catheter is used for fluid resuscitation. Once fluid resuscitation is complete, it is possible to exchange the catheter for a longer catheter that reaches the thoracic vena cava just cranial to the right atrium via the Seldinger technique (Figure 3.7a–h):

   i. The Seldinger technique uses a flexible wire that is passed distally into the catheterized vessel through the needle or catheter.

   ii. Once the wire is passed distally, the needle or catheter can be removed, leaving only the wire in the vessel.

   iii. A vessel dilator is passed over the wire to facilitate placement of a larger catheter. The dilator is then removed, again leaving only the wire.

   iv. Finally, the central venous catheter is fed over the wire into the vessel and the wire is then removed.

e. If there is a concern for intracranial trauma, the jugular vein should not be used for catheterization, as even transient compression of the jugular vein can markedly increase intracranial pressure and result in patient deterioration (see Chapter 7: Traumatic Brain Injury).

f. In addition, if there is concern for a coagulopathy (either hypo- or hyper-coagulability), jugular venipuncture should be avoided.

   iii. Catheterization techniques:

   1. Percutaneous catheterization: most commonly used when peripheral vessels are readily visible or palpable. The catheter is inserted at a 15–30° angle into the vessel with the bevel up. When a flash of blood is noted in the catheter hub, the entire catheter and stylet should be advanced together another 1–2 mm, then the catheter fed off the stylet into the vessel.

   2. Facilitated percutaneous catheterization should be used in animals with tough or thick skin that results in burring of the catheter tip during insertion through the skin. In this approach, a needle or scalpel blade is used to make a small knick (i.e., 2–4 mm) in the skin overlying the site of catheterization allowing for less tissue drag during catheter placement. The technique for placement of the catheter is identical to the aforementioned method. This approach is recommended for jugular catheterization due to the thicker nature of the skin in this area.

   3. Venous cut down: this method can be used over either a peripheral vein or the jugular vein when hypoperfusion or swelling impairs the ability to adequately visualize or palpate the vessel:

   a. When time allows, strict aseptic procedure (clipping, skin preparation, and sterile gloves) should be used.

   b. If aseptic technique cannot be used during the cut down for catheterization, the catheter should be used for the minimal amount of time necessary, at most 24 hours, until vascular access elsewhere can be obtained. Prophylactic antibiotics (cefazolin 22 mg/kg IV Q8 hours) should be administered in this situation. Once this catheter is removed, the cut down site should be treated like any contaminated wound and surgically closed when the animal is more stable.

   c. Peripheral:

      i. The saphenous or cephalic veins are preferred for this procedure as they are larger and readily accessible.

      ii. The skin can either be tented and an incision made with the scalpel

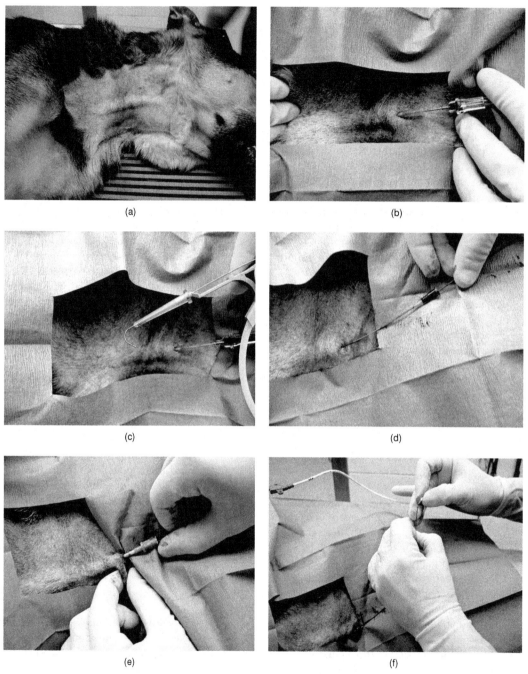

(a)

(b)

(c)

(d)

(e)

(f)

FIGURE 3.7 (a–h) Technique for placement of an intravenous catheter via the Seldinger method. (a) The animal should be placed in lateral recumbency and the hair should be liberally clipped and aseptically prepared to maintain sterility during catheter placement. (b) The jugular vein should be draped and sterile gloves should be worn. Lidocaine can be used to provide local anesthesia and a small skin incision should be made to facilitate catheter placement. In this picture, an 18 gauge, 1.5 inch over the needle catheter is inserted into the jugular vein toward the animal's heart while an assistant occludes the vein. (c): Once the catheter is inserted, the stylet is removed, and the J-wire is introduced through the catheter into the jugular vein. In order to straighten out the curve (J) in the wire, it must be retracted back into the device that holds the wire. (d): After the J-wire has been inserted, the original catheter can be removed, leaving only the wire in the vessel.

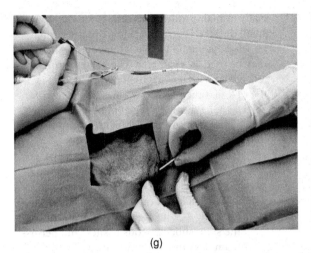
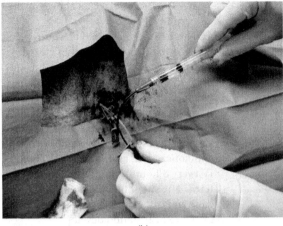

(g)   (h)

FIGURE 3.7 (*Continued*) (e): Next, the vessel dilator is fed over the J-wire and inserted into the jugular vein. There is often resistance to the dilator as it is passed through skin and into the jugular vein. The dilator is then removed, leaving only the wire in the jugular vein. Bleeding from around the jugular vein is common at this point and slight pressure with sterile gauze can be used to minimize blood loss. (f): The "permanent" intravenous catheter is then fed over the wire into the jugular vein. (g): Once the catheter is fed to the level of the skin, the J-wire is backed out until it exits the catheter at its port. (h): The catheter is then fed into the jugular vein to its desired depth, all of the ports should be checked for the ability to retrieve a blood sample, and then all ports should be flushed with sterile heparinized saline, being careful not to flush air into the jugular vein. The catheter can then be sutured in place and a soft padded bandage can be placed over the catheter. The bandage should be changed daily and the catheter site inspected for any infection or inflammation.

blade held upside down, or an incision can be made in a downward manner just lateral to the vein. Do not incise directly over the vein to avoid trauma to underlying structures.

iii. Retract the skin to expose the vein.

iv. Place the tips of Mosquito forceps directly over the vein and bluntly dissect the fascia surrounding the vein by opening/closing the jaws of the forceps in a direction parallel to the vein.

v. Once the fascia has been removed and the vein is free, pass the tips of the forceps underneath the vein to lift and stabilize the vessel for direct catheterization. Alternatively, suture can be passed around the proximal and distal portion of the vein and used as stay sutures to occlude venous flow then tied off once the catheter is in place.

d. Jugular:

i. The patient should be placed in lateral recumbency with the head and neck extended.

ii. The jugular vein should be occluded at the thoracic inlet. The skin should be incised just lateral to the vessel in line with the caudal angle of the mandible and the thoracic inlet just lateral to the vein. The incision should be approximately 1/3–1/2 of the length between these two landmarks.

iii. Subcutaneous tissue and fat should be bluntly dissected, parallel to the incision using forceps, in order to expose the jugular vein. Placement of the catheter percutaneously and then into the cut-down site and into the vessel will create a subcutaneous tunnel that may make the catheter less prone to infection rather than placing it directly through the cut-down site.

    iv. Proceed as directed above for the peripheral cut-down.

    e. These catheters should be sutured in place and the overlying skin closed with suture, a topical antibiotic ointment should be applied and the catheter wrapped in a standard fashion to secure it. Catheters placed without strict sterility should be removed as soon as better vascular access is achieved and systemic antibiotics, such as cefazolin (22 mg/kg IV every 8 hours) should be administered. The site should be monitored daily and catheters removed if signs of infection or irritation develop.

b. Intraosseous (Figure 3.8):

    i. Intraosseous catheters are underused in the traumatized and hypovolemic patient. Placement of an intraosseous catheter is a relatively easy way to gain rapid circulatory access in patients with cardiovascular collapse. Fluids and drugs administered intraosseously gain immediate access to the circulation via the sinusoids within the bone marrow cavity.

    ii. The contraindications for placement of an intraosseous catheter include localized infection or disease at the placement site, fracture of the proposed bone, and sepsis.

    iii. The biggest disadvantage to placement of an intraosseous catheter is the absolute rate at which fluids can be administered. Because bone is a nondistendable space, this limits the rate at which fluids can be accommodated. Rates as fast as 24 mL/min (1440 mL/h) can be achieved with pressurized flow. Therefore, when shock rates of fluids are needed in animals >16 kg, multiple intraosseous catheters may be needed.

    iv. The most common site for placement of an intraosseous catheter is into the proximal femur through the trochanteric fossa, similar to placement of an intramedullary pin for femoral fracture repair. Other reported sites for intraosseous catheter placement include the wing of the ilium, the ischium, the greater tubercle of the humerus, or the flat surface on the medial aspect of the proximal tibia.

    v. A variety of needles can be used for intraosseous catheterization, including styletted spinal or bone marrow needles or commer-

cially available intraosseous catheter kits. In small dogs (<7 kg), cats, and pediatric animals an 18–22 gauge 1–1$\frac{1}{2}$ inch hypodermic needle may be used as a catheter. The biggest problem associated with using a hypodermic needle is the risk that the needle becomes plugged with cortical bone during placement because of the lack of a stylet, making it difficult to impossible to flush.

    vi. Placement technique (see Figure 3.8):

    1. Aseptically prepare the skin overlying the bone.

    2. A local block can be performed by instilling 1–2 mg/kg of 2% lidocaine into the skin, subcutaneous tissues, and periosteum over the insertion site.

    3. A stab incision may be made with a scalpel where the catheter is to be inserted.

    4. Stabilize the limb in one hand with one finger running down the long axis of the bone in which you are inserting the device. With the other hand, insert the needle through the incision until the tip of the needle touches bone. For the femur, the author prefers to attempt to initially position the tip of the needle on the greater trochanter and then "walk" the tip medially until it drops into the most lateral aspect of the trochanteric fossa. This technique makes injury to the sciatic nerve very unlikely.

    5. Rotate hub of the needle back and forth 30–45° while applying firm downward pressure to seat needle into the cortical bone.

    6. Continue to drive the needle through the cortex into the medullary cavity—once you hit the medullary cavity, there is a sudden loss of resistance and the needle will feed much easier.

    7. The needle is properly placed when the hub of the needle moves with the limb and does not dislodge when the limb is moved, bone marrow can be aspirated into the needle, and when flushed with heparinized saline the fluid flows freely.

    8. If the needle does not flush you can rotate the hub of the needle 90°, back the needle out 2–3 mm or flush under pressure to attempt to dislodge any bone core

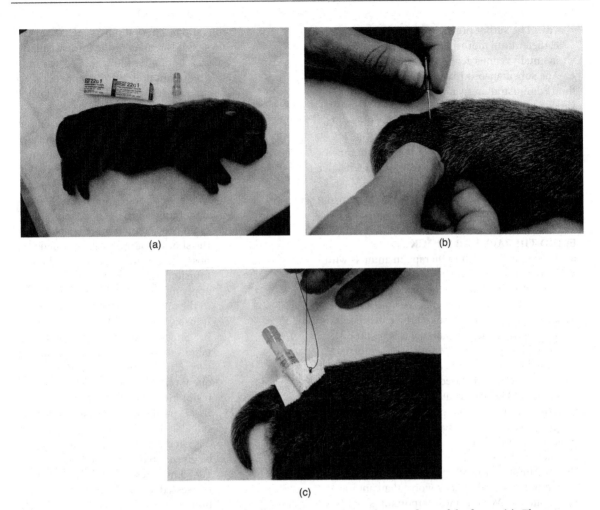

(a)

(b)

(c)

FIGURE 3.8   Technique for placement of an intraosseous catheter in the trochanteric fossa of the femur. (a): The puppy is placed in lateral recumbency and the area over the hip is clipped and aseptically prepared. In a dog of this size, a 20–22 gauge 1-inch hypodermic needle should be sufficient to penetrate into the medullary canal and deliver intravenous fluids and/or drugs. An injection cap (shown) or T-set can be connected to the needle after it is placed. (b): The femur should be stabilized with the nondominant hand near the mid-shaft. Holding the needle in the dominant hand, the needle is inserted through the skin and walked off the medial aspect of the greater trochanter to seat it in the trochanteric fossa. Gentle pressure is applied to the needle while it is rotated 30–45° on its axis. (c): Once the cortical bone has been penetrated, there will be a sudden loss of resistance and the needle should feed into the medullary canal. Aspirates on the needle should reveal marrow into the hub. The needle should be gently flushed with heparinized saline and an injection cap or T-set attached to intravenous fluids. A small piece of tape can be placed around the hub of the needle in butterfly fashion. The catheter can be secured in place by placing suture through the skin and adjacent to the wings of the butterfly tape. Alternatively, a soft bandage can be placed; however, bandages in this region area difficult to secure and may become easily soiled.

in the tip of the needle. Care should be taken to ensure fluid is not extravasating into the subcutaneous tissues.

9. The needle should be sutured in place using a tape butterfly and the area covered with a bandage/wrap.

vii. Intraosseous catheters can be left in place for at least 72 hours, similar to intravenous catheters, and could be used for longer periods of time so long as the insertion site appears clean and there is no pain associated with injection or infusion.

viii. The author prefers to only use the IO catheter until more appropriate and easier to maintain venous access can be acquired.

c. The subcutaneous route is *not* acceptable for fluid administration to animals with signs of shock:

   i. With hypovolemia, the peripheral vascular beds are vasoconstricted

   ii. This route of fluid therapy will help rehydrate the interstitial space but is not an effective way to expand the intravascular space. Most animals have normal hydration status following trauma.

8. FLUID THERAPY FOR SHOCK

a. The main goal of fluid therapy in animals with shock is to restore adequate circulation without causing excessive harm to the patient—this is a delicate balance. Overly aggressive fluid administration could potentially exacerbate the risk for hemorrhage in a bleeding animal as a result of improved blood flow to the source of hemorrhage, decreased blood viscosity, and dilution of clotting factors, as well as increased perfusion pressure. Fluids should be used cautiously in the patient with thoracic trauma and pulmonary contusions, as aggressive fluid resuscitation may exacerbate pulmonary dysfunction.

b. There is no evidence in the literature to support that one fluid resuscitation regimen (i.e., isotonic crystalloids) is any better or worse than another (i.e., colloids). What is most important is resuscitation of the patient such that delivery of oxygen to the tissues is restored.

c. Options for fluid therapy:

   i. Crystalloids:

      1. Isotonic:

         a. Isotonic crystalloids are the most readily available and familiar fluid used initially in volume resuscitation of the traumatized patient.

         b. Examples of isotonic crystalloids include 0.9% NaCl and balanced electrolyte solutions such as Normosol-R®, Plasmalyte®, Lactated Ringer's, and Ringer's Acetate.

         c. Isotonic crystalloids redistribute to the entire extracellular space, which is approximately 1/3 intravascular and 2/3 interstitial. Thus, at most, only 1/3 of these fluids remain in the intravascular space 1 hour after infusion. Because of this redistribution, the recommended volume for resuscitation with isotonic crystalloids is 3 times the volume lost.

         d. The shock dose of isotonic crystalloid solutions is 90 mL/kg in the dog and 66 mg/kg in the cat. This is the volume that one should be prepared to administer *as quickly as possible* when signs of hypovolemic shock are present:

            i. Simple concepts that facilitate rapid resuscitation include using the shortest, largest gauge catheter possible, elevating the height of the infusion relative to the patient, and applying an external pressure bag to the infusion (Clear-cuff Pressure Infusor, Medex, Dublin, OH).

            ii. Shock doses of isotonic crystalloid solutions should be administered to clinical effect, with frequent reassessment of the patient for restoration of circulation.

            iii. Typically the entire shock dose is calculated (i.e., 1800 mL for a 20-kg dog) and a portion of that fluid will be given rapidly (i.e., 600 mL over 10–15 minutes), then the patient is reassessed for adequacy of resuscitation.

            iv. Physical examination end-points of resuscitation may include normalization of heart rate, mucous membrane color, capillary refill time, peripheral pulse quality, and improvement in mentation and peripheral limb temperature.

         e. Only 1/4–1/3 of the volume infused remains in the intravascular space after one hour because of redistribution through the entire extravascular space. Therefore, the patient should be reassessed every 10–15 minutes for the first hour following their shock bolus of isotonic crystalloid, to ensure maintenance of adequate resuscitation.

2. Hypertonic:

a. Hypertonic saline solutions (HSS) are an affordable resuscitation fluid which may be beneficial in the traumatized patient with hemorrhagic shock, traumatic brain injury, and even vasodilatory shock:

   i. HSS are most commonly used at a 7.0–7.8% concentration. This fluid may be given alone or in combination with an artificial colloid.

   ii. Extremely concentrated formulations of hypertonic saline are commercially available—one common formulation is available at a 23.4% concentration (Hospira, Inc., Lake Forest, IL). *Note*: This solution should never be given directly intravenously without dilution to a lesser concentration (i.e., 7.0–7.8%) with either saline or an artificial colloid as the hypertonicity of this formulation can cause marked vascular irritation and red blood cell hemolysis.

   iii. Despite its hypertonicity, HSS is still a crystalloid fluid. Therefore, following intravascular volume expansion, it will redistribute to the entire extracellular space (interstitial + intravascular compartments) and at most 1/3 of the total volume expansion remains intravascular after 1 hour.

   iv. Combining hypertonic saline with an artificial colloid produces a synergistic effect—both the degree and duration of volume expansion obtained from the combination of these two fluids exceeds that which could be obtained by either fluid alone.

   v. The duration of volume expansion has been shown to increase 30 minutes when HSS is used alone to 3 hours when combined with an artificial colloid in dogs. The duration of volume expansion is similar whether hetastarch or dextran-70 is used in combination with hypertonic saline.

   vi. However, dextran-70 has been shown to promote a larger degree of volume expansion in combination with HSS compared to an equivalent volume of hetastarch. This is because the degree of volume expansion obtained with an artificial colloid is related to the number of molecules rather than the size of the particles present in the solution.

b. HSS are insufficient for maintenance requirements (2–3 mL/kg/h) or to replace ongoing losses. Therefore, isotonic crystalloid solutions, at rates suitable to account for those needs, are mandatory following initial shock doses of HSS.

c. Purported benefits of hypertonic saline resuscitation:

   i. Lower infusion volumes required for resuscitation compared to isotonic crystalloids and artificial colloids—this facilitates more rapid resuscitation:

      1. Experimental studies in dogs demonstrate that the volume of HSS needed for resuscitation in hemorrhagic shock was only 10% of shed blood volume, compared to 3 times the shed blood volume needed with isotonic crystalloids.

      2. The shock dose of hypertonic saline is 3–5 mL/kg for dogs and 2–3 mL/kg for cats. It is important to remember that this small volume is equivalent to giving a full shock bolus of isotonic crystalloids! Therefore, HSS should be administered "to effect" similar to the way that isotonic crystalloids are administered in shock. Not every patient will require the full shock dose.

      3. There are several different concentrations of hypertonic

saline solutions available commercially:

    a. 23.4% sodium chloride: Calculate the total dose to be administered based upon a 3–5 mL/kg dose in the dog or a 2–3 mL/kg dose in the cat. Dilute 1 part HSS into 2 parts dextran-70 or hydroxyethyl starch mixed in the same syringe to achieve the desired total dose. This will effectively make a 7.8% solution.

    b. 7.0–7.5% sodium chloride: This solution should not be further diluted with an artificial colloid. If a colloid is desired, administer a 2–3 mL/kg dose separately, rather than mixing in the same syringe.

    4. The rate of administration of HSS should not exceed 1 mL/kg/min, as vagally-mediated bradycardia and hypotension have been documented to occur at higher rates.

ii. Reduction of cerebral edema and lowering of intracranial pressure:

    1. 5 mL/kg 7.5% hypertonic saline is equiosmolar to 1.0 g/kg of Mannitol—meaning it has a similar ability to reduce cerebral edema.

iii. Minimizing vasospasm: Initially HSS promote peripheral vasodilation which reduces cardiac afterload, thus improving cardiac output. In addition, they have been shown to decrease endothelial cell swelling, which may improve local oxygen delivery to injured tissues.

iv. Minimizing excitotoxicity in the brain: Following traumatic brain injury, massive neuronal depolarization and cell membrane dysfunction result in extracellular accumulation of glutamate, an excitatory neurotransmitter which increases cerebral metabolic rate. The high sodium concentration in HSS facilitates transmembrane flux of glutamate back into the intracellular space, thus reducing further injury to the brain.

v. Reducing the inflammatory response to injury: HSS have been shown to decrease neutrophil activation and burst, reduce adhesion molecular expression in the tissues, and improve T-cell function. These properties make HSS an intriguing fluid choice in patients with brain injury, where the local inflammatory response promotes progressive neurological injury, and in the patient with the systemic inflammatory response following injury, wherein an over-exuberant inflammatory response throughout the body promotes vascular leak, vasodilation and perpetuates end-organ damage.

d. Risks associated with HSS administration:

i. HSS are not approved by the FDA for use in human patients in the United States but are approved in at least 11 other countries.

ii. HSS will promote hypernatremia immediately following administration—in fact, that is the way by which they are most effective. Despite the concern for neurological damage (central pontine myelinolysis) when sodium concentrations are rapidly raised, this has not been documented in human clinical trials involving over 1000 patients.

iii. Because HSS are so effective at rapidly increasing blood volume and pressure, there is a concern that they may promote ongoing blood loss or re-bleeding in some patients.

iv. As with other therapies used to reduce intracranial pressure (i.e., mannitol), there is always a concern that a rebound increase in intracranial pressure may result once these therapies are discontinued.

ii. Artificial colloids:

1. Artificial colloids contain large molecular weight substances which promote retention of the fluid within the intravascular space, thereby providing volume expansion at lesser doses than required for isotonic crystalloids and limiting the risk for edema formation.

   a. Hydroxyethyl starches (HES) (i.e., Hetastarch and Pentastarch):

      i. An amylopectin polymer with an average molecular weight of 400–450 kD. However, the number average molecular weight (referring to the molecular weight of the majority of the molecules in the bag) is approximately 70 kD.

      ii. Because of the larger molecular size, HES has a longer duration of action compared to Dextran-70.

   b. Dextrans:

      i. Dextran-70, a glucose polymer, has an average molecular weight of 70 kd. Because degree of volume expansion is related to the number of molecules present, rather than the size of those molecules, Dextran-70 is more effective on a per milliliter basis for volume expansion compared to HES.

      ii. Dextran-40: This artificial colloid is not recommended for use in the hypovolemic patient. While this fluid will quickly expand the vascular volume, the average size of the colloid molecules in this solution (40 kD) is such that they are rapidly filtered and lost through the kidneys and therefore are not an efficient means to maintain volume expansion. In addition, acute renal tubular necrosis has been documented with the use of this fluid.

2. Indications for artificial colloid therapy include rapid intravascular volume expansion of the hypovolemic patient and to limit edema formation in patients with hypoproteinemia (total protein <4.0 g/dL), hypoalbuminemia (albumin <2.0 g/dL), or increased vascular permeability.

3. The dose of HES or dextran-70 recommended for treatment of hypovolemic shock is 10–20 mL/kg. It is recommended that aliquots of 5–10 mL/kg in dogs, and 5 mL/kg in cats, be titrated to clinical effect.

4. The oncotic effect of artificial colloids cannot be measured with refractometry, nor does the total protein concentration accurately reflect the effective oncotic pressure in patients receiving artificial colloids. Measurement of colloid osmotic pressure (COP) with a colloid osmometer (Wescor 4420, Wescor Inc., Logan, UT) is the only way to accurately and definitively measure the effect of these products.

5. The use of both HES and Dextran-70 have been associated with increased risk for bleeding. The coagulation defects are thought to be dose related and seen with doses at or above 20 mL/kg per day. Elevations in prothrombin time (PT) and activated partial thromboplastin time (PTT) may be noted, but are usually not associated with clinical evidence of bleeding. The coagulopathy seen with HES and Dextran-70 administration is thought to occur secondary to dilution of coagulation factors, accelerated fibrinolysis, and depletion of Factor VIII/von Willebrand Factor complex. Dextran-70 impairs clotting by coating and inactivating platelets, as well.

6. Monitoring of coagulation panels is suggested when using artificial colloids at doses close to or exceeding 20 mL/kg per day and supplementation with fresh frozen plasma to correct any alterations in PT/PTT is advised when invasive procedures are planned.

iii. Hemoglobin based oxygen carriers (HBOC):

1. HBOC, such as Oxyglobin (Biopure, Cambridge, MA) can be used not only for the oxygen carrying capacity afforded from the polymerized, stroma-free hemoglobin, but also as a potent colloid, with an average molecular weight of 200 kD.

2. These products are useful for resuscitation of acute hemorrhagic shock, particularly when blood products are not readily available.

3. Doses of 10–30 mL/kg at rates up to 10 mL/kg/h have been recommended for resuscitation following acute hemorrhage in the dog. In the cat, doses of 5–15 mL/kg, at rates not to exceed 5 mL/kg/h, have been recommended. Oxyglobin should be used with caution in cats as its use is off label and cats appear to be more sensitive to volume overload with this product, resulting in pulmonary edema and/or pleural effusion. These products can be used alone or in combination with isotonic crystalloids for resuscitation.

4. Oxyglobin will discolor mucous membranes, plasma and urine, thus interfering with chromogenic biochemical monitoring techniques. With Oxyglobin use, whole blood hemoglobin concentrations should be monitored to estimate red blood cell counts, rather than measurement of packed cell volume. Multiplying the whole blood hemoglobin (g/dL) concentration by 3 will provide the equivalent hematocrit achieved by Oxyglobin administration in combination with the patient's own red blood cells.

iv. Blood products:

1. Fresh whole blood or packed red blood cells and fresh frozen plasma may all be needed for resuscitation of the traumatized patient. Transfusion of red blood cells during the early stabilizing phase after trauma offers the benefit of increasing cardiac output while preserving oxygen carrying capacity.

2. An additional benefit of early red blood cell transfusion is enhanced coagulation via release of platelet activating factor, increasing blood viscosity and promoting margination of platelets and clotting factors around the vessel wall.

3. The downside to early red blood cell transfusion is that stored blood products become depleted in 2,3-DPG making the transfused cells less readily able to release oxygen to the tissues. In addition, the cells may be damaged in storage making them less deformable in the microcirculation. Finally, transfusions can upregulate the inflammatory response.

4. As the hematocrit increases, the patient's blood will become more viscous. In low cardiac output states this may worsen cardiac output. Therefore, resuscitation with crystalloid fluids prior to or during transfusion may be optimal.

5. Massive transfusion is defined as the transfusion of more than 1 blood volume (>90 mL/kg dog, >66 mL/kg cat) in a 24-hour period or more than $1/2$ of a blood volume (>45 mL/kg dog, >33 mL/kg cat) in less than 3 hours:

a. Massive transfusions may be life-saving in patients with substantial or ongoing hemorrhage.

b. The risks associated with massive transfusion include the following:

i. Ionized hypocalcemia and hypomagnesemia:

1. The citrate which is used as an anticoagulant in blood products can bind calcium and magnesium.

2. When given in sufficient volumes, clinical signs of hypocalcemia and/or hypomagnesemia can occur:

a. Muscle weakness and tremors

b. Arrhythmias

c. Refractory hypotension

3. Treatment of transfusion-associated hypocalcemia and hypomagnesemia is warranted *only* if clinical signs are apparent:

a. Calcium gluconate (50–150 mg/kg) can be administered as a slow intravenous bolus to correct clinical signs associated with hypocalcemia.

b. Magnesium chloride is recommended over magnesium sulfate for treatment of hypomagnesemia in this scenario, as sulfates may bind calcium and potentiate the hypocalcemia.

4. Once the transfusion has been completed, the liver will metabolize the citrate and electrolyte concentrations will return to baseline.

ii. Thrombocytopenia:

1. Moderate thrombocytopenia (50,000–100,000 cells/uL) is commonly seen following massive transfusion and thought to occur secondary to dilution as stored blood products are deficient in platelets.

iii. Hypothermia:

1. Hypothermia could be caused by transfusion of cold stored blood products and room temperature crystalloid or colloidal fluids or may be occur as a result of severe systemic illness in patients requiring transfusions.

2. Commercially available in-line fluid warmers can be used to rapidly warm transfused products and other intravenous fluids at high infusion rates to reduce the incidence of hypothermia.

iv. Transfusion reactions:

1. Transient fever, vomiting, urticaria, and pruritis are the most common transfusion reactions noted when type-specific transfusions are administered to animals who have not received prior blood product transfusions. A small percentage of these reactions are related to mast cell degranulation, resulting in urticaria and pruritus, which can be treated with anti-histamines (Diphenhydramine 1–2 mg/kg IM). Nonhemolytic febrile reactions, associated with transfusion of white blood cell antigens, will not respond to anti-histamines.

2. Blood typing prior to transfusion is mandatory in cats (blood type A, B, or AB). Cats should only receive type specific blood products, as life-threatening transfusion reactions can occur quickly in cats that have never been transfused due to the presence of naturally occurring antibodies to other blood types:

   a. When blood typing is not possible, a major and minor cross-match must be performed to ensure a compatible transfusion.

3. Because dogs lack clinically significant naturally occurring antibodies to blood types other than their own, a first blood transfusion should never result in an acute hemolytic transfusion reaction. Despite this, blood typing should be performed in dogs prior to transfusion therapy in order to administer the most compatible blood product and limit the risk for allo-antibody production to the most antigenic blood group (DEA 1.1). When blood typing is not readily available, DEA 1.1 negative products should be used.

4. Crossmatching of type-specific blood products to any animal who has been previously transfused can help to minimize transfusion reactions.

v. Documented in human medicine but not documented in veterinary patients to date:

1. Hyperkalemia (dogs, other than Akitas and other Far Eastern dog breeds do not store substantial amounts of potassium inside red cells)

2. Coagulopathy due to hemodilution

3. Transfusion related acute lung injury (TRALI)

9. END-POINTS OF RESUSCITATION

a. A simple physical examination during and after resuscitation from shock is often useful to determine adequacy of resuscitation. Normalization of heart, mucous membrane color, capillary refill time, pulse quality, blood pressure, and urine output are all indicators of an improved circulatory status.

b. Despite the aforementioned clinical targets for resuscitation, it has been documented in hypovolemic human patients that more than 80% who are resuscitated to a normal heart rate, blood pressure and urine output may be under-resuscitated based upon the presence of ongoing anaerobic metabolism and tissue acidosis.

c. Measurement of global markers of anaerobic metabolism, such as lactate and base deficit, and assessment of oxygen extraction via mixed or central venous oxygen saturation, may be more sensitive markers of adequate resuscitation in the patient with shock:

    i. Lactate: Persistent elevation of lactate concentration following resuscitation likely indicates ongoing anaerobic metabolism, as the liver rapidly clears lactate from circulation once it is no longer being produced in excess. A normal lactate concentration in cats and dogs is less than 2.0 mmol/L. Persistence of hyperlactatemia has been associated with worsened outcome in human trauma patients.

    ii. Base deficit: In the absence of other causes of a high anion gap metabolic acidosis (i.e., diabetic ketoacidosis, uremic acidosis, or toxic acidosis as occurs with ethylene glycol ingestion), the base deficit can be used from standard blood gas analysis as an estimate of lactic acidosis and presence of ongoing anerobic metabolism. A normal base deficit is +4 to −4 mmol/L in dogs and +2 to −2 mmol/L in cats.

    iii. Mixed/central venous oxygen saturation: Mixed (measured from the pulmonary artery) or central (measured from the right atrium) venous oxygen saturation measurements can be used as an additional end-point of resuscitation. These measurements are available on most blood gas analyzers. With decreased oxygen delivery, the oxygen extraction ratio increases such that there is less oxygen remaining in the venous blood. Mixed and central venous oxygen saturations above 70% may indicate adequate resuscitation and restoration of normal tissue oxygen.

10. CORTICOSTEROID ADMINISTRATION FOR SHOCK IN TRAUMA PATIENTS

a. Corticosteroids are no longer recommended as a first line of therapy in traumatized patients.

b. Corticosteroids are not indicated for use in patients with hypovolemic shock.

c. Corticosteroids are not indicated for use in patients with traumatic brain injuries (see Chapter 7: Traumatic Brain Injury).

d. Corticosteroids use is questioned in patients with traumatic spinal cord injuries (see Chapter 9: Traumatic Spinal Injury).

11. HYPOTENSIVE RESUSCITATION

a. Hypotensive resuscitation refers to fluid resuscitation strategies that focus on early control of ongoing hemorrhage. In all of these strategies, the traditional end-points of resuscitation that focus on restoration of tissue perfusion and systemic blood pressure, are intentionally *not* met until after the source of hemorrhage has been controlled:

    i. Delayed resuscitation: in this strategy, no fluid resuscitation is performed until after hemorrhage has been controlled.

    ii. Limited volume resuscitation: in this strategy a conservative volume of fluids may be given, often to a preset subnormal arterial blood pressure, prior to control of hemorrhage. The target blood pressure for limited volume resuscitation is not well defined; however, a systolic blood pressure of 60 mm Hg has been used in some human clinical studies.

    iii. Early control of hemorrhage is paramount in this resuscitation scheme—in human medicine, this is most often accomplished by surgical control of hemorrhage. The one study (Bickell et al., 1994) which demonstrated a survival benefit using delayed resuscitation accomplished surgical control of hemorrhage within 80 minutes of the traumatic incident.

b. Purported benefits to hypotensive resuscitation focus predominantly on the volume of blood products needed in these patients. If lower pressures are accepted, then there is less hydrostatic pressure at the site of hemorrhage, which likely facilitates clot formation and strengthening. In addition, lower infusion volumes will cause less of a dilutional coagulopathy. This, in turn, limits the need for valuable, costly, and possibly risky blood product transfusions to the patient.

c. Contraindications for hypotensive resuscitation:

    i. Hypotensive resuscitation is *never* acceptable in animals with traumatic brain injuries, particularly when there is a concern for increased intracranial pressure:

    1. In the presence of increased intracranial pressure, any decrease in systemic blood pressure can hamper cerebral blood flow leading to increased brain injury. (see Chapter 7: Traumatic brain injury).

d. Possible risks with hypotensive resuscitation:

    i. Hypotensive resuscitation subjects the patient to prolonged organ hypoperfusion and possibly damage. The one study which supports hypotensive resuscitation in human literature left the patients hypotensive for less than 80 minutes on average from the time of injury to the surgical control of hemorrhage. It is not known if durations of time longer than this would be safe in any traumatized patient.

    ii. Hypotension and hypovolemia will persist (or possibly worsen due to blunting of the catecholamine response) during induction of anesthesia and in the early phases of surgery. This makes the patient less stable for general anesthesia and may make the surgical procedure more stressful to the patient, the anesthetist and the surgeon.

e. Application to veterinary medicine:

    i. If one is to employ the use of hypotensive resuscitation in veterinary trauma patients, it should be done with the knowledge that early surgical control of hemorrhage is the end-point, followed by full resuscitation of the patient.

    ii. Considering that few patients with traumatic intra-abdominal hemorrhage require surgical intervention for control of bleeding, one should question whether or not this resuscitation strategy should be used in veterinary patients following trauma.

BIBLIOGRAPHY

Bickell WH, Wall MJ, Pepe PE, et al. Immediate versus delayed fluid resuscitation for hypotensive patients with penetrating torso injuries. N Engl J Med 1994; 331: 1105–1109.

Bilkovskia RN, Rivers EP, Horst HM. Targeted resuscitation strategies after injury. Curr Opin Crit Care 2004; 10: 529–538.

Boysen SR, Rozanski EA, Tidwell AS, et al. Evaluation of a focused assessment with sonography for trauma protocol to detect free abdominal fluid in dogs involved in motor vehicular accidents. J Am Vet Med Assoc 2004; 225: 1198–1204.

Brady CA, Otto CM, Van Winkle TJ, et al. Severe sepsis in cats: a retrospective study of 29 cases (1986–1998). J Am Vet Med Assoc 2000; 217: 531–535.

Hauptman JG, Walshaw R, Olivier NB. Evaluation of the sensitivity and specificity of diagnostic criteria for sepsis in dogs. Vet Surg 1997; 26: 293–297.

Hughes D, Rozanski EA, Shofer FS, Laster LL, Drobatz KJ. Effect of sampling site, repeated sampling, pH, and pCO_2 on plasma lactate concentration in healthy dogs. Am J Vet Res 1999; 60: 521–524.

Hughes D, Beal MA. Emergency vascular access. Vet Clin North Am Small Anim Pract 2000; 30: 491–507.

Jutkowitz LA, Rozanski EA, Moreau JA, Rush JE. Massive transfusion in dogs: 15 cases (1997–2001). J Am Vet Med Assoc 2002; 220: 1664–1669.

Lagutchik MS, Ogilvie GK, Wingfield WE, Hackett TB. Lactate Kinetics in veterinary Critical Care: a review. J Vet Emerg Crit Care 1996; 6: 81–95.

Okano S, Yoshida M, Fukushima U, et al. Usefulness of systemic inflammatory response syndrome criteria as an index for prognosis judgment. Vet Record 2002; 150: 245–246.

Otto CM, Kaufman GM, Crowe DT. Intraosseous infusion of fluids and therapeutics. Compend Contin Educ Pract Vet 1989; 11: 421–430.

Purvis D, Kirby R. Systemic inflammatory response syndrome: septic shock. Vet Clin North Am Small Anim Pract 1994; 24: 1225–1247.

MONITORING THE TRAUMA PATIENT

Dana L. Clarke and Andrew J. Brown

1. INTRODUCTION

a. Stabilization of the emergent trauma patient requires rapid identification of problems, appropriate therapeutic measures to correct these problems, and intensive monitoring to assess resolution of problems or deterioration in the patient's condition.

b. Monitoring the trauma patient includes thorough and repeated physical examinations in conjunction with more objective measures of patient status.

c. The trauma patient requires frequent reassessment and intensive monitoring to detect changes related to the primary problem as well as assessing response to therapeutic measures that have been instituted.

d. The trauma patient is dynamic and can decompensate rapidly. The monitoring parameters and modalities discussed in this chapter will play a crucial role in the early detection of problems. Immediate reaction to and treatment of these problems that maximize the likelihood of a positive outcome.

e. Treatment orders should be written that allow for close monitoring of the trauma patients. Specific "call-orders" should be given to enable technicians and nurses to inform the clinician of a change in status of the trauma patient.

2. RESPIRATORY MONITORING

a. The respiratory system should be closely monitored in any animal following trauma due to the high incidence of thoracic injury in the polytrauma patient.

b. Deterioration in ability to oxygenate and/or ventilate adequately occurs commonly in the trauma patient. The patient's condition may worsen due to progression of the primary injury or secondary to therapeutic and diagnostic measures.

c. Animals that initially present with mild to no respiratory distress may deteriorate and require supportive measures.

d. Animals with more severe respiratory compromise at presentation should be monitored for response to therapy.

e. Respiratory rate, effort, and pattern should be frequently reassessed in the trauma patient.

f. If the patient has increased respiratory rate and/or effort, more intensive patient monitoring is necessary.

g. If there is *any* concern about the ability of the trauma patient to adequately oxygenate, supplemental oxygen should be provided. Common methods of oxygen support include flow-by, mask, nasal oxygen prongs and catheters, and placement of the patient in an oxygen cage (see Chapter 2: Triage and Primary Survey).

Manual of Trauma Management in the Dog and Cat, First Edition. Edited by Kenneth J. Drobatz, Matthew W. Beal and Rebecca S. Syring.
© 2011 John Wiley & Sons, Inc. Published 2011 by John Wiley & Sons, Inc.

h. Visual assessment of the respiratory system:

   i. Trauma patients should be observed frequently for signs of developing respiratory distress. These signs include postural changes such as neck extension and elbow abduction, paradoxical abdominal breathing, restlessness, and increased or decreased respiratory rate. It is important to remember that patients demonstrating these signs are at their limit of physiologic reserves. It is essential to minimize patient stress so as to avoid respiratory and/or cardiac arrest.

   ii. Respiratory rate:

     1. Normal respiratory rate in veterinary patients is considered to be 24–48 breaths per minute.

     2. Increased respiratory rate (tachypnea) in dogs and cats is generally considered to be above 50 breaths per minute.

     3. Other causes of tachypnea should be considered in trauma patients since an increase in respiratory rate does not always indicate compromise, but respiratory compromise should always be assumed until proven otherwise. Pain, fever, hyperthermia, stress/fear, and compensation for metabolic acidosis will all elicit an increase in respiratory rate.

   iii. Respiratory effort:

     1. Normal respiratory effort involves perceivable chest excursions with a minimal component of motion from the abdominal musculature.

     2. Increased respiratory effort (dyspnea) is characterized by increased chest and abdominal musculature motions and is perceived as labored or difficulty in breathing. Signs of increased respiratory effort include extension of the head and neck and abduction of the elbows. Nostril flare may be observed during inspiration. Open-mouthed breathing may be a sign of severe respiratory distress in cats but may also occur due to injury to the nasal passages and sinuses. An increase in respiratory effort in the trauma patient can be seen with pleural space disease (e.g., pneumothorax, hemothorax, or diaphragmatic hernia), pulmonary parenchymal disease (e.g., pulmonary contusion), chest wall injury, and upper airway obstruction or injury.

     3. Decreased respiratory effort is less commonly seen, and is characterized by decreased chest and abdominal muscle movement. Disease processes associated with decreased respiratory effort include head and spinal injury and end stage respiratory fatigue.

     4. Abnormal respiratory patterns seen in trauma patients include paradoxical respiration and flail segment motion:

       a. Paradoxical respiratory motion occurs when the chest wall expands with inspiration and the abdominal muscles and diaphragm are pulled inward. Causes of paradoxical respiration in the trauma patient include upper airway obstruction, diaphragmatic injury (rupture or paralysis secondary to the cervical spinal cord or phrenic nerve injury), and severe decreases in pulmonary compliance (as may occur with severe pulmonary contusion).

       b. Flail chest occurs following fracture of two or more adjacent ribs in two or more locations. The fractured segment of the chest wall is drawn inward on inspiration due to negative pressure generated within the thorax and the free-floating nature of the fractured segment. Similarly, the segment will move outward on expiration. For a more in-depth discussion of flail chest, see Chapter 6: Trauma-Associated Thoracic Injury.

i. Auscultation of the respiratory system:

   i. The emergency clinician should regularly listen to the trauma patient to permit early detection of changes in the patient's condition.

   ii. Abnormal breath sounds in trauma patients include those heard from a distance and those that require the aid of a stethoscope:

     1. Abnormal sounds of breathing heard from a distance, such as stridor (high pitched sounds of upper airway origin) or stertor (lower pitched sounds of pharyngeal origin) should be noted and investigated further:

       a. Stridor occurs where there is damage or obstruction to the upper airways.

       b. Stridorous sounds often cause referred upper airway noise on thoracic auscultation. Caution must therefore be exercised to prevent the noise being inaccurately attributed to intrathoracic pathology. Laryngeal and tracheal auscultation will aid in localization of the noise.

2. The thorax should be regularly ausculted in a systematic manner. Auscultation should be more frequent if the patient has increased respiratory rate and/or effort:

a. Each hemithorax should be divided into dorsal, middle, and ventral lung fields. Within each field, depending on the size of the patient, there should be two to three cranial to caudal zones of auscultation within each third of the thorax.

b. Each lung field should be ausculted and compared to the adjacent and contralateral fields.

c. A decrease in, or absence of lung sounds (in one or both sides of the thorax) in the trauma patient is consistent with pleural space disease. This may be secondary to air (pneumothorax), fluid (hemo- or chylothorax), or organ displacement (e.g., diaphragmatic hernia). The detection of clinically significant pleural space disease is a physical examination diagnosis; imaging techniques should NOT be necessary.

d. Dull lung sounds heard dorsally on auscultation are consistent with pneumothorax. This is a common injury in trauma patients and may be unilateral or bilateral. Thoracocentesis, to remove the air, is both diagnostic and therapeutic.

e. Dull lung sounds heard ventrally on thoracic auscultation are consistent with fluid in the pleural space. In the acute trauma patient, this fluid is usually blood; thoracocentesis is both diagnostic and therapeutic. Accumulation of chyle due to rupture of the thoracic duct also may cause these physical examination findings 24–96 hours after trauma occurs.

f. Patients with a diaphragmatic hernia may present with dull lung sounds ventrally and/or dorsally. Auscultation may also be normal, depending on the extent of organ herniation into the thorax. Imaging techniques such as survey radiography, positive contrast peritoneography/celiography, ultrasound, and CT or MRI may be necessary to confirm a diagnosis. Following patient stabilization, emergent surgical intervention is indicated.

g. Crackles heard on thoracic auscultation in the trauma patient are indicative of pulmonary contusion(s). Since contusions often progress before they resolve, frequent reassessment through auscultation and objective assessment of oxygenation is important.

h. Dyspneic trauma patients with both pleural space disease AND pulmonary contusion may have normal lung sounds.

j. Mucous membrane assessment:

i. Mucous membranes should be assessed during and following patient stabilization, and then every 2–6 hours thereafter, depending on the patient's condition.

ii. Membranes may be pale secondary to vasoconstriction (hypoperfusion, pain/catecholamines) or anemia.

iii. Blue mucous membranes (cyanosis) are seen with *severe* hypoxemia (when there is at least 5 g/dL of deoxygenated hemoglobin), and indicate a profound deficiency in the oxygen saturation of hemoglobin. Significant hypoxemia must therefore occur before a patient's mucous membranes become cyanotic, and the absence of cyanosis does not rule out significant respiratory compromise and hypoxemia:

1. The detection of cyanosis is dependent upon the concentration of erythrocytes (and therefore hemoglobin) within the blood.

2. Because cyanosis is only detected after 5 g/dL of hemoglobin is deoxygenated, cyanosis will more likely be observed in patients with greater hemoglobin concentrations.

3. In a normal dog or cat, with a hematocrit of 45% (or 15 g/dL of hemoglobin), approximately 1/3 of hemoglobin must be desaturated before cyanosis is detectable. This corresponds to an oxygen saturation of 66%, or a PaO_2 of 37–40 mm Hg.

4. It is almost impossible for cyanosis to be detected when anemia is present due to low hemoglobin concentrations in anemic patients:

a. For example, in a dog or cat with a hematocrit at or below 15% (or 5 g/dL of hemoglobin), all of its hemoglobin would have to be desaturated in order to demonstrate cyanosis, which is incompatible with life. Therefore, anemic animals may be significantly hypoxemic but may never demonstrate cyanosis.

k. Objective measures of respiratory monitoring:

i. More objective measures, such as pulse oximetry, arterial blood gas analysis, and end-tidal capnography are important adjuncts to the physical examination for monitoring respiratory status.

ii. Serial monitoring of these objective measurements provides valuable information regarding improvement or rapid detection of a deteriorating ability to oxygenate.

iii. Pulse oximetry:

1. Pulse oximetry provides a convenient and technically easy modality to estimate the percentage of hemoglobin saturated with oxygen in arterial blood (SpO_2).

2. A light signal using two different wavelengths is emitted from a phototransmitter and conducted through the tissues.

3. A detector measures the difference in light absorbance of oxygenated and reduced hemoglobin during pulsatile flow.

4. The value derived (SpO_2) is expressed as the percentage of hemoglobin saturated with oxygen.

5. The probe of the pulse oximeter can be placed on any area of nonpigmented, non- or thinly-haired skin. The most commonly used sites include the lip, tongue, toe, interdigital skin, ear margin, ventral abdomen, and vulva. If needed, hair can be clipped over the site intended for pulse oximetry monitoring.

6. Common causes of error include heavily pigmented skin, motion, high ambient light, and excessive peripheral vasoconstriction that prevents the generation of a detectable pulse. Measurements taken from sites that move in conjunction with respiration are also error-prone. These include the prepuce and ventral abdomen.

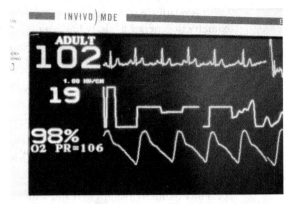

FIGURE 4.1   An example of a good pulse oximetry waveform. In this picture, the pulse rate detected by the pulse oximeter (bottom tracing) closely approximates true heart rate as detected by the ECG (top tracing) and a symmetric, repeatable waveform is created by a strong signal. The middle tracing in the picture represents the patient's respiratory rate.

7. Pulse oximetry is not reliable in patients with methemoglobinemia or carboxyhemoglobinemia.

8. For the pulse oximetry reading to be considered a reliable approximation of the percentage of saturated hemoglobin, the pulse rate generated must match that of the patient, and a consistent waveform must be produced (Figures 4.1 and 4.2).

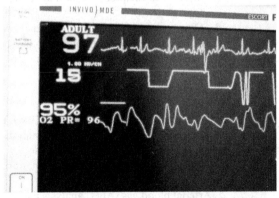

FIGURE 4.2   An example of a poor tracing from a pulse oximeter. The heart rate (generated from the top ECG tracing) and pulse rate (as detected by the pulse oximeter in the bottom tracing) are closely approximated and there is an acceptable value generated for the patient's oxygen saturation; however, the tracing is irregular and asymmetrical. The middle tracing in the picture represents the patient's respiratory rate.

9.   It is relatively common for pulse oximetry to generate a falsely low reading, underestimating oxygen saturation. Conversely, it is uncommon for it to generate a falsely elevated reading. Therefore, in the absence of methemoglobinemia or carboxyhemoglobinemia, the clinical impression is that the highest value generated by the pulse oximeter with a strong waveform and pulse rate matching that of the patient should be considered the percentage of hemoglobin saturated with oxygen.

10.   Pulse oximetry readings greater than 92% (corresponding to a PaO_2 just above 60 mm Hg) are generally considered to be acceptable and the patient probably does not require oxygen supplementation:

  a.   Patients with readings less than 92% should receive supplemental oxygen.

  b.   When the patient is already receiving oxygen supplementation, the value should be considered in light of their level of supplementation and underlying disease process to determine if more or less oxygen support is necessary. For example, oxygen should be supplemented much more aggressively in animals with head trauma to limit the risk for perpetuating brain injury (see Chapter 7: Traumatic Brain Injury).

11.   Oxygen saturation of hemoglobin should be serially or continuously monitored in any trauma patient with a concern regarding oxygenation.

iv.   Arterial blood gas analysis:

1.   By measuring the partial pressure of carbon dioxide ($PaCO_2$) and oxygen (PaO_2) in the arterial circulation, blood gas analysis provides an objective assessment of the effectiveness of ventilation and oxygenation respectively.

2.   Arterial blood gas (ABG) analysis may be utilized as a screening test for pulmonary gas exchange abnormalities in the patient that has sustained pulmonary trauma. Through the alveoloar-arterial oxygen gradient calculation, the severity of the gas exchange abnormality and thus lung injury can be quantified. Additional ABG analysis may be performed to detect improvement or deterioration in lung function.

3.   In the absence of an arterial blood gas, venous PCO_2 ($PvCO_2$) can be used as a surrogate marker for assessment of ventilation. In the cardiovascularly stable patient, $PvCO_2$ is typically 4–6 mm Hg higher than $PaCO_2$. However, when peripheral tissue perfusion is impaired, $PvCO_2$ may be substantially higher than $PaCO_2$.

4.   The most common sites for arterial blood collection are the dorsal metatarsal artery (Figure 4.3) and the femoral artery (Figure 4.4). Other sites used include the ventral tail artery, median or radial (carpal branch) arteries, and the auricular artery.

5.   In most dyspneic or compromised patients, the risk associated with the restraint needed to obtain an arterial sample often outweighs the value of information obtained from an arterial blood sample. For this reason, arterial blood gas sampling in the dyspnic patient, is sedated/anesthetized or has an indwelling arterial catheter.

6.   Obtaining an arterial blood gas:

  a.   The area should be clipped and aseptically prepared.

  b.   The pulse of the artery is palpated with the nondominant hand.

  c.   A commercially available arterial blood gas syringe kit (Smith's Medical ASD, Inc., Keene, NH) can be used:

    i.   These kits are pre-heparinized, self-filling, and contain a rubber stopper to isolate the sample from atmospheric gases. While these kits are not absolutely necessary for obtaining arterial blood gas samples, they are convenient and useful.

    ii.   The barrel of the syringe should be pulled back to the volume of blood that will be required for analysis prior to obtaining the sample. Once the artery has been punctured, the syringe will self-fill to the desired volume. Other commercial arterial blood gas syringes do not require withdrawal of the plunger prior to arterial puncture.

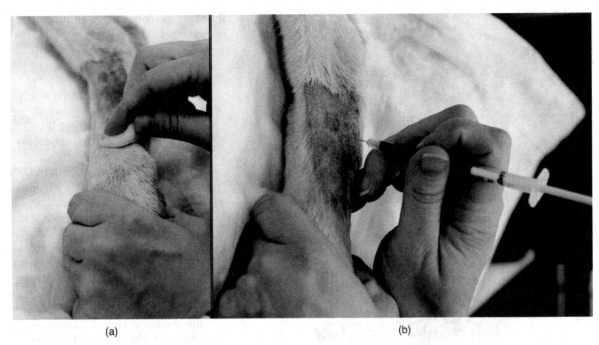

(a)   (b)

FIGURE 4.3 Obtaining an arterial blood gas from the dorsal metatarsal artery in a dog. The dog's foot is being held with the clinician's left hand and the hock is at the top of the picture. (a) shows the aseptic preparation of the dorsomedial aspect of the metatarsus after the hair has been clipped. (b) shows puncture of the dorsal metatarsal artery using the right hand by positioning the needle at approximately a 30° angle with respect to the foot. The syringe will fill automatically due to pressure within the artery and the design of the syringe within the arterial blood gas kit. Once the sample has been collected all air should be expelled from the syringe and the needle inserted into a foam/rubber stopper.

iii. Alternatively, one can manually aspirate the barrel of the syringe once the artery has been punctured, although this is more technically challenging.

iv. When an arterial blood gas kit is not available, a 1 cc syringe attached to a 25 gauge needle can be used. The needle and syringe should be coated with heparin and the plunger of the syringe will need to be manually aspirated following arterial puncture.

d. The needle of the arterial blood gas syringe is introduced through the skin and directed parallel to the long axis of the palpated arterial pulse. Adequate restraint is required; arterial blood sampling is an uncomfortable process due to the neurovascular bundle adjacent to the artery:

i. The syringe should be held at a 15–30° angle to the foot when sampling from the dorsal metatarsal artery (Figure 4.3). Restraint in this position is best accomplished by placing the patient's pelvis in lateral recumbency with the limb to be sampled "down." The assistant places the fingers behind the calcaneous to prevent withdrawal of the limb. The individual performing the procedure is able to grasp the distal limb with the hand not holding the syringe.

ii. The needle should be inserted perpendicular to the surface of the skin when sampling from the femoral artery (Figure 4.4).

e. Once the needle tip has punctured the artery, the syringe will fill on its own due to the pressure within the vessel (if using a self-filling syringe).

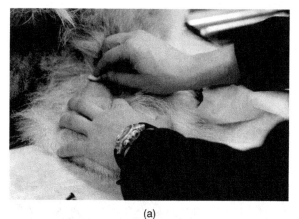

(a)

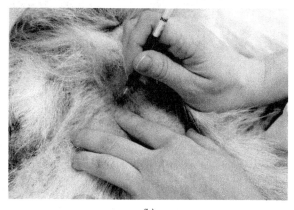

(b)

FIGURE 4.4 Obtaining an arterial blood sample from the femoral artery in a dog. (a) shows aseptic preparation of the femoral triangle, near the junction between the ventral abdomen and proximal pelvic limb. (b) shows puncture of the femoral artery by positioning the needle approximately perpendicular to the limb. The syringe will fill automatically due to pressure within the femoral artery and the design of the syringe within the arterial blood gas kit.

f.   Following collection, excess air should be evacuated from the sample and it should be protected from atmospheric gases by plugging the needle with the stopper provided in arterial blood gas kits. Alternatively, the rubber top of a blood sample vial can be used.

g.   The sample should be immediately analyzed to obtain accurate values for the blood gas both at 37°C and at patient body temperature:

   i.   If analysis cannot be performed immediately, the sample should be stored in ice water for up to 6 hours.

   ii.   With glass syringes, PCO_2 will increase and PO_2 will decrease as nucleated cells utilize oxygen the longer the sample stands from collection to analysis.

   iii. With plastic syringes, both PCO_2 and PO_2 tend to increase with time as oxygen diffuses from the plastic into the blood sample at a rate greater than its utilization.

   iv.   When heparin is utilized to coat syringes for ABG analysis, its potential effect on diagnostic results must be considered. Heparin will decrease pH and PCO_2, while increasing PO_2. Sample dilution should therefore be minimized. The amount of heparin to anticoagulate the sample should amount to 0.05–0.10 mL of 1000 unit/mL heparin per 1 mL of blood. If the needle and barrel of the syringe are coated with heparin and all of the heparin expelled by depressing the plunger (but not removing the needle), the amount remaining in the hub of the needle should be adequate for a 0.5–1.0 mL blood sample.

   v.   Following exposure to air (i.e., air not expelled from the syringe or the sample is exposed to the environment), the PCO_2 will decrease toward 0 mm Hg and PO_2 will increase toward 150 mm Hg.

7.   By evaluating deviations in pH, the partial pressures of dissolved oxygen (PaO_2) and carbon dioxide ($PaCO_2$) in arterial blood, and the patient's inspired oxygen concentration at the time of sampling, the adequacy of oxygenation and ventilation can be determined:

   a.   Hypoxemia is defined as a PaO_2 less than 80 mm Hg. When the PaO_2 is less than 60 mm Hg, strategies to increase patient oxygenation should be implemented.

b. Hypoventilation is defined as a $PaCO_2$ greater than 45 mm Hg. When a patient's $PaCO_2$ exceeds 60 mm Hg (or 45 mm Hg if traumatic brain injury) strategies to improve ventilation should be implemented.

c. The PaO_2 should be approximately five times greater than the inspired oxygen concentration.

d. Venous admixture refers to venous blood that passes to the arterial side of the circulation without being adequately oxygenated. Venous admixture occurs with pulmonary parenchymal damage or pleural space disease, and reduces the PaO_2:

   i. Deoxygenated blood from the thebesian veins and bronchial circulation enters the left side of the circulation and contributes to normal (physiologic) venous admixture.

   ii. Ventilation/perfusion mismatch secondary to pulmonary contusion and pleural space disease can cause pathologic venous admixture with resultant hypoxemia.

e. Calculation of the alveolar–arterial $(P(A-a)O_2)$ gradient provides objective information on pulmonary function by removing the influence of ventilation on PaO_2 (Table 4.1):

   i. When a patient is breathing 21% oxygen, the $P(A-a)O_2$ should be less than 10–15 mm Hg.

   ii. When a patient is breathing 100% oxygen, the $P(A-a)O_2$ should be less than 150 mm Hg.

   iii. There is increased venous admixture (and therefore evidence of pulmonary dysfunction) if the $P(A-a)O_2$ gradient is greater than 15 mm Hg while breathing 21% oxygen.

   iv. Trauma-induced pulmonary contusion and pleural space disease can cause pulmonary dysfunction and increased venous admixture, as evidenced by an increased $P(A-a)O_2$ gradient.

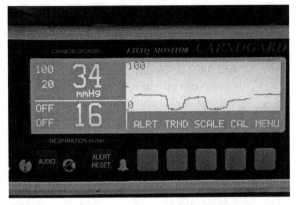

FIGURE 4.5 Tracing from end tidal capnography in an intubated patient. The top number (34) indicates the end tidal carbon dioxide concentration in millimeters of mercury and the bottom number represents the number (16) of breaths per minute. The baseline on the tracing represents the end tidal carbon dioxide and the deflection below baseline corresponds with decreased carbon dioxide upon inspiration and subsequent increase to baseline with expiration.

   v. End-tidal capnometry ($ETCO_2$):
   1. End-tidal capnometry ($ETCO_2$) is the measure of carbon dioxide in expired gas and provides an assessment of ventilation.
   2. The use of end tidal capnometry is reserved for patients who are intubated or have a tracheostomy tube in place.
   3. $ETCO_2$ provides a continuous, noninvasive estimate of dissolved carbon dioxide in arterial blood ($PaCO_2$). Figure 4.5 shows a waveform generated by an end tidal capnograph.
   4. Hypoventilation is defined as an $ETCO_2$ greater than 45 mm Hg. In the trauma patient, hypoventilation may be observed secondary to head and spinal trauma, drugs that influence respiratory drive (e.g., opiates, propofol), or severe pulmonary parenchymal/pleural space disease. When $ETCO_2$ exceeds 60 mm Hg (or 45 mm Hg if traumatic brain injury), strategies to improve ventilation should be implemented.
   5. $ETCO_2$ is usually 1–4 mm Hg lower than $PaCO_2$. A larger gradient between $ETCO_2$ and $PaCO_2$ may exist in severe pulmonary parenchymal disease because of an

increase in alveolar dead space ventilation. $ETCO_2$ should therefore be periodically correlated to a $PaCO_2$ by arterial blood gas analysis.

6. $ETCO_2$ is closely correlated to cardiac output and may be used to assess the effectiveness of chest compressions during cardiopulmonary cerebral resuscitation (CPCR).

7. An original study in healthy, sedated dogs demonstrated that end-tidal CO_2 sampled from an intranasal catheter provided an acceptable alternative for determining ventilation when compared to arterial samples. The effectiveness of this means of assessing ventilation function has not been evaluated in diseased patients (Pang et al., 2007).

3. CARDIOVASCULAR MONITORING

a. Decreased perfusion is common in the trauma patient, with hypovolemia being the most common cause of perfusion deficits. Inappropriate vasodilatation secondary to sepsis or prolonged hypotension may be delayed causes of inadequate tissue perfusion (see Chapter 3: Shock in the Trauma Patient).

b. Monitoring of the cardiovascular system centers on subjective data obtained from serial physical examinations and more objective measures that can provide continuous, real time information on cardiovascular status.

c. More intensive monitoring is indicated if cardiovascular instability is present.

d. Monitoring of the trauma patient's cardiovascular status with physical examination should focus on mentation, mucous membrane color and capillary refill time (CRT), heart and pulse rate, pulse quality, and rectal and distal extremity temperatures:

  i. Mentation:

    1. An assessment of the trauma patient's mentation should include level of consciousness and response to surroundings and manipulation.

    2. The level of mentation and responsiveness can provide an assessment of cerebral perfusion. The brain is the last organ to experience a compromise in blood flow and

is therefore a marker of significant compromise to perfusion.

    3. Decreased mentation secondary to decreased tissue perfusion will resolve following correction of cerebral perfusion. If mentation does not improve with correction of hypovolemia, or other perfusion parameters assessed are not consistent with hypovolemia, primary brain injury should be suspected.

    4. Caution should be exercised when assessing the neurologic status of the hypoperfused patient as decreased cerebral perfusion will make patients mentally depressed.

    5. For more information on the assessment of neurologic system of the trauma patient, refer to the section on neurologic monitoring below.

  ii. Mucous membrane color and capillary refill time:

    1. Assessment of mucous membrane color and capillary refill time provides information on local tissue perfusion:

      a. Mucous membranes should be assessed before, during, and after fluid therapy and every 2–6 hours thereafter.

      b. Membranes that can be assessed include the oral, vulvar, penile, preputial, and conjunctival mucosa. Extra-oral sites may be helpful in patients with heavy pigmentation in their oral cavity or are too fractious to have their oral cavity safely examined.

      c. Lighting conditions, observer subjectivity, local inflammation (such as with dental disease), and level of pigmentation will impact the determination of mucous membrane color.

      d. Normal mucous membrane color is a light pink:

        i. The normal mucous membrane color in cats is often more pale than that of dogs.

        ii. The pink color is generated by the presence of oxygenated erythrocytes within the capillaries at a normal level of vasomotor tone.

e. Pale mucous membranes indicate decreased red blood cells within the capillaries:

   i. This may be secondary to an absolute decrease in red blood cells (anemia) or peripheral vasoconstriction secondary to hypovolemia, hypothermia, pain, stress, or various medications.

f. White or gray mucous membranes are a more severe exacerbation of the causes of pale mucous membranes.

g. Red mucous membranes imply vasodilatation resulting in increased local blood flow:

   i. Vasodilatation, though uncommon in trauma patients initially, may be seen if the patient is septic or suffered prolonged hypotension.

   ii. Increased local blood flow can be seen with hyperthermia, hypertension, and severe acidosis (as is seen with severe hypercarbia secondary to hypoventilation).

h. Tacky mucous membranes are seen in dehydrated patients. It is important to remember that acutely hypovolemic patients are rarely dehydrated.

i. Capillary refill time (CRT) is defined as the amount of time it takes for blood, and therefore color, to return to the capillary bed after it has been forced out of the capillaries through digital pressure. CRT should be considered a crude indicator of cardiac output:

   i. Normal CRT in dogs and cats is 1.5–2 seconds.

   ii. Prolonged CRT (>2 seconds) results from decreased local blood flow from vasoconstriction secondary to hypoperfusion.

   iii. Shortened CRT (<1 second) results from increased local blood flow from vasodilation or hypermetabolic states.

iii. Heart rate and rhythm, pulse rate, and pulse quality should be frequently assessed. They provide information on perfusion status and pain:

a. Heart rate:

   i. Normal heart rate for dogs is 60–120 beats per minute.

   ii. Normal heart rate for cats presenting to a veterinary clinic is 160–200 beats per minute.

   iii. Tachycardia in dogs and cats is considered to be at rates greater than 120–140 beats per minutes in dogs and greater than 220 beats per minute in cats. Acute changes in heart rate should prompt further evaluation:

   1. Tachycardia is common in dogs and cats secondary to trauma and may be secondary to hypovolemia (due to blood loss), pain, stress, and/or fear.

   2. Hypovolemia secondary to acute blood loss is common in the trauma patient and will result in a decreased stroke volume.

   3. Cardiac output is the product of heart rate and stroke volume (CO = HR × SV). An acute decrease in stroke volume will precipitate a reflex compensatory tachycardia. An increase in heart rate is therefore a sensitive but nonspecific marker of hypovolemia in dogs and should be immediately addressed.

   4. Heart rate should be monitored frequently to assess response to fluid therapy and to rapidly identify acute changes in hemodynamic status. Patients with external or cavitary blood loss (thoracic, abdominal, or retroperitoneal) will often have an initial decrease in heart rate in response to fluid therapy. However, correction of hypovolemia and hypotension with aggressive fluid support may disrupt previously formed clots and bleeding may resume.

   5. Other causes of tachycardia in the trauma patient include tachydysrhythmias, hypoxemia, pain, and fear/anxiety. The cause of the tachycardia should be identified and treated.

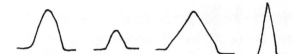

FIGURE 4.6 Line diagrams of descriptions of pulse quality, from left to right: normal pulse pressure, weak pulse, bounding pulse, and a thready/snappy pulse.

iv. Bradycardia in the average dog is considered to be a heart rate of less than 60 beats per minute and less than 140 beats per minute in cats:

   1. Causes of trauma-induced bradycardia include severe hypoxemia, electrolyte abnormalities (hyperkalemia), increased intracranial pressure (Cushing's reflex; see Neurologic section), myocardial failure, hypothermia, and shock in cats. Some medications (e.g., fentanyl) may induce a bradycardia; reversal agents and/or re-evaluation of dosages may need to be considered.

b. Pulse quality:

   i. Palpation of peripheral pulse quality provides a tangible assessment of the difference between systolic and diastolic pulse pressures (the height of the pulse wave) and the duration of the pulse waveform (the width) (Figure 4.6).

   ii. Arteries most commonly used to assess pulse quality include the femoral, dorsal metatarsal/dorsal pedal, and radial arteries.

   iii. Weak pulses have a decreased pulse pressure but normal width of the waveform, and are commonly identified in hypovolemic trauma patients.

   iv. Bounding pulses have a large pulse pressure difference and wide waveform, and are often felt with vasodilation and increased stroke volume.

   v. Snappy pulses have a normal pulse pressure but decreased waveform width, and are commonly seen with anemia.

vi. Pulse quality and rate should be frequently assessed in the trauma patient to assess response to therapy and rapidly identify new problems.

c. Body temperature and core/extremity temperature difference provide an assessment of perfusion and vascular tone:

   i. Normal rectal temperature in canine and feline patients is 99–102.5°F.

   ii. Subjective assessment of peripheral perfusion can be obtained by feeling the paws and ears for perceptible differences when compared to the patient's core temperature. A palpably discernable difference between core and extremity temperatures is consistent with peripheral vasoconstriction and shock.

   iii. A reduction in the core to extremity temperature difference is expected following restoration of normal perfusion.

e. Objective measures of cardiovascular monitoring:

   i. A more objective assessment of the cardiovascular system can be achieved with the aid of an electrocardiogram (ECG), blood pressure monitoring, and an emergency blood screen.

   ii. These tools are important adjuncts to the physical examination for monitoring cardiovascular function and assessing the trauma patient's response to therapy:

   1. The trauma patient can be closely monitored with continuous ECG and blood pressure providing the clinician with the ability to detect acute and subtle changes in the patient's cardiovascular status.

   2. Electrocardiography (ECG):

      a. ECG uses the electrical impulses generated by the cardiac conduction system to create a tracing for monitoring both heart rate and rhythm.

      b. ECG monitoring in trauma patients is important as conduction abnormalities commonly occur secondary to hypovolemia, hypoxemia, myocardial contusion, electrolyte abnormalities, variation in sympathetic tone, and the release of inflammatory mediators. In addition, ECG gives moment to moment

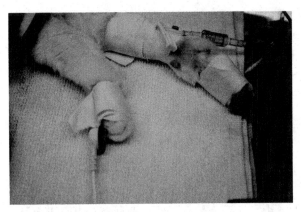

FIGURE 4.7 Adhesive ECG patches attached to a cat's front feet for continuous ECG monitoring. In this picture, the palmar surface of the metacarpal region is clipped of hair and the patches are secured in place with medical tape. Snap-on ECG leads are attached to the patches, rather than alligator clamps to the animals skin, making this procedure less painful.

information about heart rate, which can be an excellent indicator of the response of the hypovolemic patient to fluid therapy.

c. ECG is readily available and technically easy to use.

d. Metal alligator clips can be used for temporary monitoring.

e. Adhesive patches can be attached for long-term use (Ambu Blue Sensor N, Medicotest, Malaysia) (Figure 4.7).

f. Alcohol or a conducting gel placed between the patient's skin and metal clips will improve conduction. To avoid the risk of fire, alcohol should not be applied to the patient if the possibility of electrical defibrillation is considered imminent.

g. In veterinary patients, most Lead II ECG analysis is done with the patient in right lateral recumbency, although this position should be avoided if it compromises or stresses the patient.

h. Common ECG disturbances in trauma patients include sinus tachycardia, sinus bradycardia, accelerated idioventricular rhythm, premature ventricular complexes, and ventricular tachycardia. ECG manifestations of hyperkalemia (spiked

T waves, prolonged PR interval, loss of P waves, and widening of the QRS) may occur in patients with urinary tract disruption.

i. Treatment of cardiac dysrhythmias should be based on heart rate, clinical signs, evidence of perfusion abnormalities, treatment of underlying cause, and presence of multiform complexes or the "R on T" phenomenon.

j. Dysrhythmias, considered secondary to hypovolemia, hypoxemia, or excessive catecholamines should be treated by correction of the underlying cause.

k. A uniform ventricular rhythm with a heart rate of 140 beats per minute or less is considered an accelerated idioventricular rhythm. In the absence of perfusion abnormalities attributed to this rhythm, definitive treatment with an antidysrhythmic is not warranted. Maintenance of euvolemia, adequate oxygenation, and normal acid-base and electrolyte status is indicated. Figure 4.8 illustrates two examples of an accelerated idioventricular rhythm.

l. Dysrhythmias resulting in decreased perfusion as evidenced by clinical signs (e.g., depression, syncope, poor pulse quality, pale mucous membranes, cool extremities, prolonged CRT) or objective means (hypotension, hyperlactatemia) should be treated following correction of hypovolemia and hypoxemia.

3. Blood pressure monitoring:

   a. Monitoring of blood pressure is extremely useful in the trauma patient and allows fluid therapy to be tailored to a patient's needs.

   b. Arterial and central venous blood pressure can be measured, providing valuable information on volume status and perfusion.

   c. Arterial blood pressure:

      i. Patients with evidence of shock (both hypovolemic and distributive) will benefit from the monitoring of arterial blood pressure.

      ii. Animals that have incurred head trauma may develop an acute increase

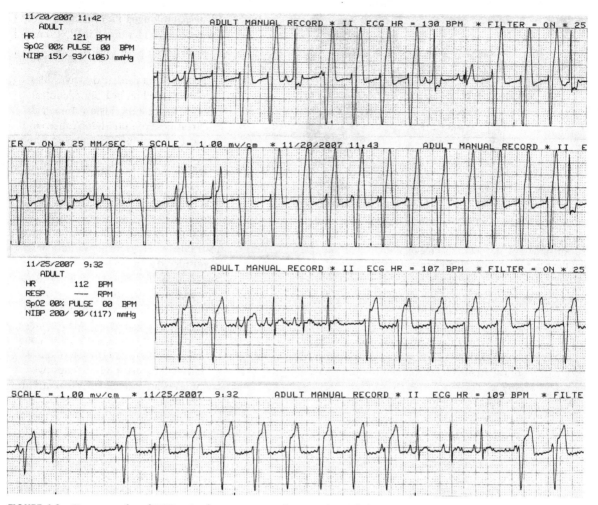

FIGURE 4.8   Two examples of ECG strips from patients with an accelerated idioventricular rhythm. This rhythm is characterized by atrioventricular junction or ventricular shaped complexes at a much slower rate (120–140 beats per minute) than ventricular tachycardia. Normal sinus beats can occur at random within runs of the accelerated idioventricular rhythm.

in mean arterial pressure and decrease in heart rate if intracranial pressure increases (Cushing's reflex) (see Chapter 7: Traumatic brain injury). Therefore, close monitoring of arterial blood pressure in head trauma patients is warranted.

iii. Blood pressure can be used as a surrogate marker of blood flow to tissues. However, intense vasoconstriction may result in "adequate" blood pressure but with minimal tissue flow. Similarly, different vascular beds may

have differing blood flow at the same blood pressure.

iv. Normal blood pressure:

1. Normal blood pressure values for dogs:

   a. Systolic pressures of 110–190 mm Hg

   b. Diastolic pressures of 55–110 mm Hg

2. Normal blood pressure values for cats:

   a. Systolic pressures of 120–170 mm Hg

b. Diastolic pressures of 70–120 mm Hg

3. Hypertension:

a. Hypertension becomes a concern when systolic pressure increases above 170 mm Hg, or diastolic pressure is greater than 110 mm Hg.

b. Following head trauma, systolic pressures of greater than 140 mm Hg (with a heart rate of less than 100 beats per minute) should raise suspicions of increased intracranial pressure.

c. Elevations in arterial blood pressure result from pain, fear, raised intracranial pressure, metabolic and endocrine diseases, renal and cardiac disease, and various medications.

4. Hypotension:

a. Systolic blood pressure of less than 100 mm Hg or mean arterial pressure of less than 70 mm Hg should be addressed.

b. In the trauma patient, low blood pressure can result from reduced cardiac output secondary to hypovolemia, myocardial failure, and dysrhythmias.

c. Decreased systemic vascular resistance due to vasodilating agents (e.g., propofol, isoflurane), systemic inflammation, and adrenergic receptor down-regulation can all result in low blood pressure even in the presence of adequate or increased cardiac output.

v. Indirect (noninvasive) blood pressure monitoring:

1. Relies on the inflation of a cuff to occlude arterial flow, followed by measurement of the pressure at which blood flow returns. The inflatable cuff is attached to a sphygmomanometer or directly to an oscillometric blood pressure monitoring system.

2. Noninvasive blood pressure monitoring is readily available, relatively cheap, and easy to use.

3. Appropriate cuff size selection is important. To select the best cuff, the width of the cuff should be 40% of the circumference of the limb:

a. Cuffs that are too large will give falsely low pressure readings.

b. Cuffs that are too small will generate falsely elevated pressure readings.

4. Doppler ultrasonographic determination of blood pressure:

a. This method is thought to provide a systolic pressure measurement and can be used in all small animals.

b. Doppler blood pressure monitoring systems are economical and reliable in dogs and cats of various sizes.

c. A 10-MHz ultrasound probe is placed over an artery distal to the cuff. The Doppler sounds become audible when pressure in the cuff is less than pressure in the artery.

d. Common arteries used for Doppler blood pressure measurement include the dorsal metatarsal, ulnar, and tail arteries.

e. The probe should be kept perpendicular to the vessel and adequate amounts of ultrasonic gel used to aid sound conduction (Figure 4.9a–c).

5. Oscillometric blood pressure monitors:

a. These monitors utilize vibrations conducted to adjacent tissues by the return of

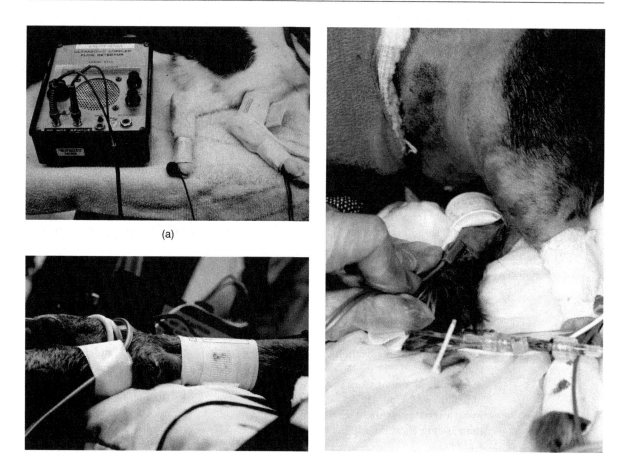

FIGURE 4.9 The placement of the Doppler probe for blood pressure monitoring. In (a) the probe is taped to the plantar surface of the cat's hind foot for long-term use. An occlusive cuff is placed above the hock. The Doppler flow detector box is on the left side of the picture connected to the Doppler probe. (b) shows the placement of the occlusive cuff on the ante-brachium of a canine patient and the Doppler probe taped over the median artery. (c) shows the placement of an occlusive cuff above the hock and Doppler probe over the dorsal metatarsal artery.

blood flow to the occluded artery to calculate systolic, diastolic, and mean arterial blood pressure.

b. Sites for placement of the oscillometric cuff are the mid-antebrachium and metatarsus (Figure 4.10a and b).

c. The cuff must fit snugly so that the oscillometric blood pressure monitor is able to detect tissue vibrations.

d. The Dinamap (Critikon, Inc., Tampa, FL) may not be reliable in cats or very small dogs.

e. The Cardell (Sharn Veterinary, Inc., Tampa, FL) has been shown to be effective at determining systolic, diastolic and mean pressures in anesthetized healthy cats (Pedersen et al., 2002) as well as dogs.

f. Accuracy is limited in vasoconstricted patients or in patients with dysrhythmias.

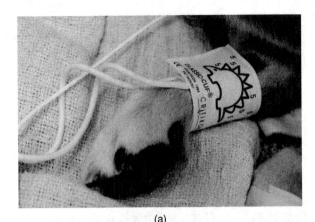

(a)

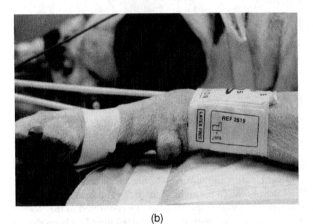

(b)

FIGURE 4.10 Sites for oscillometric blood pressure monitor cuff placement. (a) shows the cuff on the metatarsus of a canine patient. (b) shows an occlusive cuff on the antebrachium of a canine patient.

6. At least three measurements should be obtained, and the average value recorded.

7. Inappropriate cuff size is the most common source of error with noninvasive blood pressure monitoring. Other causes include overzealous patient restraint leading to increased blood pressure, operator deficiencies, deflation rate, and failure to fully deflate the cuff between readings.

vi. Direct arterial blood pressure measurement (Figure 4.11):

1. Direct arterial blood pressure measurement is the gold standard for the determination of blood pressure.

2. Direct arterial blood pressure measurement involves catheterization of a peripheral artery.

3. The arterial catheter is then connected to a pressure transducer via a fluid-filled tubing system. Noncomplaint tubing must be used to avoid dampening of the pressure signal (Transpac, Hospira, Inc., Lake Forest, IL).

4. The pressure tranducer converts the mechanical signals induced by pulsatile arterial pressure to electrical signals that are then recorded, quantitated, and displayed graphically.

5. Most commercially available arterial blood pressure recording systems provide a continuous delivery of heparinized, isotonic solution at 1–3 mL/h to prevent catheter occlusion.

6. A catheter is most commonly placed in the dorsal metatarsal artery although femoral, auricular, and arteries on the antebrachium may also be used:

   a. With over-the-wire arterial catheters (Arrow International, Reading, PA), a modified Seldinger technique is used (see Chapter 3: Shock in the Trauma Patient for the description of this technique). Conversely, standard over the needle catheters may be used as well.

   b. The site should be aseptically prepared and the patient adequately restrained.

   c. After palpation of the metatarsal pulse, the catheter should be advanced through the skin and directed toward the artery. Once the artery is punctured with the catheter

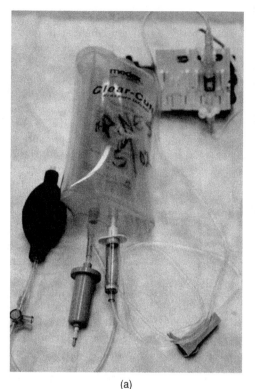

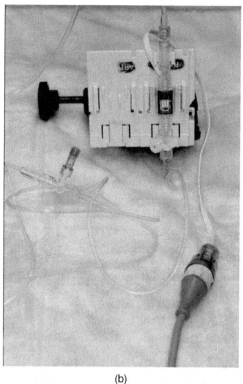

(a)   (b)

FIGURE 4.11   Overview of the necessary items for direct arterial blood pressure monitoring. On the left of (a) is the bulb for inflation of the pressurized bag, which is shown in the middle of the photo. To the right of the bulb, and below the bag, is the bag pressure indicator. Within the pressurized bag is heparinized saline with a special fluid line connected to the top of the pressure transducer, located on the right. (b) shows the pressure transducer, with the heparinized fluid line from the pressure bag at the top, a three-way stop cock in the middle (used to zero the monitor), and the fluid line, which connects to the patient, at the bottom of the photo. The pressure transducer connects to a transducer cable (gray) that connects to the patient monitor.

stylet, a flash of arterial blood will be seen in the hub of the stylet and it should fill readily due to arterial blood pressure. The entire catheter and stylet should be advanced forward 1–2 mm to allow the distal tip of the catheter to penetrate the vessel lumen. The catheter should then be advanced off of the stylet and into the artery.

d. After the catheter is in the artery, it should be connected to the pressure monitoring system or a length of low compliance IV extension tubing, flushed with saline, and occluded with an injection cap. The arterial catheter is then taped very securely and labeled as "arterial" so that it is not mistakenly used for the administration of fluids or medications (Figure 4.12).

7. Direct arterial blood pressure measurement is reliable in hypoperfused and vasoconstricted patients, though placing an arterial catheter during these situations is technically more

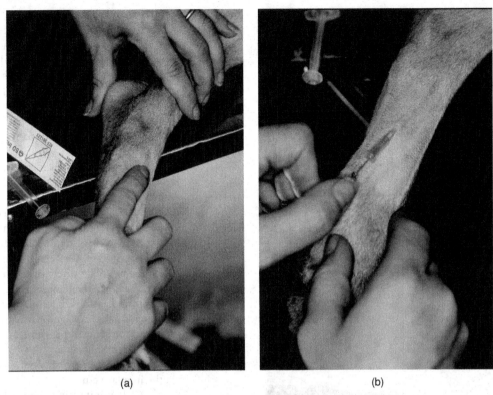

(a)　　　　　　　　(b)

FIGURE 4.12　The placement of an arterial catheter in the dorsal metatarsal artery of a dog. Pulse and vessel orientation are palpated with the clinician's right hand in (a) while the hock is stabilized with the left hand. In (b), a standard over the needle catheter is used to puncture into the skin, and the tip aimed at the metatarsal artery. The catheter is advanced into the vessel after a flash of arterial blood is seen and the needle stylet is removed once the entire length of the catheter is seated in the artery.

challenging. If necessary, a cut down to the dorsal metatarsal or femoral artery can be performed. A strict sterile technique should be practiced:

a. For the dorsal metatarsal artery, an incision is made just distal to the dorsomedial aspect of the tarsal metatarsal joint and extended 2–4 cm distally toward the paw.

b. Blunt dissection to the level of the artery is performed.

c. Once the artery is visualized, it is dissected from the surrounding fascia and elevated out of the incision for cannulation with a catheter. The catheter should first be inserted through the skin distal to the cutdown site and then advanced into the cutdown site and into the artery. Figure 4.13 shows the technique used for a dorsal metatarsal arterial cut down.

8. Arterial catheters and monitoring systems should be clearly labeled so they are not mistaken for venous catheters. Drugs and medications should never be injected into an arterial catheter. Blood that is removed from the arterial catheter prior to

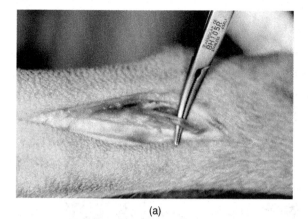

(a)

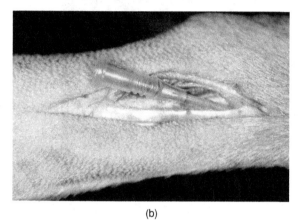

(b)

FIGURE 4.13   Cut-down to the dorsal metatarsal artery. (a) shows the general anatomy in the area—the dog's foot is to the left of the picture and hock to the right. The dorsal metatarsal artery is elevated on a mosquito hemostat. (b) shows cannulation of the dorsal metatarsal artery with a standard catheter.

obtaining a blood sample should be returned to the patient via a venous catheter or discarded.

9. Patients with arterial catheters must be closely monitored to ensure they do not dislodge any connections or displace the catheter; both of which could lead to substantial blood loss.

10. An arterial catheter may be used to obtain blood for arterial blood gas determination.

4. Central venous pressure (CVP):
    a. CVP represents the hydrostatic pressure in the intrathoracic vena cava and provides an assessment of right-sided preload (right ventricular end-diastolic pressure) and thus, an indirect reflection of intravascular volume.
    b. CVP measurement is most useful in the acute resuscitation of patients in hypovolemic states.
    c. Monitoring CVP in the cardiovascularly stable trauma patient may aid in the detection of acute hypovolemia.
    d. CVP is most commonly recorded following placement of a jugular catheter.
    e. In the absence of significant intra-abdominal disease, CVP can be measured via placement of a catheter into the caudal vena cava via the femoral vein.
    f. Contraindications to jugular catheter placement include coagulopathy, risk of increased intracranial pressure, and risk of thromboembolism.
    g. Placement of a central venous catheter via the jugular vein:
        i. CVP monitoring requires the percutaneous or surgical placement of a catheter. The tip of the catheter should be positioned just outside the right atrium in the cranial vena cava. Appropriate catheter length is determined by measuring from the point of insertion to the third rib. See Chapter 3: Shock in the Trauma Patient, for further description of the placement of central venous catheters using the Seldinger technique.
        ii. If the central venous catheter inserted is a double or triple lumen catheter (Arrow International, Reading, PA), other ports may be used for blood sampling and total parenteral nutrition administration as needed. The distal port should be used for monitoring of CVP.
    h. Methods of measuring CVP:
        i. The central venous catheter can be connected to a commercially available pressure transducer system as described above for arterial blood

pressure monitoring. Values obtained will typically be displayed using mm Hg units.

ii. A standard water manometer may be used for intermittent CVP measurements. Values obtained will be in cm H_2O.

iii. The transducer or manometer should be at the level of the right heart, and all measurements taken with the patient in the same position:

1. The manometer should be filled with normal (0.9%) saline and connected to the patient's central venous catheter. A three-way stop-cock can be used between the manometer and patient's catheter to facilitate filling the manometer and measuring CVP.

2. The manometer should be perpendicular to the patient with the bottom of the manometer level with the right heart.

3. Saline will move from the manometer to the patient's vein until the pressures are equilibrated. The measurement is made when the meniscus of saline stops falling and instead fluctuates slightly around a given number with each respiration.

4. The CVP should be read at end expiration to minimize the influence of changing intrapleural pressures (due to breathing).

5. Normal central venous pressure is 0–5 cm H_2O:

   a. 1 mm Hg = 1.36 cm H_2O; 1 cm H_2O = 0.73 mm Hg.

   b. Trauma-associated pathologic processes that elevate CVP readings include pleural space disease (pleural effusion and pneumothorax), cardiac tamponade, and pulmonary hypertension.

   c. A low CVP (less than 0 cm H_2O) is consistent with hypovolemia due to fluid loss or vasodilation secondary to peripheral vasodilation.

   d. A high CVP (greater than 10 cm H_2O) may indicate volume overload (or volume expansion if fluid resuscitation has occurred), right-sided heart failure, or severe pleural space disease (pleural effusion or pneumothorax).

   e. If CVP is normal, but there is still suspicion of underlying hypovolemia, a small test bolus of 10–15 mL/kg of an isotonic crystalloid solution or a 3–4 mL/kg bolus of a synthetic colloid can be given over 5 minutes:

      i. If the patient has a low CVP due to hypovolemia, the CVP will either show no change or will have a transient rise toward normal, then rapidly decrease again.

      ii. An increase of 2–4 cm H_2O with a return to baseline within 15 minutes is usually seen with euvolemia.

      iii. A large increase (greater than 4 cm H_2O) and slow return to baseline (more than 30 minutes) is seen with hypervolemia whereas a >4 cm H_2O increase in CVP with a rapid return to baseline (within 15 minutes) implies reduced cardiac compliance.

5. Diagnostic blood sampling:

   a. Packed cell volume (PCV) and total protein by refractometry (TP):

      i. Determination of PCV and TP provide information that might increase the suspicion for acute blood loss.

      ii. Packed cell volume represents the percentage of red blood cells in whole blood. It can be easily determined by filling heparinized microcapillary (hematocrit) tubes with whole blood and centrifuging. The erythrocytes will separate from the leukocytes (buffy coat) and plasma. The PCV is determined by placing the hematocrit tube against a commercially available scale to determine the percentage of red cells:

    1. Normal PCV for dog is 40–60% and 31–48% for cats.

iii. The plasma portion of whole blood is used to determine the total plasma protein (TP), consisting of albumin and globulins:

    1. Normal TP in dogs is 6.0–8.6 g/dL and 6.4–8.6 g/dL in cats.

iv. PCV and TP should be interpreted together:

    1. Immediately after acute hemorrhage, there will be no change in PCV or TP.

    2. TP will begin to decrease prior to a decrease in PCV.

    3. Initially, fluid moves from the interstitium into the vasculature, diluting proteins and reducing the measured TP and PCV in equal proportions.

    4. In the hypovolemic dog, activation of the sympathetic nervous system results in splenic contraction and the release of blood with a high PCV into the systemic circulation. The result is that the PCV tends to fall slower than the TP in acute hemorrhage.

    5. A trauma patient with acute hemorrhage may therefore have a decreased TP with a normal (or even increased) PCV.

    6. Over time, PCV and TP will both be decreased as fluid continues to shift from the interstitial space into the vasculature. Fluid therapy to correct hypovolemia will further this change (hemodilution).

    7. Increases in both PCV and TP concurrently imply hemoconcentration, which is consistent with dehydration.

    8. Normal TP in conjunction with decreased PCV implies anemia caused by something other than acute blood loss.

    9. A baseline PCV and TP value should be obtained at hospital presentation, and these values should be monitored frequently (Q1–2 hours) for changes and response to therapy until stabilized.

    10. Serial monitoring of PCV and TP is necessary to tailor a trauma patient's fluid and transfusion needs.

  b. Lactate determination:

    i. Blood lactate is considered a global indicator of tissue perfusion that can be monitored in the trauma patient to assess tissue oxygenation and response to therapy.

    ii. Lactic acid is generated during anaerobic metabolism. In the trauma patient this is most commonly secondary to decreased tissue perfusion, severe hypoxemia, or a combination thereof. Lactic acid dissociates into lactate and hydrogen ions.

    iii. Normal serum lactate concentrations in dogs have been reported to range from 0.3 to 2.5mmol/L (Hughes et al., 1999). Concentrations greater than 2.5 mmol/L are considered clinically significant.

    iv. Prolonged vessel occlusion, excessive restraint or patient struggling, and delays in sample analysis will increase the serum lactate concentration, even in animals with adequate perfusion.

    v. Lactate is most useful as a monitoring tool for gauging response to resuscitation in traumatized patients with decreased oxygen delivery to the tissues (shock).

vi. Severe anemia will result in a decreased oxygen delivery to tissues with the generation of lactic acid secondary to anaerobic metabolism. The presence of hyperlactatemia may therefore be utilized to aid in the decision to transfuse anemic patients.

vii. Lactate is measured on some commercial blood gas analyzers. In addition, handheld lactatometers (Accutrend Lactate, Roche, Manheim, Germany) are also available. These handheld devices make lactate measurement a quick, point-of-care monitoring tool requiring less than 0.5 mL of blood.

c. Coagulation assays (PT, aPTT) should be performed in the bleeding trauma patient:

i. Coagulation times are frequently prolonged in the trauma patient.

ii. Activation of the inflammatory and coagulation pathways occurs following trauma.

iii. A "lethal triad" of hypothermia, acidosis, and coagulopathy may develop with hemorrhagic shock and resuscitative measures.

iv. Coagulation factors are lost with hemorrhage, consumed through activation, and diluted through fluid therapy:

1. Crystalloids will contribute to coagulopathy via dilution (although only approximately 25% of the administered volume remains in the vasculature after an hour).

2. Synthetic colloids remain in the intravascular space longer than crystalloids, and therefore cause a greater dilutional coagulopathy per volume administered.

v. Colloids can also alter platelet function and inhibit factor VIII.

vi. Fresh frozen plasma (FFP) should be administered if clotting times are prolonged and there is evidence of ongoing hemorrhage or prior to an invasive procedure.

4. NEUROLOGICAL MONITORING

a. Monitoring of neurologic function in the trauma patient is essential.

b. The neurologic system requires frequent reassessment to monitor for deterioration or improvement of clinical signs and response to therapy.

c. A trauma patient with signs of traumatic brain injury requires more frequent assessment than the patient with appropriate neurological function.

d. Monitoring of the neurological system focuses on serial physical and neurologic examinations.

e. Mentation, body position, cranial and peripheral nerves should be frequently assessed.

f. All physical examination findings (both normal and abnormal) should be recorded.

g. Prior administration of drugs (e.g., atropine and opioids) should be considered when performing a neurological examination.

h. Levels of consciousness should be frequently monitored and described as follows:

i. Excited/agitated

ii. Normal

iii. Depressed

iv. Obtunded

v. Stupor (unconscious but responds to noxious stimuli)

vi. Coma (unconscious and does not respond to noxious stimuli)

i. If there is a change in level of consciousness, a full neurological examination should be performed.

j. An initial decrease in mentation may be secondary to hypoperfusion or a result of traumatic brain injury. If fluid therapy is indicated, the patient's neurologic status should be re-assessed after volume resuscitation to determine the extent of signs attributable to hypoperfusion.

k. Trauma patients should be monitored closely for seizure activity.

l. The patient's position should be monitored closely.

m. If there is any concern of traumatic brain injury, and following cardiovascular stabilization, the patient's head and neck should be elevated 15–30° with a flat board to decrease intracranial pressure. The jugular veins should not be occluded for blood collection or by the method of head elevation, and any stimulus that may induce sneezing (e.g., placement of nasal oxygen catheters) should be avoided.

n. Patients with possible spinal or neck trauma should be secured to a backboard.

o. The initial examination of the head should involve both an assessment of cranial nerve function as well as close visual inspection for physical evidence of head trauma.

p. The cranial nerve examination entails evaluation of all 12 cranial nerves, with particular attention to pupil size, symmetry, and direct and consensual light reactivity. The patient should be assessed for pathologic and physiologic nystagmus as well as the presence of a head tilt (only if it is safe to move the patient's neck).

q. Abnormalities of body-position seen in the trauma patient:

   i. Schiff-Sherington—forelimb extensor rigidity and hindlimb flaccidity secondary to a spinal cord lesion between T2 and L4.

   ii. Decerebrate rigidity—opisthotonus with hyperextension of all four limbs and loss of consciousness.

   iii. Decerebellate rigidity—hyperextension of the forelimbs with variable flexion and extension of the hindlimbs and appropriate level of consciousness. The prognosis for decerebellate rigidity is more favorable than that for decerebrate rigidity.

r. Spinal reflexes and assessment of deep pain should be performed for each limb. If possible, it should be performed prior to administration of opioids and any limb bandaging. This assessment may be limited in patients with cardiovascular compromise.

s. Postural reflexes, such as placing, and evaluation of hemi- or tetraparesis should be performed following assessment and stabilization of other injuries.

t. The modified Glasgow coma score (MGCS) was developed to determine the severity of neurologic injury (see Table 7.2) (Shores, 1983):

   i. It uses a combination of observed neurologic signs to ascertain patient prognosis. Scores for motor function, cranial nerve function, and level of consciousness are added to render the final MGCS.

   ii. It permits objective re-assessment of progression, through repeat scoring for comparison purposes.

   iii. In all trauma patients, regardless of whether or not the MGCS is used, frequent reassessment of neurologic status and prompt investigation of any decline in status is crucial for ensuring the best chance for patient survival and recovery.

   iv. It has been suggested that MGCS scores between 3 and 8 carry a grave prognosis, scores between 9 and 14 have a poor to guarded prognosis, and a good prognosis is assigned to patients whose score is between 15 and 18 (Platt et al., 2001). However, no large-scale prospective study has been performed in veterinary medicine to validate these outcome categories.

u. To ensure adequate delivery of oxygen to the brain, the trauma patient's respiratory and cardiovascular systems should be monitored as outlined above.

v. Heart rate and blood pressure can also provide indirect information regarding intracranial pressure:

   i. Cerebral perfusion pressure (CPP) is equal to mean arterial pressure (MAP) minus intracranial pressure (ICP) (CPP = MAP − ICP).

   ii. Increased intracranial pressure results from cerebral edema, cerebral hemorrhage, and space occupying lesions such as fractures or subdural hematomas.

   iii. When intracranial pressure increases, mean arterial pressure must also increase to maintain cerebral perfusion pressure. The resultant increased mean arterial pressure and reflex bradycardia is called the Cushing's reflex.

   iv. Heart rate and blood pressure must therefore be frequently monitored in the trauma patient with suspected brain injury.

w. To ensure adequate oxygenation of the blood, oxygen saturation should be frequently monitored by pulse oximetry. SpO_2 should be maintained >95%.

x. Body temperature should be closely monitored to prevent the development of hyper- or hypothermia.

y. Blood glucose should be closely monitored in the neurological trauma patient.

   i. Hyperglycemia has been associated with the severity of head trauma in dogs and cats (Syring et al., 2001).

   ii. Normal blood glucose is considered to be between 65–112 g/dL in dogs and 67–168 g/dL in cats.

5. **URINARY MONITORING**

a. Signs of urinary tract compromise may not be apparent at initial presentation. Serial monitoring will allow the clinician to detect a problem before it becomes a life-threatening complication.

b. Injury to the kidneys, ureters, bladder, and urethra can all occur in the trauma patient.

c. Questioning the owner regarding ability to urinate since the trauma, and closely monitoring the patient's urine output will provide information about urinary tract integrity. However, patients with renal pelvis injury, ureter rupture, or a small bladder tear will still be able to urinate. The ability to urinate, therefore, does not ensure integrity of the entire urinary system.

d. Because urinary tract trauma is not often evident on presentation, serial physical examinations should be performed:

    i. Bruising along the ventrum or perineal and inguinal regions, and identification of pelvic fractures should raise the index of suspicion for urinary tract trauma.

    ii. Serial abdominal palpation will aid identification of abdominal pain, abdominal effusion, and the presence or absence of a bladder.

    iii. Palpation of a bladder does not completely rule out urinary tract disruption.

    iv. Perineal and hind-limb swelling may develop secondary to a urethral tear.

e. Monitoring of blood work and urinalysis performed before, during, and after patient resuscitation will aid identification of urinary tract trauma:

    i. Differentials for trauma patients presenting with azotemia:

        1. Pre-renal from dehydration and impaired renal perfusion.

        2. Renal azotemia from renal disease related to the trauma, or pre-existing renal disease.

        3. Postrenal azotemia from disruption of the urinary tract.

        4. Urine specific gravity (prior to fluids) can help differentiate the origin of azotemia.

    ii. Differentials for trauma patients that develop azotemia:

        1. Pre-renal azotemia from inadequate fluid therapy.

        2. Renal azotemia from renal injury, ischemia, or thromboembolic event.

        3. Postrenal azotemia from damage to the lower urinary tract.

f. Monitoring cardiovascular parameters is important to determine renal perfusion and effectiveness of fluid resuscitation efforts:

    i. Blood pressure monitoring helps determine adequacy of renal perfusion.

    ii. The kidney is unable to autoregulate blood flow when the mean arterial pressure (MAP) is less than 60 mm Hg. This will increase the risk for renal ischemia and acute renal failure.

    iii. Central venous pressure can be helpful to guide fluid therapy. It is especially useful in oliguric or anuric patients or if there is concern of preexisting heart disease.

g. Diagnostic imaging techniques are important in monitoring of the urinary tract in trauma patients:

    i. Ultrasonography can be used to detect free abdominal fluid in the trauma patient.

    ii. The focused assessment with sonography for trauma (FAST) is a rapid yet sensitive technique for detecting fluid, and can be performed reliably by emergency veterinarians with minimal ultrasound training:

        1. The FAST method involves placement of patients in lateral recumbency and using both the longitudinal and transverse views in four locations: immediately caudal to the xiphoid process, midline along the bladder, and the most dependent portions of the right and left flank (see Chapter 3: Shock in the Trauma Patient, Figure 3.5).

        2. Monitoring of the trauma patient includes frequent FAST scans to aid rapid detection of abdominal effusion that may suggest compromise to the urinary tract.

    iii. Repeat abdominal radiographs may detect the development of peritoneal or retroperitoneal fluid (see Figure 3.3), and the absence or presence of a urinary bladder.

    iv. Abdominal fluid should be collected via abdominocentesis:

        1. Abdominocentesis may be performed with ultrasound guidance or with single or four quadrant techniques.

        2. Cytology should be performed on all abdominal fluid samples. Culture should be performed if cytological evaluation reveals evidence of acute inflammation or the presence of infectious agents.

        3. Paired blood and abdominal fluid should be analyzed for potassium and creatinine:

a. In dogs, an abdominal fluid creatinine to peripheral blood creatinine ratio of greater than 2:1 and abdominal fluid potassium to peripheral blood potassium ratio of greater than 1.4:1 was diagnostic for uroperitoneum (Schmiedt et al., 2001).

b. In cats, an abdominal fluid to peripheral blood creatinine ratio of greater than 2:1 and abdominal fluid potassium to peripheral blood potassium ratio of greater than 1.9:1 was diagnostic for uroperitoneum (Aumann et al., 1998).

h. Urine output should be monitored in the trauma patient:

i. In a well-hydrated and adequately volume resuscitated patient, adequate urine production is considered to be 2 mL/kg/h.

ii. Aggressive fluid therapy can increase urine output well above 2 mL/kg/h, as can the polyuric phase of renal failure recovery and postobstructive diuresis.

iii. Oliguria is considered to be urine production less than 1 mL/kg/h. Anuria is considered to be urine production less than 0.5 mL/kg/h.

iv. Objective measures of urine output monitoring include indwelling urinary catheter placement with a closed collection system, weighing disposable plastic-backed absorbent pads, and free catching urine (if the patient is ambulatory).

v. The most accurate way to measure urine output is the placement of an indwelling urinary catheter attached to a closed collection system as it allows quantification of all urine produced.

vi. Risks associated with catheter placement include nosocomial infections, and bladder and urethral trauma.

i. Trauma patients should be weighed regularly to monitor for weight loss or gain.

BIBLIOGRAPHY

Aldrich J. Global assessment of the emergency patient. *Vet Clin North Am Small Anim Pract* 2005; 35: 281–305.

Aumann M, Worth LT, Drobatz KJ. Uroperitoneum in cats: 26 cases (1986–1995). *J Am Anim Hosp Assoc* 1998; 34: 315–324.

Boag AK, Hughes D. Assessment and treatment of perfusion abnormalities in the emergency patient. *Vet Clin North Am Small Anim Pract* 2005; 35: 319–342.

Bosiak AP, Mann FA, Dodam JR, *et al.* Comparison of ultrasonic Doppler flow monitor, oscillometric, and direct arterial blood pressure measurement in ill dogs. *J Vet Emerg Crit Care* 2010; 20: 207–215.

Boysen SR, Rozanski EA, Tidwell AS, *et al.* Evaluation of a focused assessment with sonography for trauma protocol to detect free abdominal fluid in dogs involved in motor vehicle accidents. *J Am Vet Med Assoc* 2004; 225: 1198–1204.

Hughes D, Rozanski ER, Shofer FS, *et al.* Effect of sampling site, repeated sampling, pH, and PCO_2 on plasma lactate concentration in healthy dogs. *Am J Vet Res* 1999; 60: 521–524.

Johnson RA, deMorais HA. Respiratory acid-base Disorders. In: DiBartola SP. *Fluid, Electrolyte, and Acid-Base Disorders in Small Animal Practice*. WB Saunders, St. Louis, 2006; 283–296.

Macintire DK, Drobatz KJ, Haskins SC, Saxon WD. *Manual of Small Animal Emergency and Critical Care*. Lippincott Williams & Wilkins, Baltimore, 2005.

Marino PL. *The ICU Book*. 3rd edition. Lippincott Williams & Wilkins, Philadelphia, PA: 2007.

Pang D, Hethey J, Caulkett NA, *et al.* Partial pressure of end-tidal CO_2 sampled via an intranasal catheter as a substitute for partial pressure of arterial CO_2 in dogs. *J Vet Emerg Crit Care* 2007; 17: 143–148.

Pedersen KM, Butler MA, Ersboll AK, Pedersen HD. Evaluation of an oscillometric blood pressure monitor for use in anesthetized cats. *J Am Vet Med Assoc* 2002; 221: 646–650.

Platt SR, Radaelli ST, McDonnell JJ. The prognostic value of the modified Glasgow coma score in head trauma in dogs. *J Vet Intern Med* 2001; 15: 581–584.

Proulx J. Respiratory monitoring: arterial blood gas analysis, pulse oximetry, and end-tidal carbon dioxide analysis. *Clin Tech Small Anim Pract* 1999; 4: 227–230.

Sande A, West C. Traumatic brain injury: a review of pathophysiology and management. *J Vet Emerg Crit Care* 2010; 20: 177–190.

Schmiedt C, Tobias KM, Otto CM. Evaluation of Abdominal Fluid: peripheral blood creatinine and potassium ratios for diagnosis of uroperitoneum in dogs. *J Vet Emerg Crit Care* 2001; 11: 275–280.

Shapiro BA, Peruzzi WT, Kozlowski-Templin R. *Clinical Application of Blood Gases*. Mosby, Philadelphia, PA: 1994.

Shores A. Craniocerebral trauma. In: Kirk RW, ed. *Current Veterinary Therapy X*. WB Saunders, Philadelphia, PA: 1983; 847–854.

Simpson SA, Syring R, Otto CM. Severe blunt trauma in dogs: 235 cases (1997–2003). *J Vet Emerg Crit Care* 2009; 19: 588–602.

Smith MM. Flail chest. In: King LG. *Textbook of Respiratory Disease in Dogs and Cats*. WB Saunders, St. Louis, 2004; 647–651.

Syring RS, Otto CM, Drobatz KJ. Hyperglycemia in dogs and cats with head trauma: 122 cases (1997–1999). *J Am Vet Med Assoc* 2001; 218: 1124–1129.

Syring RS. Assessment and treatment of central nervous system abnormalities in the emergency patient. *Vet Clin North Am Small Anim Pract* 2005; 35: 343–358.

Waddell LS, Brown AJ. Hemodynamic monitoring. In: Silverstein DC, Hopper K, eds. *Manual of Small Animal Emergency & Critical Care*. WB Saunders, Philadelphia, PA: 2008; 859–864.

ANESTHESIA AND ANALGESIA FOR THE TRAUMA PATIENT

Benjamin M. Brainard and Lindsey Culp Snyder

CHAPTER 5

1. PAIN PHYSIOLOGY

a. Pain is the physiologic and emotional reaction to real or perceived tissue damage. Nociception is the physiologic process that leads to the perception of pain.

b. Nociceptive nerve endings first transduce the chemical stimuli of inflammatory mediators into a nerve impulse. These impulses then transmit to the spinal cord, where they synapse onto neurons that communicate to ascending spinal tracts. These tracks carry the nociceptive signal to the brain, where pain is perceived. The types of nerves that carry the initial pain impulses are classified on the basis of myelination and size, which determines the type of pain they sense:

   i. $A\delta$ fibers transmit acute, well-localized, pin-prick pain.

   ii. C-fibers transmit more chronic, less well-localized, aching pain.

   iii. $A\beta$ fibers are associated with normal touch sensation and are ordinarily not associated with nociceptive pain. In pathologic conditions; however, their transmission may be perceived as painful.

c. Modulation of nociceptive signals occurs in the dorsal horn of the spinal cord where the nociceptive nerve fibers synapse to the spinal tracts:

   i. Descending tracts from the brain may modify pain transmission at the synapse.

   ii. Signals from local interneurons may also influence synaptic transmission.

   iii. Many analgesic drugs with spinal mechanisms of action modify nociceptive transmission by altering the polarization of the interneurons.

d. Upregulation of inflammatory or nociceptive stimuli in the periphery or in the spinal cord can magnify pain sensations:

   i. COX-2 upregulation increases PGE_2 expression, which sensitizes nerve endings to nociceptive input.

   ii. Glutamate released from afferent nociceptive neurons can upregulate spinal N-methyl-D-aspartate (NMDA) receptors, which facilitates nociceptive transmission and may contribute to a pathologic or chronic pain state.

   iii. With upregulation of spinal cord nociceptive processing, even innocuous stimuli (such as those carried by $A\beta$ fibers) may be perceived as painful (allodynia).

e. Pathologic pain states:

   i. Hyperalgesia: an exaggerated response greater than the magnitude of the nociceptive input.

   ii. Allodynia: the perception of an innocuous stimulus as painful.

   iii. Wind-up: a state where the spinal cord has an increased responsiveness to nociceptive stimuli as a result of chronic activation (e.g., from a chronic painful condition).

f. Analgesic therapy is directed against the different physiologic and pathophysiologic mechanisms of transmission of nociceptive stimuli.

Manual of Trauma Management in the Dog and Cat, First Edition. Edited by Kenneth J. Drobatz, Matthew W. Beal and Rebecca S. Syring.
© 2011 John Wiley & Sons, Inc. Published 2011 by John Wiley & Sons, Inc.

2. CATEGORIES OF PAIN SECONDARY TO TRAUMA

a. Primary tissue trauma:

   i. Direct tissue injury (e.g., laceration or tearing of skin or muscle).

   ii. Fractures or other orthopedic pain (e.g., joint pain).

b. Secondary tissue trauma (inflammation):

   i. The body's response to tissue injury involves the generation of inflammatory mediators, which act to recruit leukocytes to the site of injury to help fight infection and remove debris.

   ii. These mediators, with additional inflammation from leukocyte activation, sensitize C-fibers. Sensitization results in pain that radiates beyond the site of initial injury, producing an area of hyperalgesia.

c. Compartment syndrome:

   i. Associated with hemorrhage or fluid accumulation into a closed space.

   ii. May also be caused by large-scale tissue swelling associated with inflammation or edema.

   iii. Pressure on the tissues of the compartment and decreased oxygen delivery (due to vessel compression or disruption) causes ischemia and necrosis:

   1. Release of potassium and hydrogen ion from dying cells sensitizes nociceptors.

   2. Upregulation of COX increases tissue PGE_2 which also sensitizes nerve fibers.

   iv. Direct compression of nerves and nerve roots may also cause severe pain and neurologic deficit.

d. Crush injury:

   i. Direct destruction of muscle tissue causing cellular leakage of hydrogen and potassium, as well as myoglobin, into the circulation. Compartment syndrome may be seen after crush injury.

   ii. Systemic effects (e.g., hyperkalemia, myoglobinuria) may not be noted until circulation is returned to the injured area (reperfusion).

e. Anxiety:

   i. From initial traumatic event

   ii. Hypovolemia secondary to blood loss

   iii. Injury and transport to unfamiliar settings

   iv. Can contribute to and intensify the pain experience

3. ANALGESIC CHOICES FOR THE TRAUMA PATIENT MUST ACKNOWLEDGE THE PHYSIOLOGIC CHANGES THAT ACCOMPANY THE INJURY.

a. Cardiovascular (see Chapter 3: Shock in the Trauma Patient):

   i. Changes in blood volume (hypovolemia):

   1. Hemorrhage:

   a. With anemia secondary to hemorrhage, oxygen delivery to the tissues is compromised and may result in further physiologic changes (e.g., lactic acidosis).

   b. Hypovolemia alone will also compromise tissue perfusion and thus oxygen delivery to tissues.

   2. Relative hypovolemia:

   i. Shock states

   ii. Changes in cardiac performance:

   1. Myocardial contusions +/− direct tissue damage (e.g., from hypoxia)

   2. Arrhythmias

b. Respiratory (see Chapter 6: Trauma-Associated Thoracic Injury):

   i. Pleural space disease:

   1. Decreased functional residual capacity (FRC) results in inability to ventilate and oxygenate, as the lungs may not be fully expanded.

   2. Rib fractures may cause an additional decrease in FRC as pain prohibits a normal inspiratory effort.

   3. Pneumothorax or pneumomediastinum.

   4. Hemothorax.

   5. Chylothorax.

   ii. Pulmonary parenchymal disease:

   1. Pulmonary contusion is often the sequelae to blunt thoracic trauma, and is characterized by hemorrhage into the lung parenchyma:

   a. Depending on extent, may cause significant impairment of pulmonary function by ventilation/perfusion inequality:

   i. Hypoxemia

   ii. Hypercarbia

   2. Pulmonary edema:

   a. May result from trauma that causes a transient airway obstruction or head trauma (noncardiogenic edema).

b. May result from inadequate cardiac function (cardiogenic edema):

  i. This is a very uncommon comorbid condition in a trauma patient, although patients with compensated heart disease may decompensate secondary to trauma.

iii. Rarely, blunt chest trauma may result in avulsion of elements of the tracheobronchial tree or of the esophagus:

  1. Pneumomediastinum, pneumothorax, and/or progressive sepsis must be considered.

c. Urogenital (see Chapter 10: Trauma-Associated Urinary Tract Injury):

  i. Bladder rupture, ureteral avulsion, urethral tear.

    1. May not be immediately obvious.

    2. May need contrast urography to obtain a definitive diagnosis.

    3. Inability to eliminate urine results in life-threatening alterations of electrolytes and acid-base status:

      a. Hyperkalemia

      b. Metabolic acidosis

    4. Leakage of urine into the peritoneum or retroperitoneum is extremely inflammatory and painful.

d. Nervous system (see Chapter 7: Traumatic Brain Injury):

  i. Central nervous system:

    1. Head trauma/traumatic brain injury:

      a. May require emergent care to decrease elevated intracranial pressure, if present (see Chapter 7: Traumatic Brain Injury).

      b. May be accompanied by fractures of skull or jaw, in addition to other fractures (see Chapter 16: Trauma-Associated Musculoskeletal Injuries to the Head).

      c. Secondary injury may be progressive and cause changes in mentation during the initial hospitalization, which may make it difficult to fully assess the effects of analgesic therapy.

    2. Spinal cord trauma (see Chapter 9: Traumatic Spinal Injury):

      a. If an unstable vertebral fracture is present, patients may require sedation and/or anesthesia to prevent further damage to the spinal cord (ongoing primary injury).

  ii. Peripheral nervous system (see Chapter 8: Trauma-Associated Peripheral Nerve Injury):

    1. Brachial plexus avulsion

    2. Localized nerve injury

    3. Compartment syndrome

e. Gastrointestinal/hepatic/splenic (see Chapter 11: Trauma-Associated Abdominal Parenchymal Organ Injury and Chapter 14: Trauma-Associated Gastrointestinal Injury):

  i. Fractures or hematomas that form on the spleen or liver can cause rapid hypovolemic shock.

f. Musculoskeletal (see Chapter 18: Trauma-Associated Musculoskeletal Injury to the Appendicular Skeleton and Chapter 19: Trauma-Associated Musculoskeletal Injury to the Pelvis, Sacrum and Tail):

  i. Severe trauma can lead to hemorrhage or necrosis of muscle:

    1. Compartment syndrome possible, although rare.

    2. Danger of reperfusion injury, if blood supply is initially compromised.

4. ASSESSMENT OF PAIN

  a. In human and veterinary emergency rooms, pain is undertreated. This could be due to:

    i. Unknown/unrecognized pain

    ii. Concerns about side effects of analgesics

  b. Pain scales are useful to evaluate patients both before and after analgesic administration (Figure 5.1):

    i. The visual analogue scale (VAS) is a simple method to record the pain level of the patient (Figure 5.1a):

      1. A 100 mm line represents the patient's pain, with no pain at the 0 mm mark and excruciating pain at the 100 mm mark.

      2. The VAS may be evaluated prior to analgesic administration and following analgesia, and should result in a decrease in VAS score if analgesia is adequate.

    ii. More specific scoring systems exist for veterinary patients and many are easily adapted for clinical use:

      1. Most use a combination of physiologic parameters and clinical observations:

        a. The University of Melbourne Pain Scale (UMPS) evaluates physiological

(a)
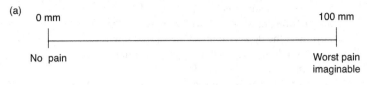

(b)
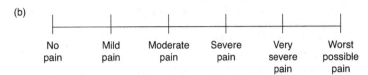

FIGURE 5.1 Three versions of pain scales that can be adapted for use in the clinical setting. All are based on the visual analogue scale (1a). The use of these scales allows for documentation of the degree of a patient's pain as well as the effect of analgesic therapy.

(c)
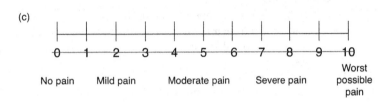

parameters (heart rate, respiratory rate, rectal temperature, etc.), activity, posture, vocalization, mental state, and, most importantly, response to palpation, which makes this an active assessment of patient pain (Firth and Haldane, 1999).
b. The Glasgow pain scale is designed for dogs, and also evaluates the patient in an interactive context (Holton et al., 1998).

5. CHOICE OF ANALGESIC DRUGS FOR TRAUMA VICTIMS
a. Analgesic drug choices are based on educated decisions that result in utilization of a drug or combination of drugs that best address the type of pain and physiologic state of the patient.
b. Multi-modal analgesia (using more than one drug with different mechanisms of action) is a wise choice:
   i. Synergism between drugs may allow equivalent analgesia at lower doses, reducing side effects.
   ii. Less likely to compromise the patient's physiology.

6. DRUG TYPES
a. Opioids:
   i. Opioids are potent, effective analgesic drugs that are frequently indicated for acute analgesia of the trauma patient.

   ii. Analgesia is provided from interactions with opiate receptors in the periphery, spinal cord, and brain.
   iii. Three major types of opioid receptors:
     1. μ (mu) receptors:
      a. Located spinally, supraspinally, and peripherally.
      b. Agonism provides analgesia.
      c. Side effects include respiratory depression, emesis, gastrointestinal ileus, and euphoria.
     2. κ (kappa) receptors:
      a. Located spinally, supraspinally, and peripherally. Their distribution varies between species.
      b. Receptors provide analgesia, especially of the viscera, and specific agonists may be useful in the treatment of intraabdominal disease.
     3. δ (delta) receptors:
      a. Provide primarily spinal analgesia.
   iv. Opioid drugs are characterized by their receptor activation profile. Knowing this profile allows for selection of appropriate drugs for each patient:
     1. Agonism at opioid receptors may have variable effects between species; notably, cats have a higher incidence of arousal and hyperactive behavior after administration of full opioid agonists.

v. Route of administration of opioids is usually flexible; most may be given by any route, although the most commonly used in companion animals are intravenous, intramuscular, subcutaneously, and transdermally.

vi. Opioids may be combined with tranquilizers (e.g., benzodiazepines, acepromazine) for neuroleptanalgesia, a synergistic interaction with sedative and analgesic properties.

vii. Full opioid agonists (agonists at mu, kappa, and delta opioid receptors):

    1. These drugs are potent analgesic agents, but administration may be associated with emesis, sedation, ileus, and panting in dogs:

      a. Morphine:

        i. May be administered as intermittent bolus or constant rate infusion (CRI).

        ii. Preservative-free solutions are available for infusion into joints, epidural space and intrathecal ("spinal" or "CSF") space.

        iii. Has been associated with histamine release when administered intravenously.

        iv. For analgesia in dogs and cats, doses range from 0.1 to 1.0 mg/kg IM or IV slow, q. 4–6 hours, or as 0.1–0.2 mg/kg/h IV CRI.

      b. Oxymorphone (Numorphan®):

        i. Semisynthetic, 10 times more potent than morphine.

        ii. For analgesia in dogs and cats, doses range from 0.05 to 0.1 mg/kg IM, IV q. 4–6 hours.

      c. Hydromorphone (Dilaudid®):

        i. Semisynthetic, 10 times more potent than morphine.

        ii. Has been associated with episodes of extreme hyperthermia when administered to some cats (Posner et al., 2007).

        iii. For analgesia in dogs and cats, doses range from 0.05 to 0.2 mg/kg IM, IV q. 4–6 hours.

      d. Fentanyl (Sublimaze®):

        i. Synthetic opioid, 100 times more potent than morphine.

        ii. Fast acting, with a duration of action of approximately 15–20 minutes.

        iii. Administered as a CRI for analgesia at 0.002–0.006 mg/kg/hr. An initial intravenous bolus of 5 μg/kg may also be given as a single dose, or as part of a protocol for induction of anesthesia in debilitated patients.

        iv. Extremely potent respiratory depressant, especially if used concurrently with tranquilizers such as phenothiazines or benzodiazepines. It should be used with caution in animals with respiratory compromise. See "Opioid Side Effects" in the following.

        v. May be administered transdermally (Duragesic® patch, and others):

          1. Depending on the species, analgesic blood levels will not be achieved for 12–24 hours, thus limiting the use of the patch for acute traumatic injuries.

          2. Patches are sized to deliver a certain mcg/hour of drug, and may be dosed in the same way (mcg/kg/hour; see Table 5.1. Recommended dosing by weight may also be found in veterinary drug handbooks.

          3. Patches may elute increased amounts of drug if they are applied to irritated or broken skin. Warming of the skin (as by a forced warm air blanket after anesthesia) may cause vasodilation and an increased uptake of drug. By the same token, inappropriate adhesion of the patch may result in much lower drug concentrations than anticipated. Animals should be routinely monitored for pain and analgesia supplemented if indicated.

          4. Patches, even when used, contain a significant amount of fentanyl, which may cause severe side effects (respiratory

TABLE 5.1
DOSES FOR ANALGESIC DRUGS IN THE CANINE AND FELINE TRAUMA PATIENT

Drug	Dose Range	Notes
Morphine	Dogs: 0.1–1.0 mg/kg IM, IV slow, q. 4–6 h 0.1 mg/kg/h IV CRI Cats: 0.1–1.0 mg/kg IM, IV slow, q. 4–6 h 0.1 mg/kg/h IV CRI	Rapid IV administration may cause histamine release. IM or SQ administration may result in emesis. Administration of opioids in cats may result in excitation.
Hydromorphone	Dogs: 0.05–0.2 mg/kg IM, IV q. 4–6 h. Cats: 0.05–0.2 mg/kg IM, IV q. 4–6 h.	IM or SQ administration may result in emesis, panting may be observed. Administration of opioids in cats may result in excitation. May cause hyperthermia in cats.
Oxymorphone	Dogs: 0.05–0.1 mg/kg IM, IV q. 4–6 h. Cats: 0.05–0.1 mg/kg IM, IV q. 4–6 h.	May cause slight sedation.
Fentanyl	Dogs: 0.003–0.010 mg/kg/h IV CRI, bolus dose 0.002–0.005 mg/kg IV 0.003–0.005 mg/kg/h transdermal (patch) Cats: 0.003–0.010 mg/kg/h IV CRI, bolus dose 0.002–0.005 mg/kg IV 0.003–0.005 mg/kg/h transdermal (patch)	Potent respiratory depressant; patients must be monitored. May take up to 24 hours for adequate analgesia after transdermal administration.
Buprenorphine	Dogs: 0.01–0.06 mg/kg IM, IV q. 6–8 h. Cats: 0.01–0.06 mg/kg IM, IV q. 6–8 h.	Longer time to onset of action. May cause less excitation in cats, while still providing adequate analgesia. Can be administered transmucosally in cats.
Butorphanol	Dogs: 0.1–0.5 mg/kg IM, IV q. 2–4 h. Cats: 0.1–0.5 mg/kg IM, IV q. 2–4 h.	Provides mild analgesia. Short duration of action.
Methadone	Dogs: 0.1–0.3 mg/kg IM,IV Cats: 0.1–0.3 mg/kg IM,IV	
Lidocaine	Dogs: following loading dose of 1–2 mg/kg, 30–50 mcg/kg/min IV CRI Cats: following loading dose of 1 mg/kg, 30–50 mcg/kg/min IV CRI	Provides analgesia in combination with opioid analgesics (plus/minus low-dose ketamine CRI); useful for treating ventricular arrhythmias. Cats are more sensitive to the toxic effects of local anesthetics.
Ketamine	Dogs: following loading dose of 0.2–0.5 mg/kg, 0.1–0.5 mg/kg/h IV CRI 0.001–0.010 mg/kg/min IV CRI Cats: following loading dose of 0.2–0.5 mg/kg, 0.1–0.5 mg/kg/h IV CRI 0.001–0.010 mg/kg/min IV CRI	May not be adequate as a sole analgesic at lower doses. Higher doses may provide analgesia and sedation.
Medetomidine	Dogs: 0.002–0.010 mg/kg IM, IV 0.001–0.002 mg/kg/h IV CRI Cats: 0.002–0.010 mg/kg IM, IV 0.001–0.002 mg/kg/h IV CRI	Use with caution in the trauma patient with cardiovascular instability.

depression, death) in humans if abused, or if eaten by animals in the house. Care should be taken to alert the owner of these possibilities when sending an animal home with a patch.

5. Patches, when removed from the patient, should be folded in half, and flushed down the toilet, or returned to the veterinarian who dispensed them, for appropriate disposal.

viii. Partial opioid agonists (agonists at mu opioid receptors):

1. Buprenorphine (Buprenex®):

a. Synthetic opioid, agonist at mu opioid receptors.

b. Binds to the receptors with high affinity and may be difficult to reverse.

c. The degree of analgesia is less than an equipotent dose of a full mu agonist; hence this drug is classified as a partial agonist.

d. Higher doses (up to 0.03 mg/kg in dogs and cats) do not necessarily result in more analgesia, but rather a longer duration of action.

e. Except in extremely ill animals, does not usually result in profound sedation or clinically significant respiratory depression.

f. May be given sublingually (transmucosally) in cats without affecting the pharmacokinetics, making it a useful analgesic that may be sent home (Robertson et al., 2005).

g. For analgesia in dogs and cats, doses range from 0.005 to 0.030 mg/kg SQ, IM, IV, and transmucosally q 6–8 hours.

ix. Opioid agonist/antagonists:

1. Butorphanol (Torbugesic®):

a. A synthetic opioid, which acts as an *ant*agonist at mu opioid receptors and an agonist at kappa opioid receptors.

b. The analgesic effect is short-lived in healthy animals (30–60 minutes):

i. This period may be prolonged in debilitated cats, which may show sedation for 4–6 hours following butorphanol administration.

ii. More frequent dosing intervals may be necessary in dogs.

iii. For analgesia in dogs and cats, doses range from 0.1 to 0.5 mg/kg IM, IV, SQ q. 2–4 hours.

iv. May also be administered as a CRI (0.2 mg/kg/h) to provide sedation and some analgesia.

c. Some moderately painful abdominal conditions may respond favorably to kappa opioid agonism, but butorphanol is not adequate for treating severe or orthopedic pain.

d. Butorphanol may also be used as an anti-emetic and anti-tussive agent.

e. Due to its antagonism at the mu receptor, butorphanol may be used as a partial reversal agent for the adverse effects caused by the mu opioid agonist drugs (e.g., excessive sedation or respiratory depression), while preserving a degree of analgesia:

i. Smaller doses of butorphanol (0.005–0.050 mg/kg IV), may be used for this effect.

ii. To preserve a degree of analgesia, the dose may be titrated to the desired effect.

x. Opioid antagonists:

1. Add to the utility of this class of drugs; if adverse effects occur, the antagonists have equally flexible routes for dosing and are rapidly effective.

2. Naloxone (Narcan®):

a. To reverse the effects of opioids in dogs and cats, doses range from 0.02 to 0.04 mg/kg IM, IV, SQ, and intratracheally, and may be repeated as necessary.

b. Naloxone has been used as a CRI (0.2 mg/kg/h) in cases of massive opioid overdose (da Cunda, 2007).

3. Butorphanol may also be used in micro doses (0.005–0.050 mg/kg) to reverse full opioids that are causing adverse effects (e.g., dysphoria) in a patient.

xi. Opioid side effects:

1. Respiratory:

a. Opioids decrease the responsiveness of the respiratory center to elevated arterial carbon dioxide levels (hyper-carbia). Consequently, hypoventilation and possibly hypoxemia may occur, especially in patients with respiratory compromise.

b. Hypoventilation is of particular concern in patients with head trauma, as hypercarbia may result in increased intracranial pressure.

c. Hypoventilation in patients with pulmonary trauma who are not receiving oxygen supplementation may result in hypoxemia.

d. Panting is a frequent side effect of opioid administration in dogs and may be related to a reset of the hypothalamic temperature set point. Often this effect is transient and is not observed when opioids are administered by constant rate infusion.

2. Cardiovascular:

a. Opioids in general are regarded as cardiovascularly sparing. Some drugs may cause a significant vagally-mediated bradycardia (e.g., fentanyl) with minimal change to the cardiac output or systemic vascular resistance, outside of the changes caused by the bradycardia.

b. Fentanyl is especially potent with regard to bradycardia and should be used with caution in animals with pre-existing high vagal tone without concurrent ECG monitoring.

c. Animals who need high heart rates to sustain cardiac output (e.g., with hypovolemia) may be more profoundly affected by the opioid-induced brady-cardia. Blood pressure and ECG monitoring should be used as indicated.

3. Gastrointestinal:

a. Full opioid agonists may result in decreased gastrointestinal motility and ileus. In animals with traumatic injuries, this may predispose to gastroesophageal reflux, possible regurgitation, and subsequent aspiration pneumonia.

b. This effect appears to be less pronounced with the partial opioid agonists or opioid agonist/antagonists.

c. The effect may be partially reversed by opioid antagonists.

d. Most full agonist opioids have a stimulatory effect on the chemoreceptor trigger zone (CRTZ) and may cause emesis (especially profound with apomorphine):

1. This effect is usually encountered only with the first dose due to subsequent opioid effects on the vomiting center.

2. Animals who have esophageal disease (e.g., foreign bodies, tears) should not receive full opioid agonists until fully anesthetized for surgical correction, which will minimize the chance of emesis.

3. Likewise, animals who have corneal defects (e.g., corneal lacerations, descemetocele) should not receive full opioid agonists, as emesis may lead to corneal rupture due to acute elevations of intraocular pressure. Opioids may be given when they are fully anesthetized for surgical correction.

b. Benzodiazepines:

i. Provide relaxation and anxiolysis, especially when combined with opioids:

1. Benzodiazepines work by potentiating the effects of gamma–amino–butyric acid (GABA) in the CNS, which causes hyperpolarization of nerve membranes and decreased transmission resulting in sedation and muscle relaxation.

2. GABA also modulates some arousal influences in the CNS. When given alone, benzodiazepines (and other GABA agonists) may disinhibit these control mechanisms and result in agitation.

ii. Diazepam (Valium®):

1. Labeled for IV or IM usage, this drug may cause pain on injection because it is dissolved in propylene glycol.

2. Doses in dogs and cats range between 0.2 and 0.5 mg/kg IV, IM.

3. May be given per rectum or intra-nasally as a treatment for status epilepticus in patients without IV access.

4. May be given as a CRI (0.25–0.5 mg/kg/h), however, the propylene glycol solution has an osmolality of over 7000 mOsm/L:

    a. The high osmolality may result in thrombophlebitis if administered through a peripheral catheter for an extended period of time.

5. Propylene glycol is metabolized to lactate, and may cause a high-anion gap acidosis in susceptible patients if administered for extended periods of time (Wilson et al., 2000; Neale et al., 2005).

iii. Midazolam (Versed®):

    1. A benzodiazepine in a water-soluble formulation, which may result in better absorption and less pain after intramuscular administration.

    2. May be given as an intermittent bolus (0.1–0.5 mg/kg) or as a CRI (0.2 mg/kg/h) for maintenance of sedation or treatment of status epilepticus, without propylene glycol related side effects.

iv. The cardiovascular and respiratory alterations caused by benzodiazepines are minimal and these are usually safe additions to anesthetic or sedative protocols for patients with unstable cardiovascular disease:

    1. Smaller doses are usually necessary to achieve similar effect in debilitated patients and some effects that are minor (e.g., the slight decrease in systemic vascular resistance from midazolam) may be more pronounced in animals with severe disease.

v. Central nervous system:

    1. The benzodiazepines are effective drugs to treat patients experiencing seizures secondary to CNS disease. They may be administered as an intermittent bolus or CRI.

vi. Benzodiazepine reversal:

    1. Flumazenil (Romazicon®):

        a. A competitive antagonist at the benzodiazepine binding site, flumazenil is useful for treatment of benzodiazepine overdose or to reverse the sedative effects after a procedure is complete.

        b. Doses in dogs and cats to reverse the effects of benzodiazepines range from 0.01 to 0.02 mg/kg IV, IM, SQ. A reversal dose ratio of 1 mg. of flumazenil for every 13 mg of diazepam or midazolam has also been proposed.

        c. The clinical duration of action is short (30–40 minutes), so multiple doses may be necessary to avoid re-sedation.

        d. Anecdotal reports have recommended flumazenil for reversal of sedation associated with hepatic encephalopathy:

            i. Endogenous benzodiazepine-like substances have been implicated in the clinical encephalopathic signs; however, flumazenil is not a definitive solution and must be followed with more specific treatment to lower blood ammonia levels.

            ii. The use of flumazenil for this purpose requires further investigation.

c. Phenothiazines:

    i. Potent anxiolytic drugs that also have antiemetic effects due to anti-dopaminergic effects at the vomiting center:

        1. Common examples include acepromazine and chlorpromazine (Thorazine®).

        2. These drugs have a potent alpha-1 antagonist effect, resulting in hypotension.

        3. A neuroleptanalgesic synergy exists, especially with opioids, which may create suitable anesthesia for minor procedures such as urinary catheterization and radiographs:

            a. Doses for this indication range from 0.005 to 0.03 mg/kg, IV/IM. It should be noted that the initial FDA-approved labeled dose is significantly higher than these equally effective doses and may be associated with adverse effects as the dose increases.

            b. If needed, the above dose can be repeated q 6–8 hours.

            c. The above combination, with the addition of a local anesthetic block and adequate restraint, could be sufficient for the repair of minor lacerations.

        4. Due to alpha-1 antagonism, may cause vasodilation and splenomegaly:

            a. Relative hypovolemia, hypotension, and apparent anemia may result.

            b. The sequestration of red blood cells in the spleen caused by this drug could also cause a significant decrease in oxygen delivery to tissues.

c. Due to the possible hypotensive effects of this drug and the inability to reverse its effects, it should be used sparingly in the trauma patient.

5. Acepromazine can reduce the respiratory rate and tidal volume, although the effects are seldom clinically significant.

6. Decreased platelet function following administration of acepromazine to dogs has been documented, although this effect was transient and not associated with clinical bleeding.

7. If acepromazine is the only available anxiolytic, it is recommended to use it sparingly; 0.005–0.010 mg/kg given intravenously may have the same sedative effect as much larger doses:

    a. These smaller doses may cause less severe, or more transient, hypotension.

8. Anecdotal reports exist of increased sensitivity to acepromazine in English boxer dogs, although this has not been assessed by controlled studies.

d. Alpha-2 agonists:

  i. Available as both less selective (e.g., xylazine) and more selective (e.g., medetomidine) drugs at the alpha-2 adrenergic receptor; these drugs have both sedative and analgesic qualities.

  ii. These drugs may be administered via many different routes (IV, IM, SQ), as well as epidurally:

    1. Doses of medetomidine for analgesia in dogs and cats can range from 0.002 to 0.03 mg/kg, depending on the use of adjunct analgesics.

    2. Systemic cardiovascular effects will be seen regardless of route of administration.

    3. Comparable doses of dexmedetomidine are 0.001–0.015 mg/kg.

  iii. Cardiovascular effects:

    1. The alpha agonist qualities of these drugs result in significant cardiovascular changes that may not be tolerated in patients that are in shock following a trauma.

    2. After administration of medetomidine, perfusion to every organ system, including the myocardium and GI tract, is decreased:

    a. These changes occur at very small doses of these drugs (as low as 0.002 mg/kg of medetomidine).

    3. Commonly, animals will experience a brief period of hypertension (due to the vasoconstrictive effects of the alpha agonism) and an associated reflex bradycardia, followed by hypotension:

    a. The hypotension results from a general decrease in sympathetic discharge from the alpha agonism in the central nervous system.

    4. While these cardiovascular events may be tolerated in healthy animals, they may cause significant compromise in an unstable animal, especially one who is initially hypovolemic or has any cardiovascular compromise.

  iv. If deemed appropriate and not contraindicated, lower doses of these drugs (e.g., 0.005–0.010 mg/kg) may be combined with opioids such as butorphanol (at 0.1–0.2 mg/kg) for good sedation with analgesia.

  v. The drug may be reversed at the end of the procedure, if necessary.

  vi. The alpha-2 drugs are not always reliable sedatives, especially when used in aggressive or excited animals; some animals that appear sedate will experience quick arousal with stimulation that may result in disruption of the procedure or bites to the care-giver. For this reason, these drugs are not frequently used in the emergency room. The authors find the dissociative anesthetics (e.g., ketamine, tiletamine) to be much more reliable sedation for aggressive or potentially dangerous animals.

e. Dissociative agents:

  i. Ketamine and Tiletamine (combined with zolazepam in Telazol®) are the most common dissociative anesthetic agents used in small animal veterinary practice.

  ii. The dissociative anesthetics have an incompletely understood anesthetic action. They are antagonists at the N-methyl-d-aspartate (NMDA) receptor in the dorsal horn of the spinal cord.

  iii. The use of dissociative agents is associated with analgesia and an anesthetic state, where the animal may retain some reflexes (e.g., control of the larynx, ocular reflexes) while being unable to react in an organized way to external stimuli:

    1. For this reason, the authors prefer these drugs in a sedation protocol for aggressive animals; combined with an opioid and/or benzodiazepine, this combination provides analgesia, sedation, and protection from bites that may result from unpredictable arousal.

    2. Analgesia is best when used in combination with an opioid.

iv. Given alone, these drugs may result in significant muscle rigidity; they are most frequently combined with a tranquilizer to provide an element of muscle relaxation:

    1. Telazol is a proprietary mixture of tiletamine with zolazepam, a benzodiazepine. The ratio of the two drugs is not able to be changed, although the concentration of the final product may be changed if desired.

v. These drugs may be incorporated into sedative protocols for short procedures when used with a tranquilizer alone, or with an opioid if more analgesia is required:

    1. There is a wide dose range for these drugs in dogs and cats (see Tables 5.1–5.3).

    2. At higher doses, these drugs may be used to induce general anesthesia.

vi. Cardiovascular effects:

    1. The dissociative agents are thought of as cardiovascularly sparing drugs, but this may not be the case in a trauma patient, especially if combined with hypovolemia or myocardial trauma.

    2. While ketamine alone is a myocardial depressant, administration will result in a concomitant sympathetic stimulus, which more than offsets the depression, in healthy patients:

        a. The sympathetic stimulus is responsible for the elevated heart rate and blood pressure occasionally seen with ketamine's use.

        b. In the trauma patient, depleted sympathetic reserve may limit the degree to which the animal can compensate for the myocardial depression; this is espe-

cially true in patients presenting with septic shock.

        c. In the hypovolemic trauma patient, the sympathetic stimulation may also fail to fully compensate for the myocardial depression.

vii. Respiratory effects:

    1. Respiratory effects of the dissociative drugs are minimal, and these are the drugs least likely to result in hypoventilation:

        a. Irregular breathing patterns characterized by periods of apnea (apneustic breathing) may occur.

viii. Central nervous system effects:

    1. While activity in some areas of the brain is depressed, it is increased in other areas, and consequently, ketamine is associated with an increased metabolic activity and oxygen consumption in the brain, which increases intracranial pressure. For these reasons, it is not recommended as an agent for patients with head trauma.

    2. Ketamine will also increase intraocular pressure and is not recommended for use in patients with ocular disease.

f. Nonsteroidal anti-inflammatory drugs (NSAIDs):

i. These drugs inhibit the cyclooxygenase (COX) enzyme, which is located in many different organ systems, and produces prostanoids (prostaglandins and thromboxanes) to maintain homeostasis in the body:

    1. COX produces prostaglandins that contribute to the tissue changes associated with inflammation.

    2. Inhibition of COX results in decreased production of both homeostatic and pro-inflammatory prostanoids.

ii. NSAIDs have relatively little effect on the cardiorespiratory system, but are contraindicated in the trauma patient with poor perfusion:

    1. The kidneys and the GI tract rely on prostaglandins to maintain blood flow and mucosal integrity during periods of hypovolemia or hypotension.

    2. Inhibition of the ability to augment blood flow from prostaglandins may result in serious side effects such as acute renal failure and gastric or duodenal ulceration.

TABLE 5.2
SEDATIVE COMBINATIONS FOR SHORT, NONINVASIVE PROCEDURES (E.G., RADIOGRAPHS, CATHETER PLACEMENT) FOR THE CANINE TRAUMA PATIENT

Drug Combination	Dose: Drug 1	Dose: Drug 2	Notes
Opioid/diazepam	Morphine 0.1–0.2 mg/kg IV IM	Diazepam: 0.3–0.5 mg/kg IV	Can substitute midazolam (IV or IM) for diazepam at the same dose.
	Hydromorphone 0.1–0.2 mg/kg IV IM	Diazepam: 0.3–0.5 mg/kg IV	Can substitute midazolam (IV or IM) for diazepam at the same dose.
	Butorphanol 0.1–0.2 mg/kg IV IM	Diazepam: 0.3–0.5 mg/kg IV	Can substitute midazolam (IV or IM)for diazepam at the same dose.
	Oxymorphone 0.05–0.1 mg/kg IV IM	Diazepam: 0.3–0.5 mg/kg IV	Can substitute midazolam (IV or IM)for diazepam at the same dose.
Opioid/acepromazine	Morphine 0.1–0.2 mg/kg IV IM	Acepromazine: 0.01–0.03 mg/kg IV IM	Caution: acepromazine is a potent hypotensive agent.
	Hydromorphone 0.1–0.2 mg/kg IV IM	Acepromazine: 0.01–0.03 mg/kg IV IM	Caution: acepromazine is a potent hypotensive agent.
	Butorphanol 0.1–0.2 mg/kg IV IM	Acepromazine: 0.01–0.03 mg/kg IV IM	Caution: acepromazine is a potent hypotensive agent.
	Oxymorphone 0.05–0.1 mg/kg IV IM	Acepromazine: 0.01–0.03 mg/kg IV IM	Caution: acepromazine is a potent hypotensive agent.
Opioid/medetomidine	Butorphanol 0.1–0.2 mg/kg IV IM	Medetomidine 0.005–0.015 mg/kg IV IM	Use with caution in the trauma patient due to cardiovascular effects.

These drugs may be combined in the same syringe for administration. These protocols may also be supplemented with *judicious* use of propofol (0.5–1 mg/kg IV slowly) as long as blood pressure and respirations are within the normal range. Always consider intubation when utilizing propofol.

3. COX in platelets is important for platelet aggregation, and some NSAIDs such as aspirin and ketoprofen, may result in decreased platelet function. The other available NSAIDs (carprofen, meloxicam, deracoxib, firocoxib) have no, or clinically insignificant, inhibitory effects on platelet aggregation.

iii. The veterinary NSAIDs are predominantly orally administered medications, with the exception of carprofen (Rimadyl®), meloxicam (Metacam®), and ketoprofen (Ketofen®), which have injectable forms:

1. Carprofen is dosed in dogs at 1–2 mg/kg IV, IM, SQ, PO q. 24 hours.
2. Meloxicam is labeled in dogs for a dose of 0.2 mg/kg PO, IV, or SC on the first day of treatment, with subsequent doses of 0.1 mg/kg q. 24. In cats, the dose is 0.2 mg/kg

TABLE 5.3
SEDATIVE COMBINATIONS FOR SHORT, NONINVASIVE PROCEDURES (E.G., RADIOGRAPHS, CATHETER PLACEMENT) FOR THE FELINE TRAUMA PATIENT

Drug Combination	Dose: Drug 1	Dose: Drug 2	Notes
Opioid/diazepam	Butorphanol 0.1–0.2 mg/kg IV IM	Diazepam: 0.2–0.4 mg/kg IV	Can substitute midazolam for diazepam at the same dose.
	Oxymorphone 0.05–0.1 mg/kg IV IM	Diazepam: 0.2–0.4 mg/kg IV	Can substitute midazolam for diazepam at the same dose.
	Hydromorphone 0.1–0.2 mg/kg IV IM	Diazepam: 0.2–0.4 mg/kg IV	Can substitute midazolam for diazepam at the same dose.
Opioid/diazepam/ketamine	May add ketamine 2–5 mg/kg IV if combinations above are not adequate		
Opioid/acepromazine	Butorphanol 0.1–0.2 mg/kg IV IM	Acepromazine: 0.01–0.03 mg/kg IV	Caution: acepromazine is a potent hypotensive agent.
	Oxymorphone 0.05–0.1 mg/kg IV IM	Acepromazine: 0.01–0.03 mg/kg IV	Caution: acepromazine is a potent hypotensive agent.
	Hydromorphone 0.1–0.2 mg/kg IV IM	Acepromazine: 0.01–0.03 mg/kg IV	Caution: acepromazine is a potent hypotensive agent.
Opioid/medetomidine	Butorphanol 0.1–0.2 mg/kg IV IM	Medetomidine 0.005–0.015 mg/kg IV IM	Use with caution in the trauma patient due to cardiovascular effects.

These drugs may be combined in the same syringe for administration, but combinations with diazepam will form a cloudy emulsion that will not affect drug potency. These protocols may also be supplemented with judicious use of propofol (0.5–1 mg/kg IV slowly) as long as blood pressure and respirations are in the normal range. Always consider intubation when utilizing propofol. The full opioid agonists have been deemphasized due to the potential for excitatory reactions.

SQ for day 1, followed by 0.1 mg/kg SQ q 24 for 2 days, followed by 0.025 mg/kg every other day.

3. Adverse effects of NSAIDs in cats and dogs can include gastric or duodenal ulceration and acute renal failure. These drugs should be used with caution, especially in animals that may have experienced hypotension as a result of trauma or subsequent anesthesia.

iv. Many patients who have experienced trauma, especially those with orthopedic fractures, can benefit from the anti-inflammatory properties of short-term NSAID administration.

v. Used alone, the NSAIDs are unlikely to be adequate for acute posttraumatic pain. It is imperative to administer these drugs to stable, normovolemic patients without signs of organ dysfunction:

1. It is frequently safer to wait at least 12–24 hours posttrauma in some patients prior to administering NSAIDs.

vi. NSAIDs are used with caution in cats; in addition to sometimes unpredictable metabolism (via hepatic glucuronidation), the possibility of subclinical renal insufficiency in many cats may predispose some patients to acute renal failure.

g. Intravenous induction agents:

   i. Although they will rapidly induce an anesthetic state that will allow endotracheal intubation, these drugs do not provide analgesia and are quickly metabolized or redistributed in the body, resulting in a relatively short duration of effect. They have recommended doses, but in practice are dosed to effect.

   ii. Propofol (Diprivan®, Propoflo):

   1. Propofol is supplied as an oil-in-water emulsion with isopropylphenol, soybean oil, egg lecithin, and glycerol. It is a white, opaque liquid for IV injection, dosed to effect at a range of 0.5–2 mg/kg or higher IV).

      a. Due to the emulsion (which can support bacterial growth), the shelf-life of the drug is limited:

         i. The unused portion should be immediately refrigerated and then discarded 6 hours after opening.

      b. There is a perception that, due to its short duration of action, propofol is a safe anesthetic agent that can be safely used in sick or compromised patients. The cardiovascular and respiratory effects of propofol *must be strongly considered* prior to utilization in sick or injured patients.

   2. Propofol has a rapid onset of effect, but is also a powerful vasodilator (especially in sick cats) and respiratory depressant:

      a. The side effects are rate and dose dependent; however, blood pressure measurement and intravenous fluids should be available when this drug is used in a patient.

      b. The respiratory effects are dose dependent and apnea is not uncommon with the administration of propofol. Endotracheal intubation and ventilation should always be anticipated.

      c. For patients sedated for long periods of time with propofol as a CRI (e.g., to control seizure activity), supplemental oxygen is indicated and intu-

bation may be necessary if there is a depressed gag reflex (to guard against regurgitation and aspiration).

   3. Propofol decreases the cerebral metabolic rate and is a good drug for use in patients who have sustained head trauma, as long as ventilation and perfusion parameters are monitored and adequate ventilation and cardiovascular support are provided.

   4. There is a possibility that repeated propofol anesthetics in cats may predispose to Heinz-body anemia.

   iii. Thiopental (Pentothal®):

   1. An ultra-short-acting barbiturate, thiopental is an effective and safe induction agent. It is available, most often, as a 2% solution that has an extremely basic pH. A typical intravenous induction dose ranges from 2 to 6 mg/kg, and is given to effect.

   2. Like propofol, the side effects of thiopental should be considered critically prior to use in critically ill or traumatized patients. Dose-related cardiovascular and respiratory depression may make this drug a poor choice for the traumatized animal:

      a. The high pH will cause damage if injected perivascularly, so an intravenous catheter should be placed prior to usage.

      b. Perivascular administration should be treated with subcutaneous lidocaine to neutralize the pH and to provide analgesia. Saline can also be used to dilute the concentration of drug.

   3. Thiopental rapidly redistributes to other body tissues; it is not metabolized rapidly and when given as a CRI or as multiple boluses, it will accumulate and delay recovery.

   4. Because metabolism occurs in the liver, this drug is contraindicated in animals with hepatic disease. It is highly protein bound, and may require lower total doses in patients that are hypoalbuminemic.

   5. Thiopental will sensitize the myocardium to catecholamine-induced arrhythmias. In trauma patients who

may already have some arrhythmias due to traumatic myocarditis or ischemia-reperfusion injury, this drug should be avoided.

6. Thiopental may also be mixed 1:1 with propofol for an effective induction cocktail that will decrease the total amount of each drug administered.

iv. Etomidate (Amidate®):

1. This drug is a water-insoluble compound and is thus delivered in a propylene glycol vehicle as a 0.2 % solution. The vehicle may cause pain on injection, and in cats may cause hemolysis due to the sensitivity of the feline red blood cell to osmotic damage.

2. Etomidate has few cardiovascular or respiratory side effects and is thus a good induction agent for patients with significant cardiovascular compromise that need to be anesthetized before adequate cardiovascular stabilization can occur.

3. At lower doses, etomidate is emetogenic, so an endotracheal tube should be available to protect the airway as soon as possible. Adequate dosing is important.

4. Etomidate interferes with the synthesis of cortisol by the adrenal glands and should be used with caution in patients with sepsis or other diseases associated with adrenocortical dysfunction. When etomidate is deemed the appropriate drug to use for anesthetic induction in these patients, a physiologic dose of corticosteroids should be administered postoperatively. One induction dose of etomidate will decrease cortisol production in the dog for approximately 8 hours.

v. Local anesthetics:

1. The most commonly used local anesthetics in small animal practice are lidocaine and bupivacaine:

a. While lidocaine may be administered IV for systemic analgesia (usually as a CRI of 0.03–0.05 mg/kg/min) or control of ventricular arrhythmias, bupivacaine should *never* be administered IV due to a much higher risk of cardiotoxicity.

b. Bupivacaine is only used for local or regional analgesia (1–1.5 mg/kg SQ q. 6–8 hours).

c. When injecting a local anesthetic, the syringe should always be aspirated prior to injection due to the risk of cardiotoxicity from inadvertent intravenous injection.

d. While there is a concern that cats may be more sensitive to the adverse cardiac effects of the local anesthetics, dosing at appropriate doses and intervals does not appear to cause an increased incidence of adverse effects.

2. The local anesthetics block the fast sodium channels in sensory nerves (and motor nerves, at higher doses) and disrupt transmission of nociceptive input:

a. They work by a similar mechanism whether given locally (subcutaneously, intra-articularly) or regionally (epidurally, brachial plexus block).

3. The most common indication for the use of lidocaine in trauma patients is for treatment of arrhythmias that occur from traumatic myocarditis or ischemia-reperfusion injury. For this purpose, higher doses (up to 0.08 mg/kg/min IV) may be used.

4. For animals that remain painful despite opioid analgesia, the addition of lidocaine, sometimes in combination with low-dose ketamine, may be used to augment analgesia.

5. When lidocaine is given IV, a loading dose of 1–2 mg/kg is initially given to achieve therapeutic plasma concentrations followed by a CRI at a dose from 0.03–0.05 mg/kg/min to provide continuous analgesia. Lidocaine may be administered at doses up to 0.08 mg/kg/min for its anti-arrhythmic effects.

6. At lower doses, lidocaine may provide a mild prokinetic effects, however at higher doses, toxicity may manifest as anorexia or nausea. These signs will happen prior to the signs of cardiotoxicity and should be monitored closely. Another sign of impending local anesthetic toxicity is seizure activity. Again, this occurs prior to the cardiac side effects, but warrants immediate discontinuation of administration of the local anesthetic.

7. Local anesthetics are frequently used to provide analgesia for patients with chest tubes. See this section for specific recommendations.

vi. Inhalant anesthetics:

1. The most commonly used inhalants in small animal practice are isoflurane and sevoflurane.

2. The inhalants produce reversible, dose-dependent CNS unresponsiveness:

   a. The potency of an inhalant is related to its minimum alveolar concentration (MAC).

   b. The MAC of an inhalant is affected by the physical state of a patient.

   c. Concurrent disease in a patient can decrease the amount of inhalant required for anesthesia.

3. Inhalants cause dose-dependent and species-specific respiratory depression:

   a. Spontaneous ventilation progressively decreases, causing $PaCO_2$ to increase, in a dose-dependent manner. Apnea occurs at high doses of either isoflurane or sevoflurane.

4. Inhalant anesthetics cause dose-dependent cardiovascular depression:

   a. A dose-dependent decrease in arterial blood pressure is observed with the use of inhalants:

      i. The decrease in arterial blood pressure primarily occurs secondary to vasodilation.

5. The inhalant anesthetics decrease cerebral metabolism:

   a. Decreased ventilation may result in an increase in cerebral blood flow, resulting in an increase in intracranial pressure. Mechanical ventilation to a normal $PaCO_2$ can decrease this effect by minimizing vasodilation of the cerebral arteries.

6. In the trauma patient, depending on the physical status of the patient, the amount of inhalant needed for general anesthesia can be greatly reduced. The use of other analgesics (e.g., opioids) will further reduce inhalant requirements.

7. Due to the dose-dependent cardiorespiratory effects of inhalant anesthetics, it is crucial to provide adequate monitoring of the cardiovascular and respiratory systems during general anesthesia. This is especially true in the debilitated, trauma patient.

8. Mask or box inductions should be avoided in the trauma patient, as a higher concentration of inhalant anesthetic is needed for intubation with this method.

vii. Common combinations for sedation (see Tables 5.2 and 5.3):

1. Opioids alone may sometimes cause anxiety or dysphoria in patients. While this is a transient effect and usually occurs only after prolonged usage, it may result in increased oxygen consumption by the patient and struggling, which may disrupt fracture sites or other injuries:

   a. Additionally, dysphoria can be difficult to distinguish from pain, making therapeutic decisions more difficult.

   b. The addition of a tranquilizer to an opioid results in a much smoother and more reliable sedation.

2. Opioid and benzodiazepine (see Tables 5.2 and 5.3):

   a. Very effective combination in debilitated patients, causing minimal cardiovascular depression.

   b. Hydromorphone with diazepam or midazolam:

      i. Lower doses (especially of the benzodiazepine) should be used in the cat.

   c. Opioid and acepromazine (see Tables 5.2 and 5.3):

      i. This combination should be reserved for patients that are cardiovascularly and hemodynamically stable, due to the vasodilation caused by acepromazine.

   d. Opioid and alpha-2 agonist (see Tables 5.2 and 5.3):
      i. Because the opioid and alpha-2 receptors are similar in structure and location in the spinal cord, a decreased dose of both drugs can be administered when used in combination.
viii. Analgesia for head trauma patients:
   1. Hypoventilation may lead to increases in intracranial pressure due to vasodilation of the cerebral circulation; respiratory rate and/or arterial or venous carbon dioxide tension should be monitored if opioids are given.
   2. Analgesic drugs may alter the neurologic examination.
   3. Opioids may result in bradycardia:
      a. It is important to monitor blood pressure to ensure that cerebral perfusion is adequate and to avoid confusion with the Cushing's reflex (see Chapter 7: Traumatic Brain Injury).
      b. Animals with head trauma may have increased vagal tone:
         i. Anticholinergics should be used sparingly to prevent severe tachyarrhythmias (this is more likely in the anesthetized patient).
      c. A fentanyl or morphine CRI may be easier to titrate to an appropriate analgesic dose, while minimizing side effects, as compared to intermittent boluses of an opioid.
   4. While alpha-2 agonists do not affect intracranial pressure in anesthetized dogs, their respiratory depressant effects in the awake animal may cause unacceptable hypoventilation that may result in elevated intracranial pressure. These drugs may also result in hypotension due to decreased sympathetic tone, which may decrease cerebral perfusion pressure in susceptible patients.
   5. Benzodiazepines are indicated as therapy for early posttraumatic seizures, as long as more directed therapy (e.g., dextrose to treat hypoglycemia) is not indicated.

   6. Phenothiazines have been associated with seizures in dogs, albeit at high doses that are not clinically relevant. A benzodiazepine may be a safer anxiolytic in patients with CNS disease.
   7. The use of inhalant anesthetics is controversial in patients with head trauma, as these compounds may cause disregulation of the normal mechanisms that maintain adequate cerebral perfusion pressure:
      a. If a patient with head trauma is in need of prolonged anesthesia, the use of a constant rate infusion of propofol (0.05–0.1 mg/kg/min) supplemented as necessary with fentanyl (0.0003–0.0007 mg/kg/min) will give a stable plane of anesthesia:
         i. Both of these drugs are potent respiratory depressants, and mechanical ventilation or intermittent assistance will be necessary to maintain normocapnia.
ix. Sedation for radiographs:
   1. Radiographs are indicated after trauma to ascertain the presence or absence of thoracic abnormalities (e.g., rib fractures, pneumothorax) or fractures of the pelvis or long bones. Contrast studies may also be of use to diagnose urinary tract trauma:
      a. Practitioners should strive toward diagnostic acumen for thoracic auscultation, as the restraint and positioning necessary for diagnostic radiographs may stress a fragile patient beyond their ability to compensate.
      b. It is imperative to stabilize patients with regard to their hemodynamic and respiratory systems prior to attempting radiographs. If thoracic auscultation is dull, it may be better to attempt a diagnostic thoracocentesis rather than stressing a patient for radiographs.
   2. If the patient is cooperative, sedation may not be necessary, although sometimes (e.g., spinal radiographs) positioning is very important to avoid misdiagnoses.
   3. Short-term sedation may be accomplished via neuroleptanalgesia,

combining an opioid, such as butorphanol, morphine, or hydromorphone, with a benzodiazepine:

    a. Both drugs can be reversed at the end of the procedure.

    b. Buprenorphine is not recommended due to its minimal sedative qualities and long latent period before onset of analgesia.

x. Short procedures:

1. If extensive surgery is anticipated to suture or debride wounds, the most expedient option is the induction of general anesthesia, as this eliminates the necessity to provide repeated "top-off" doses of an anesthetic, such as propofol.

2. If a short procedure is anticipated, especially on a distal limb, the combination of an opioid and benzodiazepine with a local block using lidocaine may be sufficient:

    a. The lidocaine may be placed as a splash block over the area to be repaired, or may be given as a ring block proximal to the area of surgery.

    b. Lidocaine is preferred because of its short onset of action, *versus* bupivacaine, which will last longer, but may take up to 30–45 minutes to provide analgesia.

    c. A 1:1 combination of lidocaine and bupivacaine may be used to provide immediate analgesia for the procedure, and a degree (usually up to 6 hours) of analgesia for the post operative time. As with all local anesthetics, the syringe should be aspirated prior to administering the drug to avoid intravascular injection.

3. If the initial neuroleptanalgesia is not adequate, slow titration of an anesthetic agent such as propofol can be used for additional immobility (recognizing that this compound does not provide analgesia):

    a. Doses of 0.5–1 mg/kg of propofol given slowly will provide immobilization (assuming that neuroleptanalgesia has been provided), with top-up doses of 0.25–0.75 mg/kg to maintain the animal adequate for procedures.

    b. Etomidate may also be used for this purpose, but may cause emesis when given as a slow titrated infusion.

    c. Thiopental, also an intravenous anesthetic, may be used for induction or for 2–3 additional doses, but should not be administered as a CRI or for an excessive period of time, as accumulation of drug will occur and result in prolonged recoveries.

    d. Whenever propofol or thiopental are used in addition to initial neuroleptanalgesia, endotracheal intubation and oxygen supplementation should be strongly considered, as significant respiratory depression may occur.

4. The combinations discussed above are also suitable for other procedures such as female urinary catheter placement and, if there is not an aspect of pain, these drugs may be reversed at the end of the procedure.

xi. Chest tube placement:

1. Chest tube placement should not be attempted under sedation; all animals having an open thorax must be intubated so that assisted ventilation can be provided as needed.

    a. General anesthesia also facilitates radiographs to verify accurate placement of the tube (especially if it needs to be replaced).

2. For emergent chest tube placement, a rapid sequence anesthetic induction is indicated. A combination of opioid and benzodiazepine, as described above, is given intravenously and followed immediately by an induction agent, such as thiopental, propofol, or ketamine. After intubation, the animal may be maintained on inhalant anesthetic or on an intravenous anesthetic infusion, as discussed above.

3. After placement of the chest tube, analgesia can be provided to the pleura by instillation of 1.5 mg/kg bupivacaine, flushed with 3–5 mL air or saline, into the chest tube every 6–8 hours. Strict asepsis must be adhered to when instilling medications into a chest tube. The local anesthetic will sting, and a small amount of sodium bicarbonate may be added in a 1:9 ratio (a white precipitate may form) prior to instillation:

a. For animals that require continuous thoracic drainage, the suction will need to be discontinued for approximately 15 minutes to allow the bupivacaine to spread beyond the immediate end of the chest tube:

i. If the suction cannot be discontinued sterilely, it may not be possible to infuse local anesthetics for analgesia.

ii. The addition of intrapleural bupivacaine should be used as an adjunct to other methods of analgesia.

4. Another method for analgesia, performed in the anesthetized patient, is a blockade of the intercostal nerves. The nerves are located on the caudal aspect of the ribs, and a small amount of the total dose of bupivacaine (1.5 mg/kg) may be divided and instilled to block the intercostal nerves two rib-spaces in front and two rib-spaces behind the entry point of the chest tube:

a. Because the intercostal arteries are also located in the same spot, it is important to aspirate the syringe to verify that the needle is not intra-arterial prior to instilling any local anesthetic.

xii. Tracheostomy:

1. The decision to place a tracheostomy is often a stressful one, especially if endotracheal intubation is not likely to be possible. Ideally, an intravenous catheter is placed, but if not, one can take advantage of the flexible (i.e., intramuscular) dosing of many anesthetic and analgesic drugs to allow the procedure to proceed.

2. In the vast majority of cases, intubation (even with an undersized tube) may be possible prior to placement of the tra-

cheostomy tube, although in many cases, it will be a difficult airway. The use of a stylet can lead to a successful intubation.

a. Polypropylene urinary catheters may be used as stylets to facilitate intubation, which can be threaded through the Murphy eye of the endotracheal tube.

b. Commercial products, such as the airway exchange adapters from Cook, are also available:

i. This product will attach to an anesthetic machine or Ambu-Bag, and allow administration of oxygen during intubation.

c. Many different endotracheal tube sizes (widths and lengths) should be available; even a small tube will allow the administration of oxygen during the procedure.

3. Preparation:

a. Prior to administration of any drugs (if there is time), it is important to preoxygenate the patient; this can delay the onset of hypoxia by minutes.

b. The patient should be preclipped and gross prepped prior to the administration of anesthetic drugs.

c. A local block using lidocaine (2–3 mg/kg SQ) can provide analgesia during this procedure.

4. Induction of anesthesia:

a. A rapid sequence induction is preferred in this case:

i. Ketamine (5–8 mg/kg) and valium (0.3–0.5 mg/kg) may be given IV or IM.

ii. Propofol (2–5 mg/kg, to effect).

iii. Propofol (1–4 mg/kg) with valium (0.3–0.5 mg/kg):

1. Use propofol cautiously, as it is a potent respiratory depressant and frequently results in apnea.

2. Providing flow-by oxygen to the patient prior to induction (if possible) will result in a longer time to the onset of hypoxemia, even if apnea ensues.

b. If the patient is difficult to restrain for venous access, intramuscular ketamine and valium (or telazol) is a rapid method to gain sedation and anesthesia to allow a fast tracheostomy. Once an airway is acquired, anesthesia may be continued using either inhalant anesthesia, or an intravenous infusion, as discussed previously.

xiii. A brief note about cardiac arrest:

1. It is uncommon, but the administration of analgesic agents to the trauma patient may result in decompensation to the point of cardiac or respiratory arrest. This may be secondary to anesthetic-related vasodilation in an animal who was already hypovolemic, or due to respiratory compromise in an animal that had a dynamic airway obstruction or a subclinical pneumothorax.

2. In addition to the usual CPR techniques involving intubation and the initiation of thoracic compressions, it is important to reverse the analgesic drugs as well. In some studies, naloxone actually had a favorable effect alone in rats after cardiopulmonary arrest. In the authors' hands, vasopressin (0.4–0.8 U/kg) is an extremely effective drug for anesthetic-related CPA. Epinephrine is an effective drug as well.

xiv. Practical aspects of drug administration by constant rate infusion (CRI):

1. Diluent fluids:

a. Opioid analgesic drugs may be incorporated into admixtures using 0.9% saline, 5% dextrose in water, or lactated Ringer's solution if necessary. Fentanyl is rarely admixed and is usually given without dilution, but is also compatible if dilution is necessary. Naloxone is also compatible for admixture with 0.9% saline. It is recommended to choose an isotonic solution (i.e., not 5% dextrose in water) for long-term IV infusion of medications.

b. Neither diazepam nor midazolam are recommended for dilution. Diazepam will cause a precipitate when added to most IV fluids unless at a very dilute concentration (e.g., 150–200 mg/L). Additionally, diazepam will adsorb to the plastic in the IV bag and tubing; a gradual loss in potency is expected with time. It is thus recommended to administer diazepam undiluted, and using a syringe pump (it has not been shown to adsorb to the plastic used to make syringes). The administration tubing should not be changed when the syringe is refilled, to prevent loss of potency. Midazolam may be diluted in 0.9% saline if necessary, but will experience a rapid loss of potency when admixed with lactated Ringer's solution. These drugs may be light sensitive as well, and it is recommended to cover the barrel of the syringe during administration:

i. Short-term administration through peripheral catheters seems to be well tolerated. Prolonged infusion, however, is preferentially infused into a central vein to minimize the possibility for thrombophlebitis.

c. Little information is available regarding dilution of medetomidine, although it is acceptable to dilute dexmedetomidine in 0.9% saline for administration as a CRI, and the authors have successfully used 0.9% saline to administer a CRI of medetomidine to small animals.

d. For intravenous administration, it is recommended to give propofol undiluted, but it is also acceptable to dilute to a solution of not less than 2 mg/mL using either 0.9% saline or lactated Ringer's solution.

e. Lidocaine may be diluted in 0.9% saline for IV administration.

f. Ketamine may be diluted in 0.9% saline for IV administration.

2. Custom dilutions:

a. These may be made up as convenient, frequently using small fluid bags (e.g., 100 mL) or syringes. This technique is recommended because the analgesic drugs may be administered (and adjusted) separately from maintenance or replacement fluid therapy.

b. By choosing a desired rate of fluid administration (e.g., 5 mL/h), a concentrated solution of analgesic drugs may be mixed and infused.

c. After choosing a rate, the duration of infusion must be calculated. The total volume is divided by the rate to determine the number of hours that the volume will last.

d. After this determination, the mg/kg/hour of drug and then the number of mg/h of drug to be delivered may be determined (by multiplying the mg/kg/hour by the animal's weight).

e. By multiplying the mg/h by the hours determined in point (c), the total number of mg of drug may be added to the bag. If this will be an amount greater than 1–5 mL of drug, it is recommended to remove the equal amount of diluent to maintain the accuracy of calculations.

f. Examples:

i. A 20-kg dog requires morphine (0.2 mg/kg/h) to be given for analgesia. You wish to mix this in a 100 mL bag and administer it at 5 mL/h. How do you make this up?

1. A 100 mL bag, at 5 mL/h, will last 20 hours (100 mL/5 mL/h).

2. The dog will need 4 mg/h of drug (0.2 mg/kg/h * 20 mg).

3. The total drug needed for the duration of the bag is 80 mg (4 mg/h * 20 hours).

4. The total mL of morphine (15 mg/mL) to add to 100 mL of saline is 5.3 mL (40 mg/15 mg/mL).

5. Prior to the addition of the morphine, 5.3 mL of saline are removed from the bag, to make the total volume after addition of the morphine exactly 100 mL.

ii. A 5-kg cat with a heart murmur requires analgesia. You choose to give morphine as a CRI at 0.1 mg/kg/h, but need to give it at a rate 1 mL/h to avoid fluid overload. You choose to use a syringe pump and a 20 mL syringe to administer the drug. How much morphine and saline need to be added to the syringe?

1. 20 mL, at 1 mL/h, will last 20 hours.

2. This cat requires 0.5 mg/h of morphine (0.1 mg/kg/h * 5 kg).

3. For the entire syringe, the cat will require 10 mg of morphine (0.5 mg/h * 20 hours).

4. The total mL of morphine (15 mg/mL) to add to the syringe is thus 0.67 mL; the remainder is made up with sterile saline, and administered at 1 mL/h.

3. Twenty-four hour infusion:

a. Determine the amount (mg) of drug required in 24 hours.

b. Dilute this amount with sterile 0.9% saline to 24 mL of solution in an appropriately sized syringe.

c. Giving 1 mL/h of this solution will provide 24 hours of analgesia.

d. Examples:

i. A 20-kg dog in pain requires an infusion of morphine (0.1 mg/kg/h) postoperatively. You would like to make up a syringe that will deliver 24 hours of pain relief to this dog.

ii. For 24 hours, the dog will need 48 mg of morphine (20 kg * 0.1 mg/kg/h * 24 hours).

iii. 48 mg of morphine (most likely 15 mg/mL, thus 3.2 mL) are added to 20.8 (24–3.2) mL of sterile 0.9% saline, and this is administered at 1 mL/hour.

4. Inclusion of analgesic drugs in maintenance fluids:

a. Calculate by determining the number of hours that will be delivered per bag. Then, calculate the necessary amount of drug (in milligrams (mg) or micrograms (mcg)) that will need to be given to the patient per hour. By multiplying the two, the total number of mg of drug to be added to the IV fluid bag is obtained.

b. Examples:

 i. A 20-kg dog is set up to receive Normosol-R (a 1 liter bag) at an IV fluid rate of 100 mL/h. To give this dog morphine at a dose of 0.1 mg/kg/h, how much morphine needs to be added to the IV fluid bag?

  1. The liter of Normosol-R will last for 10 hours (1000 mL/100 mL/h).

  2. The dog will require 2 mg/h of morphine (0.1 mg/kg/h * 20 kg).

  3. The total amount of morphine to add to 1 liter of Normosol-R is thus 20 mg. for this dog (10 h * 2 mg/h).

 ii. A 5-kg cat, receiving sodium chloride from a 500 mL bag at a rate of 30 mL/hour needs additional analgesia to supplement the opioids he is receiving. You add in ketamine, at a rate of 200 mcg/kg/h. How much do you add to the bag?

  1. The bag of fluids, at this rate, will last 16 2/3 hours.

  2. The cat will need 1000 mcg/h, which is 1 mg/h.

  3. 16.6 mg should be added to the fluid bag (16.6 hours * 1 mg/h).

c. Caution is warranted when using this technique; if a bolus of IV fluids is necessary, a new bag must be used to avoid bolusing a large concentration of analgesic drug. Also, when changing fluid rates, the administered drug dose will also change, and this must be taken into account.

5. The rule of 6 technique:

a. This is a shortcut for calculating CRI fluids that are administered as separate infusions. Using this technique, drugs to be given at 1 mcg/kg/h will be administered at 1 mL/h. This is most relevant for administration of drugs such as vasopressors and inotropes, which are administered at these doses (analgesic drugs are usually given at higher doses)

b. The body weight of the animal, in kg, is multiplied by six. This results in the number of mg that is added to 100 mL of diluent to be administered at × mL/h to give a dose of × mcg/kg/min.

c. Multiplying by 0.6 will make 1 mL/h result in a dose of 0.1 mcg/kg/min for more potent drugs, and multiplying by 60 will make 1 mL/h equivalent to 10 mcg/kg/min (0.01 mg/kg/min)

d. Example:

 i. A 5 kg cat displays hypotension, and you wish to start a CRI of dopamine at 5 mcg/kg/min. How much drug will you add to 100 mL of saline to provide this drug?

  1. The cat weighs 5 kg, so 30 mg. of dopamine will be needed (1.5 mL).

  2. This drug is added to a 100 mL bag of saline, and administered at 5 mL/h (each mL per hour is 1 mcg/kg/min).

Case Examples:

Case 1

Three-year-old male, castrated German Shepherd
HBC, multiple pelvic fractures

Presentation

In shock, stabilized with 30 mL/kg isotonic crystalloids
Blood pressure: 140/50, HR 130 in normal sinus rhythm, SpO_2 99% (room air)

Plan

Fracture repair the next morning, treat for pain overnight

Analgesic
problem list

1. Acute pain from pelvic fractures
2. Possible blood loss from fractures or adjacent structures
3. Possible trauma to the urogenital tract

Analgesic plan
Considerations

Full opioid agonist +/− low-dose ketamine CRI and/or lidocaine CRI
1. Lidocaine may also be a helpful adjunct if cardiac arrhythmias, secondary to traumatic myocarditis, are present.
2. A benzodiazepine may be added for anxiolysis as required.
3. Partial opioid agonists may not provide adequate analgesia for the degree of trauma, and/or may need to be redosed at increased frequency
4. Alpha-2 agonists provide analgesia, but the possibility of cardiac arrhythmias and hyper- and hypotension essentially contraindicate their use in the acutely traumatized patient. Their use requires close monitoring.
5. Nonsteroidal anti-inflammatories (NSAIDs) may be used as analgesics, but alone are not adequate to control acute pain. Additionally, if there is continued bleeding, the nonselective NSAIDs may inhibit platelet function and delay resolution.

Contraindications

1. Ketamine alone is unlikely to provide adequate analgesia for a patient in this scenario.
2. Acepromazine given to a patient with shock, or during active resuscitation, may result in refractory vasodilation and hypotension. Anemic patients may also sequester red blood cells in the spleen, decreasing systemic oxygen delivery. Benzodiazepines are safer anxiolytics for this patient.
3. Anesthetic drugs such as propofol or etomidate have no analgesic properties.
4. There is no indication for corticosteroids.

Case 2

Seven-year-old female, spayed DSH
Presents after a fall from four stories

Presentation

Vocalizing and anisocoria is noted. She also has a mandibular symphyseal fracture. Blood pressure: 160 mm Hg by Doppler, HR: 200 and regular, thoracic auscultation and further musculoskeletal examination is normal. Some referred upper airway sounds secondary to trauma in the nasal turbinates. Hypertonic saline (7%) is administered at 2 mL/kg for resuscitation and to decrease intracranial pressure, and neurologic signs improve.

Plan

Observation for 12–24 hours prior to anesthesia for repair of her fracture.

Analgesic
problem list

1. Mandibular fracture
2. Head trauma

Analgesic plan

For moderate pain in cats, buprenorphine (0.01–0.02 mg/kg q. 6 hours). NSAIDs as an adjunct for analgesia.

(continued)

Case 2 (continued)

Considerations
1. Some cats may develop excitation from full agonist opioids; however, a titrated administration of full opioids will provide excellent analgesia. Concerns about respiratory depression are also relevant; full opioids may have a more pronounced effect in the presence of CNS disease.
2. NSAIDs can be used provided the cat is systemically healthy (i.e., no history of renal insufficiency, and there are no episodes of hypotension.
3. Benzodiazepines may be used for anxiolysis as necessary.

Contraindications
1. Alpha-2 agonists may cause emesis in cats, which not only increases intracranial pressure, but may result in aspiration into the lungs, if the cat is unable to fully open her mouth during emesis.

Case 3
Five-year-old female, spayed miniature Schnauzer
HBC

Presentation
Dyspneic, and cyanotic. Screams with pain when thoracic auscultation is attempted, and abdominal palpation elicits the same response. Metatarsal pulses easily palpated, but the rhythm is irregular. No gross musculoskeletal problems noted.

Plan
Provide analgesia to facilitate further diagnostics

Analgesic problem list
1. Cyanosis
2. Ill-defined pain

Analgesic plan
1. In an animal presenting with cyanosis who will not tolerate even a diagnostic thoracocentesis, the best way to proceed is to induce anesthesia, intubate the patient, and ventilate with 100% oxygen. At this point, further diagnostics (thoracocentesis, blood pressure, ECG) may be performed, while anesthesia and analgesia are provided. Analgesia with a full opioid agonist after the airway is secure. Or,
2. A rapid sequence induction with IV opioid (fentanyl, hydromorphone) followed immediately with IV benzodiazepine, followed immediately with propofol, if needed, for intubation.

Considerations
1. Ideally, an intravenous catheter should be placed prior to administration of drugs, although an intramuscular approach may also be used.
2. It is important to alert the owner that the initiation of anesthesia in a dyspneic animal that may have pulmonary contusions may require a period of mechanical ventilation before they are able to be awakened from anesthesia.
3. Intravenous protocols that are appropriate include propofol, thiopental, or etomidate alone or combined with a benzodiazepine.
4. Ketamine combined with a benzodiazepine is only a secondary choice due to the suspected presence of arrhythmias. This combination is very flexible, however, and is used frequently despite the presence of myocardial contusions. It is more likely that the animal will maintain an appropriate respiratory rate with this combination.

Contraindications
1. In this case, providing analgesic drugs of any sort without the availability of intubation and oxygen may result in respiratory decompensation and death.
2. If the patient were able to be stabilized by breathing an increased inspired oxygen concentration in an oxygen cage, judicious use of easily reversed (e.g., opioid) analgesics is indicated.
3. Myocardial contusions combined with hypoxemia indicate that the oxygen supply to the myocardium is compromised. Alpha-2 agonist drugs decrease myocardial oxygen delivery even at very low doses, and so may irreversibly damage an already compromised heart.

Case 4	Ten-year-old male, intact Labrador Retriever Accidentally shot in the thoracic region while hunting.
Presentation	A number of superficial wounds over thoracic inlet and has an increased respiratory rate and effort. HR: 120 bpm, with strong, synchronous, regular pulses.
	BP: normal. SpO$_2$: 91%. Thoracocentesis: 2 liters of air removed from left hemi-thorax.
	Thoracocentesis repeated due to worsening condition two hours after first thoracocentesis.
Plan	Place thoracostomy tube under general anesthesia Debride soft tissue wounds and place drains
Analgesic problem list	1. Soft tissue trauma (mild to moderate pain expected) 2. Thoracostomy tube (moderate to severe pain expected)
Analgesic plan	1. Full opioid agonist 2. Intrapleural bupivacaine every 8 hours instilled into the chest tube +/− 1:9 ratio of sodium bicarbonate 3. Intercostal nerve block at the time of thoracostomy tube placement
Considerations	1. The full opioid agonist can be added to a premedication prior to anesthetic induction if the patient is breathing well. If air exchange is compromised due to the pneumothorax, the respiratory depressant effects of the opioid would contraindicate its use and a rapid sequence induction would be better for the patient. 2. Thoracocentesis should be performed just prior to anesthetic induction to improve the functional residual capacity. 3. Preoxegenation will help avoid cyanosis upon anesthetic induction. 4. NSAIDs will help with local tissue inflammation.
Contraindications	1. Partial opioid agonists may not be adequate for pain control in this patient. 2. Vigorous positive pressure ventilation is contraindicated in this patient, as it may worsen the pneumothorax.

Case 5	Three-year-old male, intact DSH
	HBC
Presentation	Pale mucous membranes, nonpalpable pulses
	HR: 220, with sinus tachycardia
	Fracture of right femur, surrounded by moderate swelling and bruising
	Shock: given isotonic crystalloids, hypertonic saline, and hetastarch for resuscitation.
	PCV/TS: 15/4.0
	Palpable fluid wave in abdomen—diagnostic abdominocentesis confirms blood.
Plan	Transfuse type-specific packed red blood cells and fresh frozen plasma available for transfusion during surgery. Emergency exploratory abdominal surgery due to deteriorating condition.

(*continued*)

Case 5 (*continued*)

Analgesic problem list	1. Patient not able to be adequately stabilized prior to surgery. 2. Resuscitation to continue through the surgery.
Analgesic plan	1. Rapid sequence induction of a potent opioid mixed with (or followed immediately by) a benzodiazepine, followed with a small amount of propofol or etomidate as necessary for intubation. 2. Fentanyl infusion throughout surgery to limit vasodilatory effects of inhalant anesthetics.
Considerations	1. Prior to induction, doses of pressor agents (e.g., dopamine, dobutamine) should be calculated and prepared. 2. Normotension will be difficult to maintain with the use of inhalant anesthetic. 3. Hypotension should be treated aggressively with crystalloid, colloid, and blood products as indicated, using vasopressors such as dopamine (5–12 mcg/kg/min IV) to maintain blood pressure above a mean of 70 mm Hg. 4. Once the bleeding is controlled, it will be easier to stabilize the patient. 5. The fentanyl started during surgery may be continued into the postoperative phase for analgesia.
Contraindications	1. Propofol can cause significant vasodilation and should not be used in patients that are already hypotensive. If it is the only option for induction, combination with other anesthetic/analgesic drugs (e.g., benzodiazepines) will decrease the amount necessary to achieve intubation.

BIBLIOGRAPHY

da Cunha AF, Carter JE, Grafinger M, et al. Intrathecal morphine overdose in a dog. *J Am Vet Med Assoc* 2007; 230: 1665–1668.

Firth AF, Haldane SL. Development of a postoperative pain scale in dogs. *J Am Vet Med Assoc* 1999; 214: 651.

Holton LL, Scott EM, Nolan AM, et al. Comparison of three methods used for assessment of pain in dogs. *J Am Vet Med Assoc* 1998; 212: 61–66.

Neale BW, Mesler EL, Young M, et al. Propylene glycol-induced lactic acidosis in a patient with normal renal function. *Ann Pharmacother* 2005; 39: 1732–1735.

Posner LP, Gleed RD, Erb HN, Ludders JW. Post-anesthetic hyperthermia in cats. *Vet Anaesth Analg* 2007; 34: 40–47.

Robertson SA, Lascelles BDX, Taylor PM, Sear JW. PK-PD modeling of buprenorphine in cats: intravenous and oral transmucosal administration. *J Vet Pharmacol Therap* 2005; 28: 453–460.

Wilson KC, Reardon C, Farber HW. Propylene glycol toxicity in a patient receiving intravenous diazepam. *N Engl J Med* 2000; 343: 815.

TRAUMA-ASSOCIATED THORACIC INJURY

Matthew W. Beal

1. INTRODUCTION

a. The traumatized patient represents one of the most dynamic and challenging cases for veterinarians in the field of emergency medicine. Injuries may range from mild to immediately life-threatening and most often involve multiple organs and organ systems (polytrauma).

b. Injuries to the thorax and thoracic structures are very common in the traumatized dog and cat. These injuries are a source of significant morbidity and may be fatal if not immediately identified and treated.

c. Thoracic trauma is often categorized as blunt or penetrating:

  i. Blunt thoracic trauma is most common and is most often a result of vehicular trauma. However, animal-animal interactions, human-animal interactions, and falls from a height are other common causes of blunt injury. Most blunt thoracic injuries are managed medically; however, surgical intervention may be indicated based on the type and severity of the blunt injury.

  ii. Penetrating thoracic trauma is less common than blunt trauma and most often results from animal-animal interactions, projectile injuries (gunshot or arrow), and impalements. Like penetrating injuries to other structures, penetrating injuries to the thorax are surgical emergencies once the patient has been stabilized medically.

2. ASSESSMENT OF THE DOG OR CAT WITH THORACIC INJURY

a. Initial assessment of the dog or cat that has sustained trauma begins with triage (see Chapter 2: Triage and Primary Survey).

b. Due to the dynamic nature of traumatic injuries, all patients that have sustained trauma should be immediately triaged to the treatment area for further assessment and completion of both the primary and secondary surveys.

c. Primary survey/major body systems assessment (see Chapter 2 for a full description of the primary survey):

  i. Most serious thoracic injuries are suspected or identified based on results of the primary survey. The utility of skills of physical examination and clinical observation in making clinical diagnoses in these patients cannot be undervalued.

  ii. Because most thoracic injuries result in respiratory tract embarrassment, thorough observation of respiratory rate and character coupled with auscultation will help guide further diagnostics and treatment. Figure 6.1 provides an algorithm illustrating how auscultation can guide further diagnostics and treatment.

  iii. Early identification of injuries allows for efficient delivery of life-saving care.

d. Additional assessment, diagnostics, therapeutics, and monitoring of the thoracic trauma patient

Manual of Trauma Management in the Dog and Cat, First Edition. Edited by Kenneth J. Drobatz, Matthew W. Beal and Rebecca S. Syring.
© 2011 John Wiley & Sons, Inc. Published 2011 by John Wiley & Sons, Inc.

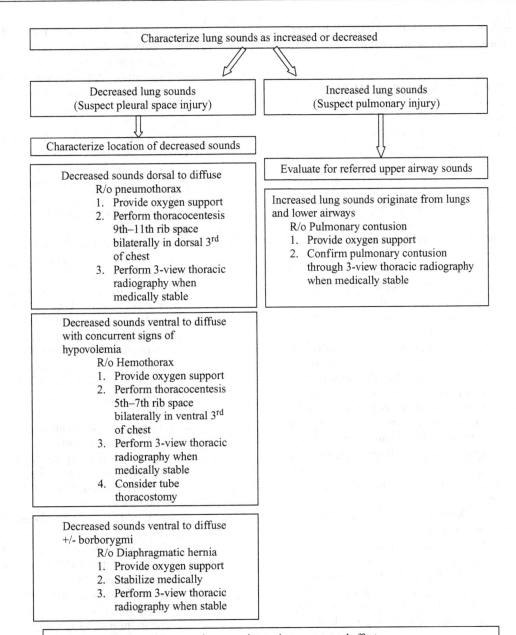

FIGURE 6.1 Auscultation algorithm for animals that have sustained *acute* trauma with clinical signs of respiratory compromise.

will be described specifically for each of the common thoracic trauma injuries below.

3. TRAUMA-ASSOCIATED PLEURAL SPACE INJURIES

a. Pneumothorax:
   i. Definition and pathophysiology:
      1. Pneumothorax is the accumulation of air in the pleural space.
      2. Pneumothorax is one of the most common trauma-associated thoracic injuries. Pneumothorax happens with such frequency that the author makes the assumption that pneumothorax is present until proven otherwise.
      3. As intrathoracic pressure increases from its normally subatmospheric level, atelectasis, ventilatory difficulty, and decreased venous return may result in respiratory and cardiovascular compromise:
         a. Tension pneumothorax results from a one-way valve effect in which air enters the pleural space during inspiration but is unable to be evacuated. The progressive increases in intra-pleural pressure result in both respiratory and cardiovascular collapse. Tension pneumothorax is a life-threatening emergency.
      4. Pneumothorax is classified as open or closed:
         a. Open pneumothorax results from penetrating injury to the thorax. Air from the environment enters the pleural space through the chest wall.
         b. Closed pneumothorax most often results from rapid compression of the chest against a closed glottis resulting in disruption of the visceral pleura. Air enters the chest directly from the pulmonary parenchyma. Additional causes of closed pneumothorax after trauma include rupture of a subpleural bleb or bulla as well as large airway or esophageal disruption resulting in pneumomediastinum and secondary pneumothorax.
         c. Closed pneumothorax is far more common than open pneumothorax.

   ii. Clinical signs/physical examination and oxygenation assessment:
      1. Respiratory rate and effort:
         a. Clinically significant pneumothorax will result in tachypnea, often characterized by shorter breaths with perceived smaller tidal volumes.
         b. Respiratory character in dogs and cats with pneumothorax is variable. In addition to tachypnea; extension of the neck, abduction of the elbows, and reluctance to lay in lateral recumbency are common. Cyanosis may be noted in pneumothorax:
            i. Animals with tension pneumothorax will display pale mucous membranes, prolonged CRT, tachycardia, and poor pulse quality (see Chapter 3: Shock in the Trauma Patient). Jugular venous distention may be noted due to decreased venous return secondary to the high intrapleural pressures. A "barrel-chest" or "sprung" appearance to the ribs may also be noted.
      2. Auscultation:
         a. Clinically significant pneumothorax is a physical examination diagnosis:
            i. With the animal positioned standing or in sternal recumbency, decreased lung sounds dorsally to diffusely will be noted.
            ii. With the animal positioned in lateral recumency (not recommended), decreased lung sounds will be noted at the top of the "arch" of the ribs.
         b. Clinically significant pneumothorax most often occurs bilaterally.
         c. Pneumothorax is often accompanied by concurrent injuries to the chest. Auscultation should be interpreted in light of the potential for concurrent injuries.
      3. Objective indicators of oxygenation:
         a. Pulse oximetry may document a decreased oxygen saturation of the arterial blood.
         b. Arterial blood gas (ABG) analysis may document hypoxemia and a decreased oxygen saturation of the arterial blood. ABG analysis should not

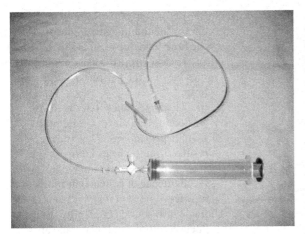

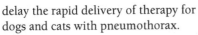

FIGURE 6.2 Equipment needed for thoracocentesis. 60 mL syringe, 3-way stopcock, IV extension tubing, needle or catheter.

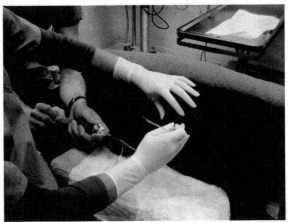

FIGURE 6.3 While maintaining contact between the hand and the chest wall, insert needle perpendicular to the chest wall staying close to the cranial edge of the rib.

delay the rapid delivery of therapy for dogs and cats with pneumothorax.

iii. Diagnostic tests:

1. Thoracocentesis:

   a. Thoracocentesis is both diagnostic and therapeutic for dogs and cats with closed pneumothorax.

   b. Equipment (assemble as indicated in Figure 6.2):

   i. 60 mL syringe.

   ii. 3-way stopcock.

   iii. IV extension tubing.

   iv. 19–21 g butterfly needle or 20–22 g needle.

   v. Some will use an 18–22 g over-the-needle catheter for thoracocentesis. The author prefers a needle because it will not collapse with respiratory motion.

   c. Procedure:

   i. Numerous techniques for thoracocentesis have been described. No single technique has been objectively evaluated and found to be superior to another.

   ii. Position the patient in sternal recumbency.

   iii. Clip and prepare the dorsal 1/2 of the thorax between the 6th and 13th ribs as if for surgery.

   iv. Use sterile technique.

   v. Landmarks for thoracocentesis for the treatment of pneumothorax are the dorsal 1/3 of the chest at the level of the 9th to 11th rib spaces.

   vi. While maintaining contact between the hand and the chest wall, insert needle perpendicular to the chest wall staying close to the cranial edge of the rib to avoid the neurovascular bundle caudally. (Figure 6.3).

   vii. Advance the needle through the skin and aspirate the syringe. Advance and aspirate in 1–2 mm increments until the pleural space is penetrated and air is retrieved.

   viii. Retrieve air until the pleural space is empty and negative pressure is achieved.

   ix. A sensation of "scratching" on the end of the needle or a small amount of blood in the hub of the needle may signify that the needle is contacting the visceral pleura of the lung. If this sensation is noted, the needle should be backed out slightly.

   x. Because pneumothorax is most often bilateral, thoracocentesis should be performed on both sides of the chest.

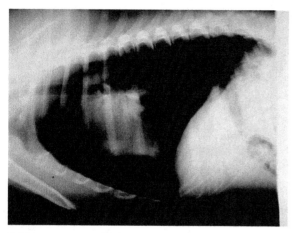

FIGURE 6.4   Lateral radiographic projection of a clinically significant pneumothorax. Note retraction of the lung from the chest wall and the hypovascular space ventral to the heart.

       xi.   Although possible, clinically significant pulmonary injury secondary to thoracocentesis is uncommon making it an excellent diagnostic and therapeutic method for the management of pneumothorax.

2. Radiography:
   a. Radiographs of dogs with clinically significant pneumothorax (Figure 6.4) probably should not exist because the problem should have been identified on physical examination and treated through thoracocentesis.
   b. Technique:
     i. Radiography is stressful. All measures to stabilize the patient prior to radiography should be undertaken:
       1. Oxygen support
       2. Fluid therapy if indicated for cardiovascular support
       3. Thoracocentesis
       4. Pain control and sedation
     ii. DV projections may be substituted for VD projections in an effort to minimize stress. Oxygen therapy should be administered while radiographs are acquired.
   c. Radiographic findings of pneumothorax:

     i. Retraction of the lung from the chest wall and increased density of the lung lobe due to consolidation.
     ii. Lack of bronchovascular markings beyond the periphery of the lung.
     iii. The appearance that the heart is "floating" on air on lateral radiographic projections. This finding results from the heart falling to the side of the atelectatic lung lobe.
     iv. Evidence of concurrent thoracic injuries.
3. Thoracic ultrasound (Lisciandro 2006):
   a. Focused ultrasound bilaterally at the 7th–9th intercostal space in the upper lateral thoracic wall reveals the "glide sign" in normal dogs. The "glide-sign" results from the "sliding" interaction between the lung margin (visceral pleura) and the thoracic wall (parietal pleura) during respiration.
   b. Lack of a "glide sign" is supportive of a diagnosis of pneumothorax.
  iv. Therapeutics:
1. Oxygen support:
   a. Oxygen support should be administered to all patients that have been sustained trauma that demonstrate increased respiratory rate and effort until specific measurement of oxygenation indices can be performed.
   b. Oxygen should initially be administered by mask, cage, or flow-by methods until nasal oxygen cannulae can be placed for longer-term oxygen support (dogs). Oxygen cages work very well for cats for longer-term oxygen support.
   c. Oxygen support may significantly speed the resolution of closed pneumothorax. By administering higher concentrations of oxygen, the concentration gradient for nitrogen between the alveoli and pleural space (pneumothorax) is increased, facilitating diffusion and thus resolution of pneumothorax. A second mechanism of resolution may include more rapid closure of the lesion in the visceral pleura. (Zierold et al., 2000) The clinical significance of this effect has

not been evaluated objectively in clinical veterinary medicine.

2. Thoracocentesis (see above) should be the initial treatment choice for management of dogs and cats with respiratory compromise secondary to pneumothorax:

　a. Thoracocentesis may be repeated if accumulation of air in the pleural space recurs.

　b. Thoracostomy tube placement should be considered as the treatment of choice for dogs and cats with recurrent pneumothorax requiring repeated thoracocentesis.

　c. Failure to achieve negative pressure necessitates thoracostomy tube placement and establishment of continuous pleural space drainage.

3. Thoracostomy tube placement:

　a. Indications:

　　i.　Sustained decompression of the pleural space in dogs and cats with pneumothorax when combined with a continuous drainage system (Figure 6.5). (Argyle Thora-Seal III Chest Drainage Unit. Tyco Health-

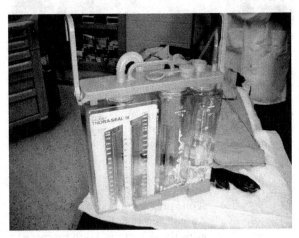

FIGURE 6.5　Continuous (3-bottle) thoracic drainage system. The chamber on the left is for the collection of fluids. The middle chamber provides a "water-seal" to prevent movement of air back into the pleural space, and the chamber on the right allows for regulation of suction. Argyle Thora-Seal III Chest Drainage Unit. Tyco Healthcare Group LP/Covidien. Mansfield, MA 02048.

care Group LP/Covidien. Mansfield, MA.)

　　ii.　Intermittent manual decompression of the pleural space in dogs and cats with pneumothorax by technical staff.

　　iii.　When combined with temporary closure of the thoracic wall, a thoracostomy tube is indicated for stabilization of dogs and cats with open pneumothorax until which time the patient is stable for definitive wound management and thoracic exploration.

　　iv.　Sustained decompression of blood or chyle from the pleural space.

　b. Equipment:

　　i.　Equipment for induction of general anesthesia

　　ii.　Equipment for preparation of a sterile field

　　iii.　Surgical pack

　　iv.　Thoracostomy tube

　　　1. Cats:

　　　　a.　8–14F chest tube (Argyle Trochar Catheter. Tyco Healthcare Group LP. Mansfield, MA) or 8–14F red rubber catheter (Kendall Sovereign Feeding tube and Urethral Catheter. Tyco Healthcare Group LP. Mansfield, MA).

　　　2. Dogs:

　　　　a.　<5 kg Dog: 8–14F chest tube (Argyle Trochar Catheter. Tyco Healthcare Group LP. Mansfield, MA) or 8–14F red rubber catheter (Kendall Sovereign Feeding tube and Urethral Catheter. Tyco Healthcare Group LP. Mansfield, MA).

　　　　b.　5–10 kg Dog: 12–16F chest tube (Argyle Trochar Catheter. Tyco Healthcare Group LP. Mansfield, MA) or 14F red rubber catheter (Kendall Sovereign Feeding tube and Urethral Catheter. Tyco Healthcare Group LP. Mansfield, MA).

c. 10–20 kg Dog: 16–20F chest tube (Argyle Trochar Catheter. Tyco Healthcare Group LP. Mansfield, MA) or 14F red rubber catheter (Kendall Sovereign Feeding tube and Urethral Catheter. Tyco Healthcare Group LP. Mansfield, MA).

d. >20 kg Dog: 20–28F chest tube (Argyle Trochar Catheter. Tyco Healthcare Group LP. Mansfield, MA) or 14F red rubber catheter (Kendall Sovereign Feeding tube and Urethral Catheter. Tyco Healthcare Group LP. Mansfield, MA).

v. #10 or #11 Scalpel blade (Bard Parker Rib-Back Carbon Steel Surgical Blade. Becton-Dickinson Acute Care. Franklin Lakes, NJ 07417).

vi. 2-0 or 3-0 nylon suture (Ethilon. Ethicon Inc.; A Johnson & Johnson Co. Somerville, NJ 08876).

c. Procedure:

i. All procedures should be performed to make thoracostomy tube placement as safe, efficient, and sterile as possible. The author prefers to completely clip and aseptically prepare BOTH hemithoraces and perform thoracocentesis immediately prior to anesthesia induction. Preoxygenation is also indicated. The author prefers to use general anesthesia for thoracostomy tube placement in all but the most urgent situations to minimize patient discomfort, maximize sterility, and allow for appropriate time for placement. Positive pressure ventilation after induction may make closed pneumothorax acutely worse.

ii. Immediately after anesthesia induction, the patient is positioned in lateral recumbency (most affected

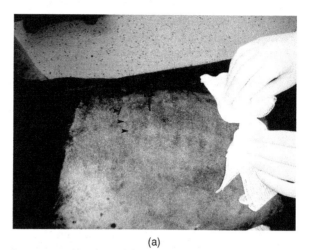

(a)

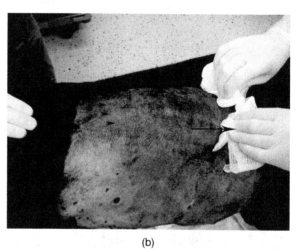

(b)

FIGURE 6.6 (a) An assistant (using sterile gauze) grips the skin at the 3–4th rib space and pulls it cranially. (b) The result is that skin that normally lies over the 12th–13th rib space is now positioned over the 9th–11th rib space. The arrow indicates the direction of tension on the skin. The arrowheads indicate the location of the 13th rib.

side up) and a final surgical antiseptic preparation is performed. An assistant (using sterile gauze) grips the skin at the 3–4th rib space and pulls it cranially. The result is that skin that normally lies over the 12th–13th rib space is now positioned over the 9th–11th rib space (Figure 6.6). Upon completion of the procedure, this maneuver will

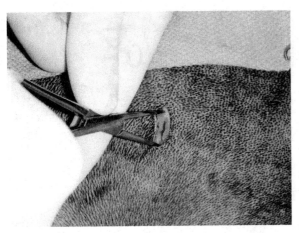

FIGURE 6.7 The sterile field over the 9th–11th rib space approximately 1/3 the distance from dorsal to ventral midline is draped. A 1–2 cm incision is created along the cranial edge of the 9th–11th rib space using the scalpel blade. Blunt dissection using a hemostat is performed both parallel to and extending to the limits of the skin incision. Blunt dissection continues until the pleural space is penetrated.

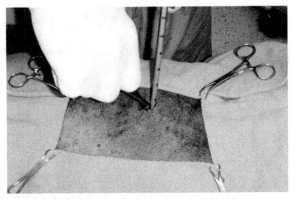

FIGURE 6.8 The hemostat is used to hold the pleura open so that the thoracostomy tube can be advanced between its jaws. The thoracostomy tube is initially directed perpendicular to the chest wall until it enters the pleural space.

create a subcutaneous tunnel through which the thoracostomy tube travels, making it resistant to infection and leakage of air around the chest tube. Finally, the sterile field over the 9th–11th rib space approximately 1/3 the distance from dorsal to ventral midline is draped.

iii. A 1–2 cm incision is created along the cranial edge of the 9th–11th rib space using the scalpel blade. Blunt dissection using a hemostat is performed both parallel to and extending to the limits of the skin incision (Figure 6.7). Blunt dissection is continued until the pleural space is penetrated.

iv. The hemostat is used to hold the pleura open so that the thoracostomy tube can be advanced between its jaws. The thoracostomy tube is initially directed perpendicular to the chest wall until it enters the pleural space (Figure 6.8). The thoracostomy tube is then directed cranially and ventrally (Figure 6.9). If the thoracostomy tube being utilized is

placed over a stylet, the tube may be advanced off of the stylet once the tube is 3–5 cm within the pleural space. Positioning of the chest tube in the cranial-ventral direction does not interfere with the ability to evacuate air from the pleural space as negative pressure will be created throughout the pleural space. The

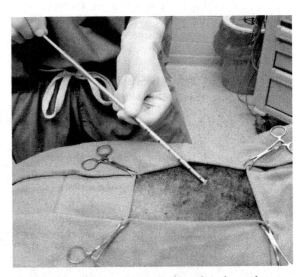

FIGURE 6.9 The thoracostomy tube is then directed cranially and ventrally. If the thoracostomy tube being utilized is placed over a stylet, the tube may be advanced off of the stylet once the tube is 3–5 cm within the pleural space.

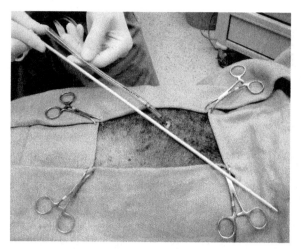

FIGURE 6.10 The stylet (if present) may be used to judge approximate location of the chest tube within the pleural space. If a red rubber catheter is utilized, a second red rubber catheter can be used to judge approximate location within the pleural space.

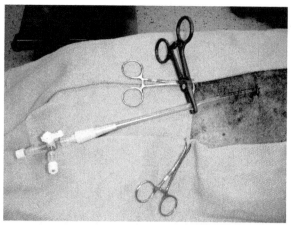

FIGURE 6.11 Connection of the thoracostomy tube to an adapter and three-way stopcock will allow the pleural space to be manually decompressed.

stylet (if present) may be used to judge approximate location of the chest tube within the pleural space (Figure 6.10). The tip of the chest tube is optimally positioned at the level of the 2nd–3rd sternebra.

v. Connection of the thoracostomy tube to a continuous pleural space drainage system or an adapter and three-way stopcock will allow the pleural space to be completely drained (Figure 6.11).

vi. Cranial skin tensioning is released and a purse-string suture and finger-trap is generally utilized to secure the chest tube in place (Figure 6.12). A sterile dressing should be placed at the insertion site. A circumferential dressing of the thorax is also recommended.

vii. The procedure is generally repeated in the opposite hemithorax because severe pneumothorax in the dog and cat is most often bilateral.

viii. Radiography is utilized to confirm chest tube placement in the cranial-ventral thorax (Figure 6.13). Radiography may be performed with

the patient anesthetized such that adjustments to tube location can be easily performed if necessary.

d. Maintenance of a thoracostomy tube:
  i. Strict sterility must be practiced when handling a thoracostomy tube. Gloves should always be utilized.
  ii. The author prefers to utilize continuous drainage systems for the

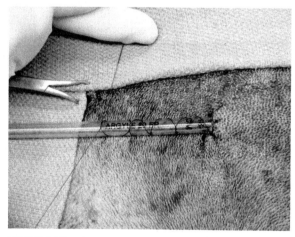

FIGURE 6.12 A purse-string suture and finger-trap is generally utilized to secure the chest tube in place. A sterile dressing should be placed at the insertion site. The site should be evaluated daily for redness, swelling, or discharge and the sterile dressing should be changed daily.

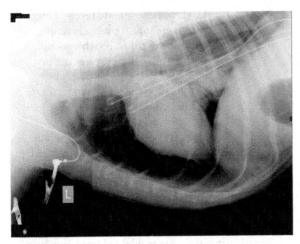

FIGURE 6.13 Radiography is utilized to confirm chest tube placement in the cranial-ventral thorax. This image reveals the presence of ongoing pneumothorax. These thoracostomy tubes were advanced an additional 2–3 cm into the pleural space.

pleural space to guarantee continuous drainage while minimizing the number of times that the chest tube must be accessed, thus decreasing the chance of contamination.

iii. Intermittent aspiration of the thoracostomy tube may be performed at a frequency necessary to maintain pleural space decompression.

iv. Antibiotic therapy is not indicated simply due to the presence of a thoracostomy tube. Early, broad-spectrum antibiotic therapy is indicated in all animals with open pneumothorax:

  1. Ampicillin/Sublactam 50 mg/kg IV TID

  2. Ampicillin 20 mg/kg IV Q6 h/Enrofloxacin 10 mg/kg IV SID (dog). Enrofloxacin 5 mg/kg IV SID (cat)

v. If persistent retrieval of air from the pleural space is recognized, all connections of the thoracostomy tube should be checked for leakage by clamping the system at the level of the skin and evaluating for ongoing retrieval of air:

  1. Inability to retrieve air after the clamp is applied implies that the air is originating at the ostomy or, more likely, within the chest.

  2. After application of the clamp at the level of the skin, ongoing retrieval of air implies that there is a leak in the system outside of the pleural space. The clamp can then be repositioned just proximal to each connection to identify the source of air accumulation.

vi. The author will remove the thoracostomy tube when retrieval of air is minimal (<10 mL/kg) or ceases completely for approximately 24 hours. Removal is performed by removing the suture(s) holding the tube in place and then pulling the tube while applying a sterile dressing and antibiotic ointment to the site. The purpose of the ointment is primarily to achieve an airtight seal at the insertion site. A circumferential thoracic dressing is applied for 12–24 hours after placement while the tract closes down.

4. Management of open pneumothorax:

a. Management of concurrent injuries should proceed in concert with management of open pneumothorax.

b. Oxygen support:

  i. Delivered by mask, flow-by, or baggie methods will improve oxygenation.

  ii. Intubation and positive pressure ventilation using cardiovascularly sparing anesthetic choices will allow for improved ventilatory function, oxygenation, pain, and wound management (see Chapter 5: Anesthesia and Analgesia for the Trauma Patient).

c. Temporary wound closure combined with thoracocentesis or thoracostomy tube placement will allow for the restoration of negative pressure in the pleural space and stabilization of the patient until which time definitive therapy can be undertaken:

    i. Skin can be sutured over the open wound.

    ii. Place gelatinous lubricant (Surgilube, E. Fougera and Co., a division of Altana Inc., Melville, NY) around the wound edge combined with a sterile dressing impermeable to air placed over the wound and around the thorax (Opsite, Smith & Nephew Medical Ltd., Hull, England).

d. Broad-spectrum antibiotic therapy should be initiated immediately:

    1. Ampicillin/Sublactam: 50 mg/kg IV TID

    2. Ampicillin 20 mg/kg IV Q6 h/Enrofloxacin 10 mg/kg IV SID (dog). Enrofloxacin 5 mg/kg IV SID (cat)

e. Definitive wound management:

    i. Thoracic exploration via lateral thoracotomy or ventral sternotomy.

    ii. Debridement of any damaged or devitalized tissues.

    iii. Copious lavage of the pleural space and the wound(s).

    iv. Acquisition of culture samples from the pleural space and the external wound.

    v. Placement of a thoracostomy tube.

    vi. Closure of the thoracic wall, thus isolating the pleural space from the external wound.

    vii. Closure of the external wound using appropriate drainage techniques.

f. Penetrating wounds to the thorax often exhibit the "iceberg effect". Surface wounds are often less-severe than thoracic wall and intrathoracic injury.

5. Pneumothorax and CPCR:

a. If pneumothorax has resulted in cardiac arrest, open chest CPCR is indicated immediately:

    i. Opening the chest will help decrease intrapleural pressures from what are likely supra-atmospheric levels to atmospheric levels. This may help improve venous return and lung expansion (when coupled with positive pressure ventilatory support).

    ii. Opening the chest will facilitate cardiac compressions.

6. Analgesia and sedation:

a. Dogs and cats that sustain thoracic trauma are very likely to be painful in the chest wall as well as from other concurrent injuries.

b. Appropriate analgesia will decrease pain and improve the patient's ability to take deeper (larger tidal volume), slower breaths. Larger tidal volumes may help prevent atelectasis.

c. See Chapter 5: Analgesia and Anesthesia for the Trauma Patient.

v. Monitoring:

1. Physical examination coupled with oxygenation indices are the cornerstones of monitoring patients with traumatic pneumothorax. Physical examination findings consistent with recurrence of pneumothorax or progressively declining oxygenation indices (oxygen saturation (SpO_2) and the partial pressure of oxygen in the arterial blood (PaO_2) as determined by ABG) should trigger decompression of the pleural space through repeat thoracocentesis or evacuation of a thoracostomy tube.

2. Use of a continuous underwater drainage system allows for real-time monitoring of ongoing leakage of air as evidenced by bubbling in the "water seal" chamber of the system (Figure 6.5).

vi. Prognosis:

1. Closed traumatic pneumothorax carries a good to excellent prognosis. Almost all dogs with closed traumatic pneumothorax respond to conservative therapy. Surgical intervention is rarely necessary, but is indicated in cases of suspected tracheal avulsion/rupture or when the accumulation of air in the pleural space is not abating over 3–4 days.

2. Open traumatic pneumothorax carries a more guarded prognosis that is more dependent on the presence of concurrent injuries that are common to animals with this pathology. Surgical management is indicated for repair of concurrent injuries, debridement of damaged/diseased tissues, and lavage.

b. Hemothorax:

i. Definition and pathophysiology:

1. Hemothorax is the accumulation of blood within the pleural space.

2. Hemothorax results from disruption of vasculature of the chest wall, lungs, or mediastinal structures including the great vessels. Concurrent diaphragmatic hernia and hemoabdomen may also result in hemothorax.

3. Clinically significant hemothorax is relatively uncommon. It is the clinical impression of the author that subclinical hemothorax occurs with greater frequency.

4. Clinically significant hemothorax will result in both cardiovascular and respiratory dysfunction. However, evidence of hypovolemia will precede evidence of respiratory distress assuming no additional pleural space or pulmonary injuries are present:

a. Cardiovascular compromise in patients with hemothorax results from hypovolemia.

b. As intrathoracic pressure increases from its normally subatmospheric level, atelectasis (resulting in ventilation-perfusion mismatch) and hypoventilation may contribute to hypoxemia.

5. The presence of concurrent hypovolemia and dyspnea generally results from four possible syndromes of injury:

a. Clinically significant hemothorax

b. Tension pneumothorax

c. Diaphragmatic hernia with a dilated stomach entrapped in the pleural space

d. Concurrent thoracic injury (most commonly, pneumothorax and/or pulmonary contusion) and acute blood loss elsewhere in the body

ii. Clinical signs/physical examination and oxygenation assessment:

1. Hypovolemia secondary to blood loss into the pleural space will result in a spectrum of clinical signs. Most often, pale mucous membranes, prolongation of the CRT, tachycardia, and poor pulse quality are recognized.

2. Respiratory rate and effort:

a. Clinically significant hemothorax will result in tachypnea, often characterized by shorter breaths with perceived smaller tidal volumes.

b. Respiratory character in dogs and cats with hemothorax is variable. In addition to tachypnea; extension of the neck, abduction of the elbows, and reluctance to lay in lateral recumbency may occur.

3. Auscultation:

a. Clinically significant hemothorax is a physical examination diagnosis.

i. With the animal positioned standing or in sternal recumbency, decreased lung sounds ventrally to diffusely will be noted.

b. Clinically significant hemothorax often occurs bilaterally.

c. Hemothorax may be accompanied by concurrent injuries to the chest. Auscultation should be interpreted in light of the potential for concurrent injuries.

4. Objective indicators of oxygenation:

a. Pulse oximetry may document a decreased saturation of the arterial blood with oxygen.

b. Arterial blood gas analysis may document hypoxemia and a decreased saturation of the arterial blood with oxygen. ABG analysis should not delay the rapid delivery of therapy for dogs and cats with hemothorax.

iii. Diagnostic tests:

1. Thoracocentesis:

a. Thoracocentesis is both diagnostic and therapeutic for dogs and cats with hemothorax.

b. Equipment (Figure 6.2):

i. 60 mL syringe

ii. 3-way stopcock

iii. IV extension tubing

iv. 19 g butterfly needle or 18–20 g needle. Note that larger thoracocentesis needles are utilized when pleural effusion (hemothorax or chylothorax) is suspected over pneumothorax. The reason for this is because of the increased viscosity of the pleural effusion compared to air. A larger radius needle or catheter will result in more rapid decompression of the pleural space.

   v.   Some will use an 18–22 g over-the-needle catheter for thoracocentesis. The author prefers a needle because it will not collapse with respiratory motion.

c. Procedure:

   i.   Position the patient in sternal recumbency.

   ii.   Clip and prepare the ventral 1/2 of the thorax between the 3rd and 9th ribs as if for surgery.

   iii.   Use sterile technique.

   iv.   Landmarks for thoracocentesis for the treatment of hemothorax are the ventral 1/3 of the chest at the level of the 5th–8th rib spaces.

   v.   While maintaining contact between the hand and the chest wall, insert needle perpendicular to the chest wall staying close to the cranial edge of the rib to avoid the neurovascular bundle caudally.

   vi.   Advance the needle through the skin and aspirate the syringe. Advance and aspirate in 1–2 mm increments until the pleural space is penetrated and blood or other fluid is retrieved.

   vii.   Retrieve effusion until the pleural space is empty and negative pressure results.

   viii. A sensation of "scratching" on the end of the needle or a small amount of air in the hub of the needle may signify that the needle is contacting the visceral pleura of the lung. If this "scratching" sensation is noted, the needle should be backed out slightly.

   ix.   Because hemothorax is most often bilateral, thoracocentesis should be performed on both sides of the chest.

   x.   Hemo-pneumothorax is also possible. Thoracocentesis for hemo-pneumothorax will result in retrieval of both air and blood from the pleural space. If hemopneumothorax is suspected using thoracocentesis, assessment of the collection system for leaks should be performed to ensure the accuracy of the hemopneumothorax diagnosis.

2. Fluid analysis:

a. Initially, any hemorrhagic fluid collected from the pleural space should be placed in a tube for the determination of serum chemistries (red-top) to evaluate for evidence of clotting:

   i. Any fluid that has been within the pleural space for any appreciable period of time will not clot.

b. Cytological evaluation should be performed on all hemorrhagic pleural fluid samples collected after trauma:

   i.   Peracute hemorrhage may reveal PCV/TS similar to that of peripheral blood. In addition, occasional platelets may be identified in the fluid.

   ii.   Erythrophagocytosis may indicate greater chronicity to the hemorrhage.

   iii. The pleural fluid should be evaluated for any evidence of sepsis. Although rare, the presence of a septic pleural effusion (pyothorax) should trigger additional diagnostic testing to identify the source of the infectious agents. Rapid surgical intervention is indicated for pyothorax once patient stability is achieved.

   iv. The pleural fluid should also be evaluated for the presence of chyle; see below.

3. Radiography:

a. Radiographs of dogs with clinically significant hemothorax probably should not exist because the problem should have been identified on physical examination and treated through thoracocentesis.

b. Technique:

i. Radiography is stressful. All measures to stabilize the patient prior to radiography should be undertaken:
1. Oxygen support
2. Fluid therapy if indicated for cardiovascular support
3. Thoracocentesis
4. Pain control and sedation

ii. DV projections may be substituted for VD projections in an effort to minimize stress. Oxygen therapy should be administered while radiographs are acquired.

c. Radiographic findings of hemothorax:
i. Retraction of the lung from the chest wall
ii. Fluid density between the lung margin and the thoracic wall
iii. Leafing of lung lobes
iv. Evidence of concurrent thoracic injuries

4. Thoracic ultrasound:
a. Use of ultrasound as a diagnostic for hemothorax offers, in a minimally invasive fashion, the advantage of confirmation of pleural effusion prior to diagnostic and therapeutic thoracocentesis.
b. Focused ultrasound bilaterally at the 4th–8th intercostal space on the ventrolateral thoracic wall reveals fluid density in the pleural space. An additional location for focused ultrasound for the detection of intrapleural accumulations of fluid is the subxyphoid position. The fluid is hypoechoic in contrast to the surrounding structures; however, cellular debris (red blood cells) may be visualized within the fluid.
c. Thoracic ultrasound facilitates the diagnosis of pleural effusion in animals with thoracic trauma. Thoracocentesis is necessary to further elucidate the type of fluid within the pleural space.

iv. Therapeutics:
1. Volume expansion:
a. Volume expansion is critical to the management of dogs and cats with hemothorax.

b. See Chapter 3: Shock in the Trauma Patient.

2. Thoracocentesis:
a. See 3. b. iii. 1. for additional information.

3. Thoracostomy tube placement in dogs and cats with hemothorax:
a. Indications:
i. The author places a thoracostomy tube in dogs and cats with hemothorax when >10 mL/kg of hemorrhagic fluid is retrieved from the pleural space after trauma:
1. Placement of a thoracostomy tube allows for sustained decompression of the pleural space helping alleviate respiratory compromise.
2. Placement of a thoracostomy tube allows for assessment of ongoing blood loss into the pleural space. Knowledge of this information will help guide fluid, colloid, and blood product support.
3. Sterile collection of blood from the pleural space from animals with no evidence of penetrating chest injury may be utilized to provide oxygen carrying capacity and albumin in the form of autotransfusion; see Chapter 11.

b. Equipment:
i. See 3. a. iv. 3. b. above for additional information.

c. Procedure:
i. The technique for thoracostomy tube placement for the management of hemothorax does not differ from that described for pneumothorax.
ii. See 3. a. iv. 3. c. above for additional information.

d. Maintenance:
i. See 3. a. iv. 3. d. above for additional information.

4. Surgical intervention:
a. Persistent ongoing hemorrhage should trigger surgical intervention.
b. The author will strongly consider surgical intervention when blood loss into the pleural space approaches

20–25 mL/kg and the patient is neither coagulopathicn or profoundly hypothermic.

c. Coagulopathy should be treated with fresh frozen plasma prior to surgical intervention.

d. Hypothermia should be prevented in the trauma patient whenever possible through the administration of warm IV fluids and blood products and the utilization of forced warm air and conductive warming measures whenever possible. Every effort should be made to achieve normothermia prior to surgical intervention in the patient with hemorrhage due to the deleterious effects of hypothermia on primary and secondary hemostasis.

e. Surgical intervention is always indicated when hemothorax results from a penetrating injury.

f. The patient should always be rapidly (<1–2 hours) stabilized medically (if possible) prior to surgical intervention.

5. Hemothorax and CPCR:
   a. If hemothorax has resulted in cardiac arrest, open-chest CPCR is indicated immediately.
   i. Opening the chest will help decrease intrapleural pressures from what are likely supraatmospheric levels to atmospheric levels. This may help improve venous return and lung expansion (when coupled with positive pressure ventilatory support).
   ii. Opening the chest may allow for surgical hemostasis.
   iii. Opening the chest will facilitate cardiac compressions and aortic compression to improve coronary and cerebral perfusion pressures.

6. Analgesia and sedation:
   a. Dogs and cats that sustain thoracic trauma are very likely to be painful in the chest wall as well as from other concurrent injuries.
   b. Appropriate analgesia will decrease pain and improve the patient's ability to take deeper (larger tidal volume), slower breaths. Larger tidal volumes may help prevent atelectasis.

v. Monitoring:
   1. Physical examination coupled with oxygenation indices and hemodynamic monitoring are the cornerstones of monitoring patients with traumatic hemothorax.
   a. Physical examination findings consistent with hypovolemia (see 3. b. ii. above).
   b. Progressive increases in respiratory rate and effort and auscultation consistent with pleural effusion (see 3. b. ii. above).
   2. Hemodynamic monitoring:
   a. Decreasing central venous pressure and decreasing arterial blood pressure are consistent with blood loss.
   3. Oxygenation indices:
   a. Declining oxygenation indices (SpO_2 and PaO_2 on ABG) may indicate progression/recurrence of hemothorax.
   4. Use of a continuous three-bottle drainage system allows for real-time monitoring and quantification of ongoing blood loss.
   5. Evidence of recurrence or progression of traumatic hemothorax should trigger volume expansion and pleural space decompression as described above (see 3. b. iv. above.

vi. Prognosis:
   1. Prognosis in dogs with hemothorax is dependent on the underlying and concurrent injuries.
   2. It is the author's opinion that most dogs with traumatic hemothorax will respond favorably to measures to both expand intravascular volume and decompress the pleural space.

c. Chylothorax:
   i. Definition and pathophysiology:
   1. Chyle is composed of lymph and chylomicrons (triglycerides). Chyle is absorbed from the intestine and carried to the cisterna chyli. The thoracic duct arises from the cisterna chyli and returns chyle to the venous system.
   2. Traumatic chylothorax may occur secondary to rupture of the thoracic duct. This injury is relatively uncommon:

a. Clinically significant chylothorax will result primarily in respiratory dysfunction.

b. As intrathoracic pressure increases from its normally subatmospheric level, atelectasis (resulting in ventilation-perfusion mismatch) and hypoventilation may contribute to hypoxemia.

ii. Clinical signs/physical examination and oxygenation assessment:

1. Chylothorax is not a peracute manifestation of thoracic trauma but is usually noted within days of the traumatic event.

2. Respiratory rate and effort:

    a. Clinically significant chylothorax will result in tachypnea, often characterized by shorter breaths with perceived smaller tidal volumes.

    b. Respiratory character in dogs and cats with chylothorax is variable. In addition to tachypnea; extension of the neck, abduction of the elbows, and reluctance to lay in lateral recumbency may occur.

3. Auscultation:

    a. Accumulation of a clinically significant volume of chyle (or any other type of pleural effusion) should be identified based on physical examination:

        i. With the animal positioned standing or in sternal recumbency, decreased lung sounds ventrally to diffusely will be noted.

    b. Clinically significant chylothorax often occurs bilaterally.

    c. Chylothorax may be accompanied by concurrent injuries to the chest. Auscultation should be interpreted in light of the potential for concurrent injuries.

4. Objective indicators of oxygenation:

    a. Pulse oximetry may document a decreased saturation of the arterial blood with oxygen.

    b. Arterial blood gas analysis may document hypoxemia and a decreased saturation of the arterial blood with oxygen. ABG analysis should not delay the rapid delivery of therapy for dogs and cats with chylothorax.

iii. Diagnostic tests:

1. Thoracocentesis:

    a. Thoracocentesis is both diagnostic and therapeutic for dogs and cats with chylothorax.

    b. Thoracocentesis should be performed bilaterally.

    c. Thoracocentesis is performed using identical technique to that used for hemothorax; see 3. b. iii. above for a description.

2. Fluid analysis of suspected chylous effusion:

    a. Chylous effusion usually appears grossly "milky" in appearance.

    b. Cell counts and protein content of chylous effusions are variable. The effusion is composed primarily of mature lymphocytes primarily with a mild acute to chronic inflammatory component. The effusion may have evidence of hemorrhage, especially in the acute traumatic setting.

    c. Triglyceride concentration of the pleural fluid should be higher than that in the peripheral blood.

3. Radiography:

    a. All radiographic precautions, techniques, and findings are identical to those described above for "hemothorax"; see 3. b. iii. 3. above.

4. Thoracic ultrasound:

    a. All ultrasound techniques and findings are identical to those described above for "hemothorax"; see 3. b. iii. 4. above.

iv. Therapeutics:

1. Stabilization through pleural space decompression via thoracocentesis or thoracostomy tube placement coupled with oxygen therapy should be the initial priority.

2. Traumatic chylothorax is rare. Conservative management is indicated based on experimental studies of thoracic duct injury in dogs in which laceration or transection of the thoracic duct resulted in self-limiting chylothorax of 5–10 days duration. (Hodges et al., 1993):

    a. Conservative management consists of maintaining pleural space decompression through thoracocentesis or thoracostomy tube placement.

b. The value of additional conservative treatment strategies such as a low-fat diet and rutin therapy are unknown in traumatic chylothorax.

c. Prospective clinical studies evaluating conservative versus surgical intervention in traumatic chylothorax in the dog and cat do not exist.

d. If chylothorax fails to resolve over two weeks, thoracic duct ligation +/− cysterna chili ablation may be considered.

3. Analgesia and sedation:

a. Dogs and cats that sustain thoracic trauma are very likely to be painful in the chest wall as well as from other concurrent injuries.

b. Appropriate analgesia will decrease pain and improve the patient's ability to take deeper (larger tidal volume), slower breaths. Larger tidal volumes may help prevent atelectasis (see Chapter 5: Anesthesia and Analgesia for the Trauma Patient).

v.   Monitoring:

1. Monitoring of dogs with chylothorax is focused on both physical examination and oxygenation indices as described for pneumothorax above.

2. Quantifying ouput of chyle via thoracostomy tube or repeated thoracocentesis will allow the attending clinician to determine whether the patient is improving.

vi. Prognosis:

1. Prognosis for dogs and cats with traumatic chylothorax is unknown.

2. Experimental studies suggest that a good prognosis can be given with appropriate supportive measures.

d. Diaphragmatic hernia:

i.   Definition and pathophysiology:

1. Diaphragmatic hernia refers to the movement of abdominal viscera through the diaphragm into the pleural space.

2. Traumatic diaphragmatic hernia is hypothesized to occur secondary to rapid compression of the abdomen with the majority of energy dissipation in the cranial direction resulting in disruption of the diaphragm. In addition, direct trauma to the caudal thorax and insertions of the diaphragm on the body wall may lead to diaphragmatic hernia.

3. Diaphragmatic hernia most often results in respiratory dysfunction:

a. As intrathoracic pressure increases, atelectasis (resulting in ventilation-perfusion mismatch) and hypoventilation may may contribute to hypoxemia.

b. On occasion, the stomach will become entrapped and severely distended within the pleural space resulting in rapidly progressive respiratory and cardiovascular collapse. Cardiovascular collapse occurs due to high intrapleural pressures interfering with normal venous return (similar to tension pneumothorax).

4. The most common organs herniated into the thorax (in order) are (Gibson et al., 2005):

a. Liver

b. Small bowel

c. Stomach

d. Spleen

e. Omentum

f. Large bowel

g. Gall bladder

h. Pancreas

ii. Clinical signs/physical examination and oxygenation assessment:

1. Respiratory rate and effort:

a. Some dogs with diaphragmatic hernia have no clinical signs. In addition, dogs may have a rent in the diaphragm without herniation of abdominal viscera into the chest.

b. Injuries to the diaphragm with resultant herniation of abdominal viscera into the pleural space will often result in tachypnea, characterized by shorter breaths with perceived smaller tidal volume.

c. Paradoxical abdominal movement (PAM) refers to inward movement of the abdomen during inspiration. PAM is a sign of diaphragmatic hernia.

d. Respiratory character in dogs and cats with diaphragmatic hernia is variable. In addition to tachypnea; extension of the neck, abduction of the elbows, and reluctance to lay in lateral recumbency may occur.

2. Auscultation:

   a. Diaphragmatic hernia may be suspected based on physical examination:

      i. With the animal positioned standing or in sternal recumbency, decreased lung sounds ventrally to diffusely will be noted. Depending on the location of the diaphragmatic rent and the viscera herniated, one side of the chest may demonstrate a greater decrease in lung sounds.

      ii. Borborygmi may be identified during auscultation of the chest.

   b. Diaphragmatic hernia may be accompanied by concurrent injuries to the chest. Auscultation should be interpreted in light of the potential for concurrent injuries.

3. Additional physical examination findings:

   a. Some abdominal organs may not be palpable if they have herniated into the pleural space.

   b. Physical examination findings and clinical signs referable to concurrent injuries and entrapped abdominal viscera may be identified. Example: Vomiting in a dog with small bowel entrapment within the thorax.

4. Objective indicators of oxygenation:

   a. Pulse oximetry may document a decreased saturation of the arterial blood with oxygen.

   b. Arterial blood gas analysis may document hypoxemia and a decreased saturation of the arterial blood with oxygen as well as hypoventilation. ABG analysis should not delay the rapid delivery of therapy for dogs and cats with thoracic trauma.

iii. Diagnostic testing:

1. Diaphragmatic hernia is an injury that may be suspected based on the history of trauma and physical examination findings;

however, it is confirmed through diagnostic imaging.

2. Survey radiography:

   a. All radiographic precautions and techniques are identical to those described above for "pneumothorax". See 3. a. iii. 2. above.

   b. Survey radiography may confirm diaphragmatic hernia or it may yield a high index of suspicion (Figure 6.14):

      i. Radiographic findings confirming diaphragmatic hernia include the presence of segments of the gastrointestinal system, liver, or spleen within the pleural space.

   c. Concurrent pleural effusion can obscure herniated abdominal viscera because both fluid and soft tissue have similar radiographic densities. Concurrent pleural effusion should be eliminated through thoracocentesis or thoracostomy tube placement prior to radiography, if possible.

   d. Right and left lateral projections should be acquired along with a DV or VD projection. Animals with respiratory compromise may not tolerate VD positioning. Additional radiographic views/techniques such as horizontal beam radiography may facilitate diagnosis if pleural effusion is obscuring suspected abdominal viscera. Abdominal radiographs may also help demonstrate an absence of various abdominal organs within the peritoneal space.

3. Positive contrast peritoneography:

   a. Positive contrast peritoneography involves the infusion of 1.1–2.2 mL/kg of a sterile iodine based contrast agent (Iohexal 240–300 mgI/mL) diluted 1:1 with saline into the peritoneal space at the level of the umbilicus while observing for any radiographic evidence of migration of contrast material into the pleural space with manipulation and gentle massage of the abdomen.

   b. The presence of contrast material within the pleural space confirms the presence of a diaphragmatic hernia (Figure 6.15).

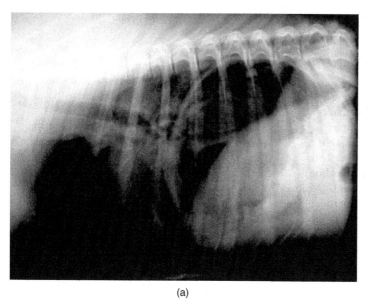

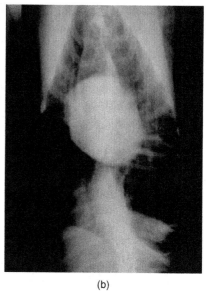

(a)   (b)

FIGURE 6.14 Lateral (a) and dorsoventral (b) radiographic projection of a dog with diaphragmatic hernia. Note that the stomach is herniated into the pleural space. A small volume pneumothorax is also visible. On the dorsventral projection, the stomach can be noted in the left hemithorax.

4. Ultrasound:
   a. Diagnostic ultrasound is a very operator-dependent diagnostic test.
   b. When imaging from the subxyphoid position, mirror image artifact can give

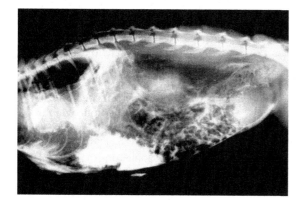

FIGURE 6.15 Positive contrast peritoneogram in a cat demonstrating an accumulation of iodinated contrast medium within the pleural space and thus the presence of diaphragmatic hernia. Note the accumulation of contrast medium within the falciform fat. Injection of contrast medium caudal to the umbilicus might have avoided this effect. (Courtesy Dr. Kenneth Drobatz, University of Pennsylvania School of Veterinary Medicine, Philadelphia, PA.)

the illusion of hepatic parenchyma on the thoracic side of the diaphragm and should not be mistaken for a diaphragmatic hernia (Figure 6.16).
   c. The presence of abdominal viscera within the pleural space confirms diaphragmatic hernia.
5. Computed tomography (CT):
   a. Noncontrast and contrast enhanced CT are a minimally invasive mechanism for accurate imaging of the abdomen and chest. It is the author's opinion that CT is an excellent diagnostic test for confirming the presence of diaphragmatic hernia when simpler imaging modalities are inconclusive.
   b. Based on the experience in humans, CT appears to be 50–100% sensitive and 100% specific for the diagnosis of diaphragmatic hernia. (Killeen et al., 1999; Nchimi et al., 2005).
iv. Therapeutics:
   1. Initial stabilization should be focused on the major body systems:
      a. Oxygen should be administered to maximize SpO$_2$. If oxygen administration by mask, flow-by, cage, or nasal

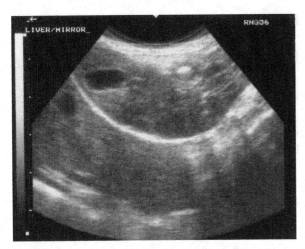

FIGURE 6.16 Mirror image artifact in a ferret. Note the illusion of hepatic parenchyma on the thoracic side of the diaphragm. This ultrasonographic finding should not be mistaken for diaphragmatic hernia.

cannulae cannot maintain SpO_2 above 90%, intubation and positive pressure ventilation should be considered.

b. Evacuation of concurrent pleural effusion or pneumothorax via thoracocentesis will help maximize SpO_2 and relieve respiratory difficulty.

c. Fluid therapy should be administered to achieve and maintain euvolemia.

2. Placing the animal on a slight incline (15–30°) once cardiovascular stability is achieved may prevent further movement of abdominal viscera into the pleural space and may facilitate movement of abdominal viscera back into the peritoneal space.

3. Gastric decompression:

   a. Herniation of the stomach into the pleural space with subsequent dilation of the stomach with gas can cause acute, catastrophic respiratory and cardiovascular embarrassment similar to that observed in tension pneumothorax. Decompression of the stomach is an absolute emergency in this scenario.

   b. Trans-thoracic gastrocentesis using the identical equipment and technique utilized for thoracocentesis can be used to rapidly decompress the stomach.

   c. Nasogastric or orogastric intubation may facilitate gastric decompression, but these techniques are associated with a greater potential for stress.

4. Surgical intervention:

   a. Surgical intervention for dogs and cats with diaphragmatic hernia should proceed as soon as patient stability has been achieved or maximized:

   i. It was once widely held that patients should undergo >1 day of stabilization prior to surgical intervention for diaphragmatic hernia.

   ii. A more recent study evaluating surgical intervention in dogs and cats within 24 hours of admission demonstrates very good patient survival rates (89.7%) (Gibson et al., 2005).

   iii. Absolute indications for immediate surgical intervention for dogs and cats with diaphragmatic hernia (after rapid stabilization) include the following:

   1. Evidence of gastric and small bowel obstruction

   2. Fever of unexplained origin

   3. Gastric herniation and dilation

   4. Vomiting

   5. Icterus

   6. Evidence of devitalized bowel

   7. Other surgical indication

   b. Surgical goals:

   i. Reposition abdominal viscera within the abdomen (Figure 6.17a).

   ii. Repair the rent in the diaphragm. In most cases of acute diaphragmatic hernia, the diaphragm can be closed in a simple, continuous suture pattern using an absorbable, monofilament suture material such as PDS (Ethicon Inc, Somerville, NJ) (Figure 6.17b). Autologous materials or synthetic/xenograft materials are rarely necessary to close the defect in the diaphragm in acute diaphragmatic hernia.

   iii. Placement of a thoracostomy tube for pleural space decompression

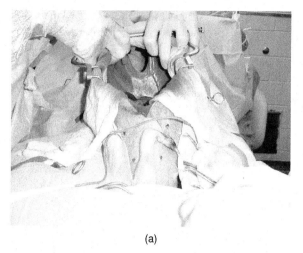

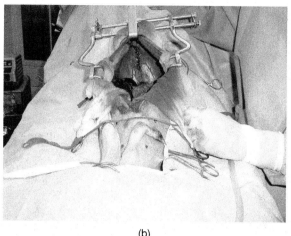

(a)   (b)

FIGURE 6.17   (a) Diaphragmatic rent in a dog after removal of abdominal viscera. (Courtesy Dr. Chick Weisse, The Animal Medical Center, New York, NY.) (b) Surgical closure of a diaphragmatic hernia in a dog using a simple continuous suture pattern. (Courtesy Dr. Chick Weisse, The Animal Medical Center, New York, NY.)

when the diaphragm is closed. Some surgeons prefer to simply perform transdiaphragmatic thoracocentesis after closure of the diaphragm. The author prefers proper thoracostomy tube placement that will allow for ongoing pleural space decompression due to the potential for penumothorax and pleural effusion accumulation in the postoperative period.

   c. Anesthetic considerations:

     i. Once the abdomen is open in dogs and cats with diaphragmatic hernia, the thorax is also open. Positive pressure ventilation will be necessary to maintain oxygenation and ventilation.

     ii. Reexpansion pulmonary edema is not a well-established clinical disease process in clinical small animal medicine and surgery. Reexpansion pulmonary edema involves what is believed to be an acute permeability pulmonary edema occasionally seen after rapid reexpansion of chronically atelectatic lung lobes. The pathophysiology is incompletely under-

stood but is thought to involve an inflammatory response induced by mechanical injury from acute reexpansion coupled with reperfusion injury. A lung-protective strategy for ventilation utilizing small tidal volumes, low peak airway pressures, and a higher than normal respiratory rate should be pursued (Sherman, 2003).

   d. Postoperative care should proceed as is routine for any major thoracic or abdominal procedure. Additional attention to monitoring of oxygenation indices to identify hypoxemia is appropriate.

5. Analgesia and sedation:

   a. Dogs and cats that sustain thoracic trauma are very likely to be painful in the chest wall as well as from other concurrent injuries (see Chapter 5: Anesthesia and Analgesia for the Trauma Patient).

   b. Appropriate analgesia will decrease pain and improve the patient's ability to take deeper (larger tidal volume), slower breaths. Larger tidal volumes may help prevent atelectasis.

v. Monitoring:

1. Monitoring of the dog or cat that has undergone treatment for diaphragmatic hernia should focus on the major body systems.

2. Frequent monitoring of oxygenation indices will help detect hypoxemia.

3. Additional monitoring should be directed toward concurrent injuries and should proceed as for any routine major thoracic or abdominal procedure.

vi. Prognosis:

a. Prognosis for the management of acute diaphragmatic hernia is good. Approximately 90% survival is expected when surgery is carried out in a referral setting within 24 hours of admission/trauma (Gibson et al., 2005).

4. TRAUMA-ASSOCIATED PULMONARY INJURIES

a. Pulmonary contusion:

i. Definition and pathophysiology:

1. Pulmonary contusion refers to a lesion of the lung that occurs after a compression-decompression injury to the chest wall that results in hemorrhage and edema leading to alveolar collapse and lung consolidation (Trinkle et al., 1973; Allen and Coates, 1998).

2. Pulmonary contusion is the most common injury identified after blunt chest trauma in people and is very commonly recognized in animals that have undergone thoracic trauma (Cohn, 1997; Powell et al., 1999).

3. Pathophysiologic mechanisms for pulmonary contusion include (Cohn, 1997):

a. The Spalling effect: Shearing or bursting effect at gas/liquid (in the alveolus) interfaces.

b. Inertial effect: Due to different rates of acceleration of the hilar and alveolar tissues resulting in stripping of alveolar tissue from the higher density hilar structures.

c. Implosion effect: Results from rebound or overexpansion of gas bubbles after a pressure wave passes.

4. Various types of pulmonary contusion have been described (Wagner et al., 1988).

5. All of the above forces and types of contusion culminate in the development of hypoxemia due to ventilation/perfusion mismatch, shunt, diffusion impairment, and occasionally hypoventilation (Hackner, 1995).

ii. Clinical signs/physical examination/oxygenation assessment

1. Clinical signs and physical examination findings may manifest soon after the trauma occurs and may worsen over the initial 24 hours.

2. Respiratory rate and effort:

a. Clinically significant pulmonary contusion will result in tachypnea.

b. Respiratory character in dogs and cats with pulmonary contusion is variable. In addition to tachypnea; extension of the neck, abduction of the elbows, and reluctance to lay in lateral recumbency are common. Cyanosis may be noted in pulmonary contusion.

c. A soft, moist cough +/− hemoptysis may be noted historically or observed during physical examination.

3. Auscultation:

a. Clinically significant pulmonary contusion is a physical examination diagnosis:

i. As a general rule, auscultation findings in dogs and cats with pulmonary contusion most often range from increased lung sounds to crackles. On rare occasions when contusion is focally very severe, decreased lung sounds may be noted. These findings may manifest unilaterally or bilaterally and will not be evenly distributed.

b. Clinically significant pulmonary contusion most often occurs bilaterally.

c. Pulmonary contusion may be accompanied by concurrent injuries to the chest. Auscultation should be interpreted in light of the potential for concurrent injuries:

i. Example: A dog that is hit-by-car that demonstrates severe dyspnea with relatively normal lung sounds may have both pneumothorax (decreasing lung sounds) and pulmonary contusion (increasing lung sound). In this example, oxygen should be administered immediately and diagnostic thoracocentesis should be performed.

4. Additional physical examination findings:

   a. Rib fractures should serve as a "flag" for pulmonary contusion. The chest wall is a resilient structure and, as such, significant trauma is necessary to fracture the ribs. As these forces are transmitted to the chest wall, they are also transmitted through the chest resulting in pulmonary contusion. For a more complete discussion of rib fractures; see below.

   b. In severe cases of pulmonary contusion, pulmonary compliance may be severely decreased and paradoxical abdominal movement may be identified.

5. Objective indicators of oxygenation:

   a. Pulse oximetry may document a decreased saturation of the arterial blood with oxygen.

   b. Arterial blood gas analysis may document hypoxemia and a decreased saturation of the arterial blood with oxygen. An increased alveolar-arterial oxygen gradient (A-a gradient) indicating a pulmonary gas exchange abnormality will be observed. The author utilizes the arterial blood gas (A-a Gradient) to document the presence of a pulmonary gas exchange abnormality in dogs with pulmonary contusion and to monitor for improvement or progression over time. Normal A-a gradient ranges from <15–22 mm Hg (see Chapter 4: Monitoring of the Trauma Patient). ABG analysis should not delay the rapid delivery of therapy for dogs and cats with pneumothorax.

iii. Diagnostics:

   1. Clinically significant pulmonary contusion is a physical examination diagnosis

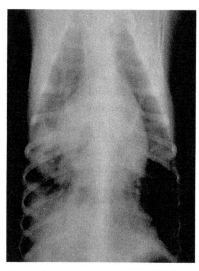

FIGURE 6.18 Pulmonary contusion in a dog that was hit by a car. Note the patchy interstitial and alveolar densities located bilaterally. An air bronchogram is visible in the right caudal lung lobe.

that is confirmed through radiographic imaging.

   2. Diagnostic imaging should be delayed until patient stability is achieved.

   3. Radiographic findings in dogs and cats with pulmonary contusion may include the following:

      a. Patchy interstitial to alveolar densities (Figure 6.18).

      b. Other radiographic findings consistent with thoracic trauma.

      c. Radiographic findings may lag slightly behind clinical signs:

         i. Clinically significant pulmonary contusion (those severe enough to cause respiratory compromise) will be radiographically evident independent of time.

   4. Pulmonary contusion is easily identified using CT.

iv. Therapeutics:

   1. Treatment of dogs and cats with pulmonary contusion is largely supportive in nature and consists of optimizing oxygenation through supplemental oxygen support, pain control, judicious fluid therapy, good nursing practices, management of concurrent injuries, and positive pressure

ventilatory support if indicated, based on arterial blood gas analysis and clinical signs. Despite popular belief, there are no specific medications that are likely to improve outcome in dogs and cats with pulmonary contusion.

2. Optimize oxygenation:

a. Supplemental oxygen support (cage, nasal cannulae) should be administered to maintain SpO_2 above 90% (approximate $PaO_2 = 60$ mm Hg).

b. Indications for positive pressure ventilatory (PPV) support in dogs and cats with pulmonary contusion:

i. Inability to maintain SpO_2 >90% or $PaO_2 > 60$ mm Hg with supplemental oxygen support (FiO_2 <0.6 = 60% inspired oxygen).

ii. Inability to maintain $PaCO_2 < 60$ mm Hg. Because carbon dioxide diffuses very easily across the alveolar membranes, hypercarbia is a relatively uncommon reason to initiate PPV in dogs and cats with pulmonary contusion.

iii. Increases in respiratory rate and effort that are unlikely to be sustainable or that do not allow the patient to sleep/rest.

iv. Older literature suggests that dogs and cats that require PPV for the management of pulmonary contusion have approximate survival rates of 30% (Campbell and King, 2000; Powell et al., 1999). However, it is the authors' impression that our ability to manage pulmonary contusion using PPV has improved significantly in the past 10 years and a much better prognosis can be given.

3. Analgesia and sedation:

a. Dogs and cats that sustain thoracic trauma are very likely to be painful in the chest wall as well as from other concurrent injuries (see Chapter 5: Anesthesia and Analgesia for the Trauma Patient).

b. Appropriate analgesia will decrease pain and improve the patient's ability to take deeper (larger tidal volume), slower breaths. Larger tidal volumes may help prevent atelectasis.

4. Nursing care:

a. Many dogs and cats that have sustained pulmonary contusion also sustain additional injuries including major orthopedic injuries. These patients are often unable or reluctant to turn themselves or walk:

i. Patients that are unable to walk should be turned every two hours. The author uses a rotation of right lateral, right sternal, sternal, left sternal, and left lateral recumbencies to help prevent dependent atelectasis.

ii. If the patient can stand but is unable to walk, he/she should be placed in a standing position every 4 hours and turned as described above.

iii. Short walks can be accomplished even if the patient is oxygen-dependent using portable oxygen cylinders and flow regulators.

b. Immobility contributes to atelectasis, which can worsen pulmonary function in patients with lung injury. Varying body position, standing, and short walks may help combat atelectasis and recruit alveoli to participate in gas exchange.

5. Fluid therapy in the patient with pulmonary contusion:

a. Much debate exists as to the optimum fluid therapy choice for dogs and cats with pulmonary contusion. Some argue that synthetic colloids or hypertonics offer advantages because they provide smaller volume resuscitation. Others argue that the *intravascular* volume expanding effect of synthetic colloids is the same as crystalloids because the colloids will draw fluid from the interstitial space:

i. In a pig model of pulmonary contusion, 7.5% hypertonic saline (4 mL/kg) afforded no advantages with regard to arterial oxygen tensions, wet-to-dry lung weights or CT scan injury volume when compared to a group receiving 0.9% saline (90 mL/kg) (Cohn et al., 1997).

b. Principles that should guide fluid therapy in the dog or cat with pulmonary contusion are as follows:

   i. Fluid should be administered to manage hypovolemia (see Chapter 3: Shock in the Trauma Patient).

   ii. Fluid should be administered to provide for maintenance and ongoing losses.

   iii. Excessive fluid administration should be avoided. Increased pulmonary vascular permeability secondary to disruption of alveolar-capillary membranes will facilitate fluid movement into the interstitium and alveoli.

   iv. In the absence of hypovolemia, fluids should be administered sparingly to dogs and cats with pulmonary contusion.

6. Specific treatment:

   a. Numerous medications have been traditionally administered to dogs and cats with pulmonary contusion with little evidence to support their use. Despite the paucity of clinical trials evaluating any of these therapies in small animals with pulmonary contusion, we are able to draw some information from the human clinical experience and trials in laboratory animals. In many of these studies, neither clear advantages nor disadvantages of these medications can be identified. If a specific advantage of a given medication cannot be identified, there is no indication for its use.

   b. Furosemide:

   i. Furosemide is traditionally administered for the purpose of decreasing preload in hydrostatic pulmonary edema situations (congestive heart failure).

   ii. Furosemide is not indicated for the management of pulmonary contusion unless inadvertent fluid overload has occurred.

   iii. The author finds that the administration of furosemide simply com-

plicates fluid therapy by adding another factor into fluid therapy balance.

   c. Bronchodilators:

   i. Bronchodilators are traditionally administered to animals with reactive small airway diseases such as chronic bronchitis or feline asthma. These conditions are characterized by reactive small airways, smooth muscle thickening of the small airways, and increased mucous production.

   ii. Dogs and cats with pulmonary contusion do not demonstrate increased reactivity of the small airways or other pathology associated with small airway diseases and as such, do not benefit from the administration of bronchodilators.

   d. Corticosteroids:

   i. Corticosteroids offer no clear advantage in the management of pulmonary contusion.

   ii. Corticosteroids impair bacterial clearance in the lung.

   iii. Corticosteroids are associated with gastrointestinal ulceration.

   iv. Corticosteroid usage was evaluated retrospectively in a single small animal study of pulmonary contusion. Dogs that received corticosteroids did not have shortened hospitalization or duration of oxygen support when compared to dogs that had not received corticosteroids. The limitations of retrospective studies must be considered when interpreting these conclusions (Powell et al., 1999).

   v. Corticosteroids cannot be recommended for the management of any traumatic condition with the potential exception of acute spinal trauma (see Chapter 9: Traumatic Spinal Injury).

   e. Antibiotics:

   i. The incidence of bacterial pneumonia in clinical small animal patients with pulmonary contusion (not undergoing positive pressure ventilatory support) is exceedingly low (Powell et al., 1999).

    ii. Due to the low incidence of bacterial pneumonia, antibiotics cannot be recommended for the prevention of pneumonia after pulmonary contusion.

    iii. Antibiotics may be indicated for the management of other traumatic conditions such as lacerations, open fractures, etc.

  v. Monitoring:

    1. Oxygenation and lung function:

      a. Oxygen saturation should be monitored every 2–4 hours to ensure adequate oxygenation (>90%). Supplemental oxygen support should be adjusted as needed.

      b. Arterial blood gas analysis may be utilized to calculate the alveolar-arterial oxygen gradient. A-a gradient should begin to improve within 24–48 hours of the initial trauma. Acute deterioration in lung function should prompt a search for a secondary condition such as pulmonary thromboembolism, pneumothorax, aspiration pneumonia, etc.

    2. Respiratory effort should be monitored to ensure that the patient is able to rest and is unlikely to become exhausted from the increased work of breathing.

    3. Additional monitoring should be performed to address major body systems and concurrent injuries.

  vi. Prognosis:

    1. Prognosis for dogs and cats with pulmonary contusion is good. In a single retrospective study, 82% of dogs with pulmonary contusion survived (Powell et al., 1999).

    2. Due to the nature of thoracic injury, prognosis in dogs and cats with pulmonary contusion is often impacted by concurrent injuries.

b. Blebs and bullae:

  i. Definition and pathophysiology:

    1. A pulmonary bleb is defined as a small pocket of air located within the visceral pleura. It likely occurs due to damage to alveoli with rupture and leakage of air into the interstitium and dissection into the pleura.

    2. A pulmonary bullae is similar to a bleb, but is associated with the pulmonary parenchyma. It results from the breakdown/rupture of adjacent alveoli.

  ii. Clinical signs/physical examination/oxygenation assessment:

    1. Most often, there are no clinical signs, physical examination findings or variation in oxygenation indices in dogs and cats with trauma-associated bullae or blebs.

    2. Thoracic trauma may result in bulla or bleb formation. Bullae and blebs can rupture acutely after trauma or at a later date. Rupture of a bleb or bullae results in pneumothorax; see 3a for a full discussion of pneumothorax.

  iii. Diagnostics:

    1. Survey radiography will often document the presence of bullae or blebs:

      a. Additional radiographic findings consistent with thoracic trauma may be identified.

      b. Radiographic evidence of pneumothorax may be associated with rupture of bullae or blebs.

    2. Computed tomography may reveal the presence of bullae or blebs:

  iv. Therapeutics:

    1. Unless bullae or blebs are associated with pneumothorax, specific treatment is not indicated.

  v. Monitoring:

    1. Animals with radiographic evidence of bullae or blebs should be monitored for the onset of respiratory distress resulting from pneumothorax.

  vi. Prognosis:

    1. Prognosis for animals with bullae or blebs is likely good. Subjectively, it is the authors experience that the later development of pneumothorax in dogs with trauma-associated bullae or blebs is quite low.

5. TRAUMA-ASSOCIATED THORACIC WALL INJURIES

a. Rib fractures:

  i. Definition and pathophysiology:

1. Rib fractures may result from blunt or penetrating thoracic trauma.

2. The canine and feline thorax is a relatively resilient structure. Rib fractures should serve as a "flag" for concurrent thoracic injury.

3. Pulmonary contusion is commonly associated with rib fractures.

4. Sequelae of rib fractures include the following:

   a. Pain: Thoracic wall pain will make the patient reluctant to breathe deeply. The resultant decreased tidal volume may predispose to hypoxemia secondary to atelectasis and hypoventilation.

   b. Pneumothorax: Pneumothorax may occur if the broken rib(s) penetrate the visceral pleura.

   c. Hemothorax: Disruption of the intercostal arteries and veins may result in hemorrhage into the pleural space. Hemothorax may occur if the broken rib(s) penetrate the visceral pleura and disrupt the pulmonary vasculature.

ii. Clinical signs/physical examination and oxygenation assessment:

   1. Clinical signs:

   a. Animals with isolated rib fractures may not display any overt clinical signs.

   b. At times, the pain associated with rib fractures will make the patient breathe in a more rapid, shallow fashion. Large tidal volume breaths cause greater movement and distortion of the chest wall and may be associated with more pain.

   c. Clinical signs referable to other thoracic injuries may be noted.

   2. Physical examination findings:

   a. Gross distortion (inward or outward displacement) of the normal thoracic wall contour may be evident on gentle palpation.

   b. A palpable rubbing or grinding of the fracture site may be noted on palpation of minimally displaced rib fractures.

   c. Young animals with isolated rib fractures and adjacent soft tissue injury may demonstrate paradoxical movement of the affected area resulting from the flexibility of the costochondral junction.

   d. Pain on palpation of sites of rib fracture is generally easy to elicit.

   e. Physical examination findings referable to other thoracic injuries may be noted.

   3. Objective indicators of oxygenation:

   a. Isolated rib fractures are unlikely to affect oxygenation (SpO_2 and PaO_2).

   b. Concurrent thoracic injuries such as pulmonary contusion and pneumothorax may cause hypoxemia.

   c. Severe chest wall injury may result in hypoventilation induced hypoxemia. In addition, concurrent atelectasis may result in hypoxemia due to ventilation-perfusion mismatch.

iii. Diagnostics:

   1. Many rib fractures are diagnosed based on physical examination.

   2. Survey (3-view) thoracic radiography may demonstrate additional rib fractures not identified on physical examination:

   a. Occasionally, review of thoracic radiographs in an inverted position aids in the identification of rib fractures.

   3. Some rib fractures are probably not identified on either physical examination or thoracic radiographs.

iv. Therapeutics:

   1. Most rib fractures do not require specific treatment beyond pain control:

   a. Systemic:

   1. A multimodal analgesic protocol consisting of both opioids and nonsteroidal anti-inflammatory drugs will provide good analgesia for patients that have thoracic wall injury; see Chapter 5 for a complete discussion of analgesia for the trauma patient.

   b. Intercostal nerve blocks have a role in the management of thoracic wall pain:

   i. Bupivicaine 0.75% diluted to 0.25% with saline and administered just caudal to the rib, both above and below the fracture site using a 22–25 g needle. The intercostal nerve both in front of and behind the fracture site should also be blocked. Total dose should not exceed 1.5 mg/kg in the dog and 1 mg/kg in the cat (Conzemius et al., 1994; Curcio et al., 2006).

ii. The intercostal muscles are secondary muscles of respiration. Intercostal nerve blocks could predispose to hypoventilation if performed in excess. The author does not perform intercostal nerve blocks on more than 4–5 sites.

2. Surgical intervention is critical when rib fractures are associated with penetrating thoracic injury.

3. Rib fractures that are displaced inward and are associated with ongoing pneumothorax or hemothorax or those that are associated with severe soft tissue injury to the thoracic wall require surgical intervention. Surgical intervention will most often consist of debridement of damaged or devitalized tissues, lavage, and closure with intrapleural +/− thoracic wall drainage.

v. Monitoring:
  1. Animals with rib fractures should be monitored for discomfort and pain should be controlled as needed.
  2. Because pneumothorax is a complication of rib fracture, acute deterioration in respiratory status in a patient with known rib fractures should prompt a search for pneumothorax or other concurrent injuries.
  3. Monitoring appropriate for concurrent thoracic injuries should be undertaken.

vi. Prognosis:
  1. Animals with isolated rib fractures have an excellent prognosis.
  2. Prognosis is best dictated by the presence of concurrent injuries.

b. Flail chest:
  i. Definition and pathophysiology:
    1. Flail chest is defined as "paradoxical movement of a floating thoracic segment" or the "fracture of two or more consecutive ribs in two places (ventral and dorsal)" (Sweet and Waters, 1991; Suter, 1984).
    2. Flail chest may be the result of either blunt or penetrating thoracic trauma.

3. The respiratory distress and respiratory dysfunction associated with flail chest was initially thought to occur secondary to flail segment associated pendulous airflow, decreased vital capacity, decreased functional residual capacity, decreased pulmonary compliance, and increased airway resistance (Olsen et al., 2002).

4. Subsequent investigation suggests that underlying pulmonary and pleural space injury coupled with severe pain are greater contributors to respiratory distress and dysfunction in patients with flail chest.

ii. Clinical signs/physical examination and oxygenation assessment:
  1. Flail chest is a physical examination diagnosis:
    a. During inspiration, as intrapleural pressure becomes more negative, the chest wall moves outward and the flail segment moves inward in the direction of negative pressure.
    b. During expiration, as intrapleural pressure becomes less negative, the chest wall recoils and the flail segment moves outward.
  2. Additional physical examination findings consistent with thoracic trauma may be noted.
  3. Objective indicators of oxygenation:
    a. Flail chest causes hypoxemia via multiple methods:
      i. Associated concurrent injuries such as pulmonary contusion and pleural space injuries are the primary causes of hypoxemia in patients with flail chest.
      ii. Thoracic wall pain may predispose to small tidal volumes with resultant hypoventilation and secondary atelectasis and hypoxemia.
      iii. Mechanical dysfunction of the chest wall may also contribute to hypoxemia via hypoventilation.

iii. Diagnostics:
  1. Flail chest is a physical examination diagnosis.
  2. Radiographic imaging will reveal multiple adjacent ribs broken in multiple

locations (generally dorsal and ventral) creating a "floating" thoracic segment.

iv. Therapeutics:

1. Following the trends in human medicine, most cases of flail chest are treated conservatively:

a. Treatment of animals with flail chest must be directed toward management of concurrent pleural space injuries and pulmonary contusion as described above.

b. Pain control appropriate for animals with multiple organ system injury and thoracic wall injury is recommended; see Chapter 5 and 5. a. iv. 1. b. i.

c. Positive pressure ventilatory support may be necessary in patients with severe respiratory dysfunction characterized by persistent hypoxemia in the presence of oxygen support, hypoventilation, or severe increases in respiratory effort as described above under Pulmonary Contusion above. PPV in animals with flail chest creates a functional brace because both the thoracic wall and flail segment move synchronously.

d. In a recent retrospective study of flail chest, dogs and cats without penetrating injury were treated conservatively almost 2:1 compared to dogs managed surgically. The survival rate for dogs managed conservatively was 93% (Olsen et al., 2002).

2. Various methods for external stabilization of the flail segment via creation of an external thoracic brace of animals have been described (Anderson et al., 1993; McAnulty, 1995).

3. Surgical intervention is absolutely indicated for animals with flail chest secondary to penetrating thoracic injury:

a. Patients with flail chest without evidence of penetrating injury may undergo surgical intervention if there is suspicion of severe concurrent soft tissue injury. Patients should always be medically stabilized prior to surgical intervention.

b. Surgical intervention is directed at debriding damaged tissues, lavage,

establishing drainage, and closure. Internal thoracic wall stabilization may be performed using IM pins, interfragmentary wires, suture approximation, or bone plates.

4. Analgesia for patients with flail chest will be similar to that described above for rib fractures 5. a. iv. 1. see Chapter 5 for a full discussion of analgesic techniques in the patient that has sustained trauma.

v. Monitoring:

1. Animals with flail chest should be monitored for discomfort and pain should be controlled as needed.

2. Because pneumothorax is a complication of rib fractures, acute deterioration in respiratory status in a patient with known rib fractures should prompt a search for pneumothorax or other concurrent injuries.

3. Monitoring appropriate for concurrent thoracic injuries should be undertaken. The general focus of monitoring will be on surveillance for hypoxemia, hypoventilation, and pain.

vi. Prognosis:

1. Prognosis for animals with flail chest is variable and is most likely impacted most significantly by the presence of concurrent injuries and their respective prognoses.

2. In a recent retrospective study in which dogs and cats with flail chest were treated both surgically and conservatively, survival ranged from 66 to 93% (Olsen et al., 2002).

c. Penetrating thoracic injury:

i. Definition and pathophysiology:

1. Bite wounds are the most common cause of penetrating thoracic injury in the dog and cat. Additional injuries include gunshot wounds, impalements, knife wounds, as well as other causes of trauma.

2. Very often, the external wound is merely the "tip of the iceberg". Severe underlying tissue injury is likely.

ii. Clinical signs/physical examination and oxygenation assessment:

1. Clinical signs:

a. Some penetrating thoracic injuries are quite obvious.

i. Direct visualization of intrathoracic structures implies penetrating injury.

ii. Air may be heard moving into and out of the pleural space creating a "sucking" sound.

b. Very often, there is no external evidence that a wound over the thorax penetrates into the pleural space.

2. Physical examination:

a. Penetrating thoracic trauma often results in a variety of concurrent injuries. Physical examination can be used to identify most of these injuries; see the aforementioned segments for a complete approach to these injuries:

  i. Open pneumothorax
  ii. Hemothorax
  iii. Diaphragmatic hernia
  iv. Rib fractures
  v. Flail chest
  vi. Pulmonary contusion

b. External wounds will be identified over the thorax.

c. Animals with penetrating thoracic injury should be closely evaluated for evidence of abdominal trauma as well as other injuries.

3. Objective indicators of oxygenation:

a. Oxygen saturation and PaO_2 may be normal or significantly decreased in dogs with penetrating thoracic injury due to open pneumothorax and/or other concurrent injuries.

iii. Diagnostics:

1. The diagnosis of penetrating thoracic injury may be made based solely on physical examination, or may require additional diagnostic testing. The presence of concurrent clinically significant pneumothorax, hemothorax, and pulmonary contusion should be identified based on physical examination.

2. Thoracic radiography will not definitively determine if a wound over the thorax is penetrating into the pleural space:

a. The presence of pneumothorax and an external thoracic wound makes penetrating thoracic injury very likely.

b. The absence of pneumothorax does not preclude penetrating thoracic injury.

c. Thoracic radiographs are valuable for characterizing concurrent injuries.

d. Three radiographic views should be acquired.

3. Surgical wound exploration is the diagnostic test of choice for the definitive diagnosis of penetrating thoracic injury. Surgical wound exploration should be performed as soon as the patient has been stabilized and can safely be placed under general anesthesia:

a. All wounds over the chest should be surgically explored:

  i. When concurrent injuries are stabilized, the patient should be placed under general anesthesia. Dogs and cats with penetrating thoracic injury very often have open pneumothorax. Positive pressure ventilatory support will likely be necessary.

  ii. All wounds and a very wide surrounding area to include the entire hemithorax should be clipped free of hair and prepared for surgery.

  iii. The author prefers to create an elliptical skin incision around the wound to excise damaged or diseased tissue while concurrently enlarging the wound for appropriate exploration. The damaged tissue planes should be followed until they end or until they penetrate the pleural space. Damaged tissues should be debrided appropriately; see 5. c. iv. (Therapeutics) for definitive wound management.

b. Simple probing of wounds with a hemostat IS NOT an adequate test for determination of whether a wound penetrates the pleural space. Various tissue planes move over one another making penetration in a straight line into the pleural space unlikely.

iv. Therapeutics:

1. Stabilization of concurrent thoracic and major body system injuries is critical to the management of animals with penetrating thoracic injuries:

    a. Oxygen therapy

    b. Volume expansion as needed

    c. Decompression of pneumothorax/hemothorax

    d. Provide appropriate analgesia and sedation

    e. Stabilization for transport:

      i. Animals with severe thoracic wall injury and obvious penetrating injury may need to be referred to a specialty hospital for definitive therapeutics.

      ii. Reestablishing negative intrapleural pressure will help stabilize the patient:

        1. Rapidly clip and surgically prepare the wound edges.

        2. Place a thoracostomy tube through a segment of normal thoracic wall; see 3. a. iv. 3.

        3. Two options exist for "closing" the thoracic cavity:

          a. Close the skin over the large thoracic wound to create an airtight seal.

          b. Place a large, sterile, adhesive drape (Op-Syte, Smith & Nephew Medical Ltd., Hull, England) or Ioban (3 M Healthcare, St Paul, MN)) over the wound.

          c. Place a thin layer of antibiotic ointment around the clipped open defect and apply thin plastic material (plastic wrap) over the wound.

        4. Evacuate the thoracostomy tube or perform thoracocentesis if a thoracostomy tube was not placed.

        5. Rapidly transport for definitive therapeutics.

2. Early, broad-spectrum antibiotic therapy is indicated when penetrating thoracic injury is suspected:

    a. Ampicillin 20 mg/kg slow IV TID-QID/Enrofloxacin 5–10mg/kg slow IV SID

    b. Ampicillin 20 mg/kg slow IV TID-QID/Cefoxitin 20 mg/kg slow IV QID

    c. Ampicillin/Sublactam 50 mg/kg IV TID

3. All wounds over the thorax should be explored as described above (see Diagnostics). Surgical wound exploration is diagnostically useful to determine if wounds over the thorax penetrate the pleural space. Therapeutic goals of surgical exploration include the following:

    a. Debridement of damaged, diseased, or infected tissues

    b. Vigorous lavage

    c. Collection of specimens for culture and sensitivity testing to direct definitive antibiotic therapy

    d. Establishment of pleural drainage

    e. Closure of thoracic wall defect

    f. Establishment of thoracic wall drainage

    g. Closure of the soft tissue layers of the thoracic wall

4. Analgesia:

    a. Thoracic wall injuries are likely to be associated with significant patient discomfort.

    b. An aggressive analgesic protocol that addresses patient discomfort yet facilitates early movement is indicated.

5. Postoperative care routine for a major thoracic procedure is indicated:

    a. Thoracostomy tubes should be removed when the volume of pleural fluid is <5 mL/kg per day and the cytological characteristics of the fluid do not suggest evidence of ongoing infection.

    b. Thoracic wall drains can be removed when drainage decreases to what the clinician believes to be acceptable values.

    c. Additional postoperative care is directed toward the management of concurrent injuries.

  v. Monitoring:

    1. Once the thoracic wall defect is closed successfully, all monitoring is directed toward the management of concurrent injuries.

  vi. Prognosis:

    1. The prognosis for dogs and cats with penetrating thoracic injury is largely dictated by the presence and severity of concurrent injuries.

6. TRAUMA-ASSOCIATED CARDIAC INJURIES

a. Traumatic-associated cardiac arrhythmias:
  i. Definition and pathophysiology:
    1. Cardiac arrhythmias are common in the traumatized patient:
      a. Sinus tachycardia associated with hypovolemia, pain, stress, and other factors is most commonly recognized. Treatment is directed at the cause of the arrhythmia.
      b. Premature ventricular contractions, accelerated idioventricular rhythms, and ventricular tachycardia are widely recognized.
      c. Other arrhythmias may be identified in the trauma patient:
        i. Third-degree atrioventricular block
    2. Pathophysiology:
      a. Cardiac arrhythmias may result from direct blunt or penetrating trauma to the heart (myocardial contusion).
      b. Cardiac arrhythmias in the trauma patient may be seen associated with high sympathetic tone, hypoxemia, metabolic acidosis, or electrolyte disturbances (hypokalemia/hypomagnesemia).
      c. Cardiac arrhythmias may result secondary to ischemia-reperfusion injury.
      d. Arrhythmias may be identified acutely after trauma or in a more delayed fashion (12–36 hours post-trauma).
  ii. Clinical signs/physical examination and oxygenation assessment:
    1. Clinical signs:
      a. Most often, cardiac arrhythmias have few outward clinical signs beyond lethargy and depression. Severe arrhythmias may result in evidence of cardiovascular instability.
      b. Clinical signs relating to concurrent thoracic and other organ system injuries may be identified.
    2. Physical examination:
      a. Tachycardias and bradycardias may be identified through auscultation and concurrent palpation of peripheral pulses.
      b. Irregular cardiac rhythms on auscultation with concurrent pulse deficits most commonly suggest ventricular arrhythmias.
      c. Clinical signs of poor peripheral perfusion (pale mucous membranes, prolonged CRT, poor peripheral pulse quality, cool extremities) may be noted if the arrhythmia is affecting cardiac output.
    3. Oxygenation assessment:
      a. Because cardiac arrhythmias may result from hypoxemia, oxygen saturation, or arterial blood gas should be assessed and oxygen should be provided as needed to maintain $SpO_2 > 90\%$.
  iii. Diagnostics:
    1. Electrocardiography (ECG):
      a. Cardiac arrhythmias are definitively identified based on ECG.
  iv. Therapeutics:
    1. Ventricular arrhythmias:
      a. The decision to treat ventricular arrhythmias in the trauma patient is best based on the clinical effect of the arrhythmia, overall rate, perfusion status, and likelihood that the arrhythmia will degenerate into a terminal arrhythmia (ventricular fibrillation). Because prospective studies have not been performed to evaluate various treatment strategies, many treatment decisions are based on personal experience and opinion.
      b. Life-threatening ventricular arrhythmias should be treated immediately:
        i. Indications that a ventricular arrhythmia may be life threatening include the following:
          1. Rates > 180 bpm in dogs. Above 180 bpm, diastolic filling time and thus stroke volume and cardiac output are compromised. The author treats dogs with rates >140 bpm to minimize myocardial work and energy consumption as well as to facilitate patient comfort.
          2. R on T phenomena.

3. Arrhythmia that is compromising perfusion or causing hypotension.

4. Some believe multiform (arrhythmias that appear electrocardiographically different) and multifocal (arrhythmias originating at different sites) to be life-threatening. This requires further evaluation in the dog.

ii. Lidocaine:

  1. Dogs: 2 mg/kg IV bolus (repeated up to 3 times) followed by CRI at 40–80 μg/kg/min will control most ventricular arrhythmias.

  2. Cats: 0.5–0.8 mg/kg IV bolus (repeated up to 2 times) followed by a CRI at 10–40 μg/kg/min.

  3. Lidocaine can cause ataxia and seizures. Lidocaine-induced seizures should be treated with diazepam and should prompt cessation or dose modification of lidocaine therapy.

  4. Lidocaine can cause nausea and vomiting.

iii. After the patient has stabilized, evaluate as described in (c) below.

c. Evaluate for the presence of factors that could contribute to arrhythmias:

  i. Evaluate oxygenation. If hypoxemic, initiate oxygen therapy.

  ii. Evaluate acid-base status. Treat the underlying condition contributing to acid base abnormalities. For example, metabolic acidosis secondary to the generation of lactate and hydrogen ion implies decreased oxygen delivery to the tissues. Oxygen delivery to the tissues should be restored.

  iii. Evaluate blood pressure. Treat hypotension.

  iv. Evaluate electrolyte status. Acute electrolyte abnormalities are very uncommon in the trauma patient. However, electrolyte abnormalities may occur hours or days into management. Specifically evaluate for hypokalemia, hypomagnesemia, and hypocalcemia.

  v. Evaluate patient comfort. Pain can contribute to upregulation of the sympathetic nervous system. Appropriate analgesia should be provided as soon as possible.

d. Anti-arrhythmics for the management of ventricular tachycardia:

  i. Lidocaine (see above)

  ii. Procainamide:

    1. Ventricular arrhythmias refractory to lidocaine may respond to procainamide.

    2. Dog: 6–8 mg/kg over 1–2 minutes followed by 25–50 μg/kg/min CRI.

    3. Procainamide can cause hypotension when administered too rapidly.

  iii. Most trauma-associated cardiac arrhythmias respond well to lidocaine and procainamide. Additional pharmacologic considerations in refractory arrhythmias include the following:

    1. Esmolol: It is an ultra-short acting beta blocker. Side effects include decreased contractility, bradyarrhythmias, and bronchoconstriction, and the possibility of hypotension:

      a. 50–100 mcg/kg IV over 1 minute repeated up to 5 times. Then, CRI 50–200 mcg/kg/min.

    2. Amiodarone: It is a Class III antiarrhythmic commonly used to treat both ventricular and supraventricular arrhythmias. Side effects may be significant and include hypotension:

    3. Consultation with a veterinary cardiologist should be considered when animals have arrhythmias refractory to lidocaine and procainamide.

v. Monitoring:

  1. ECG:

    a. Continuous ECG monitoring should be performed on all

patients with arrhythmias after trauma.

b. Response:

    i. Complete resolution of trauma-associated cardiac arrhythmias is uncommon.

    ii. Rate control for ventricular tachyarrhythmias and elimination of life-threatening arrhythmias is the focus of therapy:

        1. Overall heart rate < 140 bpm (dog)

        2. No evidence of R on T

2. Monitoring for side effects associated with anti-arrhythmic therapy should be performed and medications adjusted as needed.

3. Additional monitoring as is appropriate for concurrent injuries.

vi. Prognosis:

    1. Most trauma-associated cardiac arrhythmias resolve over 3–5 days.

    2. Ultimate prognosis is dictated by the severity of concurrent injuries.

b. Traumatic pericardial effusion:

i. Definition and pathophysiology:

    1. Pericardial effusion refers to the accumulation of fluid in the pericardial space.

    2. Pericardial effusion is an exceedingly rare complication of blunt or penetrating thoracic trauma (Witt et al., 2000).

    3. Blunt trauma may result in atrial disruption or vascular disruption with secondary hemorrhage into the pericardial space.

    4. Cardiac tamponade occurs when intrapericardial pressure approaches and exceeds right-sided diastolic pressures. The results of cardiac tamponade are evidence of right-sided heart failure.

ii. Clinical signs/physical examination and oxygenation assessment:

    1. Clinical signs:

        a. No specific clinical signs of acute pericardial effusion will be evident immediately after trauma.

        b. Extreme lethargy and collapse may be identified.

2. Physical examination:

    a. Physical examination evidence of hemodynamic compromise will predominate. This includes pale mucous membranes, prolonged CRT, tachycardia, and decreased pulse quality. In addition, pulse quality may vary with the phase of respiration (pulsus paradoxus).

    b. Muffled heart sounds may be identified.

    c. Jugular venous distention may be noted. Hypovolemia is expected to be the cause of hemodynamic compromise in most trauma patients. Hypovolemia will cause flattening of the jugular veins. Cardiac tamponade will result in distended jugular veins +/− jugular pulses.

    d. Longer-standing cardiac tamponade (hours to days) will result in abdominal effusion.

iii. Diagnostics:

    1. Because pericardial effusion is an uncommon acute manifestation of trauma, it is not often suspected solely based on physical examination.

    2. Echocardiography:

        a. Echocardiography from the right cardiac notch will definitively identify the presence of pericardial effusion.

        b. A hypoechoic region surrounding the heart and bordered by the hyperechoic pericardium suggests pericardial effusion.

    3. ECG:

        a. Electrocardiographic manifestations of pericardial effusion include decreased QRS amplitude (<1 mV in dogs) and electrical alternans (alternating amplitude of R-wave from beat to beat).

    4. Coagulation assessment:

        a. All patients with pericardial effusion should have their ACT or PT/aPTT profiles evaluated. Coagulopathy can cause hemopericardium and the "suspected trauma patient" may not have sustained trauma after all.

iv. Therapeutics:

    1. Pericardiocentesis is the treatment of choice for stabilization of dogs with traumatic pericardial effusion:

    a. Pericardiocentesis will reveal non-clotting blood. In peracute pericardial effusion with ongoing bleeding, clotting blood may be retrieved from the pericardium.

    b. Pericardiocentesis may improve patient stability temporarily, however, hemorrhage may rapidly reaccumulate and puncture of the pericardium may facilitate leakage into the pleural space.

    c. The author prefers to place an indwelling pericardial drain using the Seldinger technique in dogs with pericardial effusion. The drain allows for ongoing decompression of the pericardium while definitive management is pursued. If a locking-loop multifenestrated drainage catheter is unavailable, a multilumen central venous catheter is an excellent substitute.

  2. Animals with traumatic pericardial effusion and ongoing hemorrhage will require emergency surgical intervention.

  v. Monitoring:

    1. Monitoring should focus on hemodynamic status. Heart rate is an excellent monitoring parameter for dogs with pericardial effusion. As effusion recurs, heart rate generally elevates.

    2. Repeat echocardiography will help identify additional fluid accumulations.

    3. Central venous pressure will increase as intrapericardial pressure increases (signaling increased fluid volume within the pericardium).

  vi. Prognosis:

    1. Traumatic pericardial effusion due to rupture of a coronary vessel or cardiac chamber carries a guarded prognosis. Surgical intervention will be necessary to attempt to save the patient's life.

7. TRAUMA-ASSOCIATED MEDIASTINAL INJURIES

  a. Tracheal avulsion:

    i. Definition and pathophysiology:

      1. Tracheal avulsion refers to the traumatic disruption of the trachea between the tracheal rings.

      2. Tracheal avulsion is hypothesized to occur due to a rapid hyperextension of the head and neck.

      3. Tracheal avulsion is more common in the cat than the dog (White and Burton, 2000).

      4. Tracheal avulsion in the cat most often occurs at the 2nd–4th intercostal space.

      5. Tracheal avulsion causes acute pneumomediastinum with a "pseudoairway" maintained via reflections of mediastinal tissue. Pneumothorax may also occur acutely.

      6. If tracheal avulsion is not diagnosed acutely, stenosis of the severed ends of the trachea occurs, resulting in fixed airway obstruction. These animals often present in severe respiratory distress several days after the initial traumatic insult.

    ii. Clinical signs/physical examination and oxygenation assessment:

      1. Clinical signs:

        a. Although a rare injury, acute dyspnea is observed in animals with tracheal avulsion.

        b. Pneumomediastinum may lead to subcutaneous emphysema.

        c. Clinical signs related to concurrent injuries may be identified.

      2. Physical examination:

        a. There are few physical examination findings directly attributable to tracheal avulsion.

        b. Animals with tracheal avulsion may demonstrate severe dyspnea. Appropriate sedation and analgesia should be utilized to facilitate atraumatic handling and diagnostic testing in these patients.

      3. Oxygenation assessment:

        a. Hypoxemia resulting from concurrent injuries may be seen acutely in animals with tracheal avulsion

        b. Hypoxemia secondary to hypoventilation may be seen in animals with longer-standing tracheal avulsion and airway obstruction.

    iii. Diagnostics:

      1. Radiography:

        a. Thoracic and cervical radiographs are generally adequate for the diagnosis of tracheal avulsion.

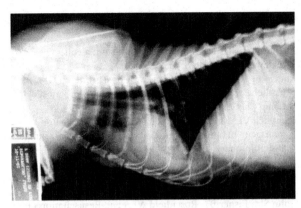

FIGURE 6.19 Tracheal avulsion in a cat. Note the discontinuation of the tracheal silhouette at the level of C7-T1.

b. Loss of continuity of the tracheal wall coupled with pneumomediastinum is consistent with tracheal avulsion (Figure 6.19).
2. Tracheoscopy:
    a. Tracheoscopy will facilitate the diagnosis of tracheal avulsion if survey radiography is not definitive. In addition, tracheoscopy may also facilitate intubation of the distal tracheal segment; see Therapeutics.
iv. Therapeutics:
    1. Anesthetic considerations and surgical considerations:
        a. Dogs and cats with tracheal avulsion are very high-risk anesthetic candidates.
        b. Most often, only the proximal tracheal segment can be intubated initially. Attempts to blindly intubate the distal segment may result in severe pneumomediastinum (due to disruption of the mediastinal reflections that are maintaining the airway), pneumothorax, and acute decompensation and death.
        c. A full surgical team should be on standby from the onset of anesthesia. The patient should be surgically clipped prior to anesthetic induction:
            i. The proximal tracheal segment should be intubated and the patient allowed to breathe normally ($FiO_2 = 1.0$).
            ii. Endoscopy-aided intubation of the distal segment was not successful in one series of cats due to the degree of stenosis or acute trauma to the proximal segment (White and Burton, 2000).
            iii. Rapid thoracotomy and intubation of the distal tracheal segment via the surgical site will allow for ventilatory support while the tracheal anastamosis is performed.
    2. Tracheal resection and anastamosis is the treatment of choice for dogs and cats with tracheal avulsion.
v. Monitoring:
    1. Monitoring of animals with tracheal avulsion is directed primarily toward the respiratory system. Indices of oxygenation along with respiratory rate and effort should be frequently assessed.
    2. Postoperative monitoring should proceed as is appropriate for any patient undergoing a major thoracic procedure.
vi. Prognosis:
    1. Animals with tracheal avulsion managed surgically had a very good prognosis in one case series (White and Burton, 2000). However, anesthesia and surgery are both technically challenging.
b. Mainstem bronchial rupture:
    i. Definition and pathophysiology:
        1. Left mainstem bronchial rupture has been reported in a cat (White and Oakley, 2001).
        2. Management is consistent with the management of animals with tracheal avulsion.
c. Pneumomediastinum:
    i. Definition and pathophysiology:
        1. Pneumomediastinum is the accumulation of air in the mediastinal space.
        2. Pneumomediastinum may occur secondary to a variety of injuries:
            a. Tracheal rupture.
            b. Tracheal avulsion.
            c. Other large airway rupture/avulsion.
            d. Esophageal disruption.
            e. Cervical lacerations. The subcutaneous space in the neck is continuous with the mediastinum.

f. Blebs. Air from blebs can track back into the mediastinum.

g. Pneumomediastinum is often seen concurrently with subcutaneous emphysema.

3. Pneumomediastinum is a radiographic finding that should prompt a search for concurrent injuries.

4. Tension pneumomediastinum is possible.

ii. Clinical signs/physical examination and oxygenation assessment:

1. Most clinical signs, physical examination findings, and hypoxemia are attributed to the underlying cause of pneumomediastinum and concurrent injuries.

iii. Diagnostics:

1. Thoracic radiographs reveal pneumomediastinum:

a. Pneumomediastinum gives negative contrast to the mediastinal space allowing for direct visualization of the aortic arch, brachycephalic trunk, tracheal and esophageal walls.

2. Radiographic evidence of pneumomediastinum should prompt a search for the underlying cause of pneumomediastinum:

a. Complete physical examination should evaluate for penetrating injury over the chest or cervical region.

b. Tracheoscopy to evaluate for tracheal and mainstem bronchial injury.

c. Esophagoscopy to evaluate for esophageal injury.

iv. Therapeutics:

1. Pneumomediastinum does not require specific treatment but can progress to pneumothorax. Treatment should be directed toward the underlying disease process.

v. Monitoring:

1. Pneumomediastinum does not require specific monitoring but can progress to pneumothorax. Monitoring should be directed toward the underlying disease process and the development of pneumothorax.

vi. Prognosis:

1. Prognosis for patients with pneumomediastinum is best dictated by the underlying disease process.

BIBLIOGRAPHY

Allen GS, Coates NE. Pulmonary contusion: a collective review. *Am Surg* 1998; 62: 895–900.

Anderson MA, Payne JT, Mann FA, Constantinescu GM. Flail chest: pathophysiology, treatment, and prognosis. *Comp Cont Ed Pract Vet* 1993; 15: 65–74.

Campbell VL, King LG. Pulmonary function, ventilator management, and outcome of dogs with thoracic trauma and pulmonary contusions: 10 Cases (1994–1998). *J Am Vet Med Assoc* 2000; 217: 1505–1508.

Cohn SM. Pulmonary contusion: review of the clinical entity. *J Trauma* 1997; 42: 973–979.

Cohn SM, Fisher BT, Rosenfield AT, et al. Resuscitation of pulmonary contusion: hypertonic saline is not beneficial. *Shock* 1997; 8 (4): 292–299.

Conzemius MG, Brockman DJ, King LG, Perkowski SZ. Analgesia in dogs after intercostal thoracotomy: a clinical trial comparing intravenous buprenorphine and interpleural bupivacaine. *Vet Surg* 1994; 23: 291–298.

Curcio K, Bidwell LA, Bohart GV, et al. Evaluation of signs of postoperative pain and complications after forelimb onychectomy in cats receiving buprenorphine alone or with bupivicaine administered as a four point regional nerve block. *J Am Vet Med Assoc* 2006; 228(1): 65–68.

Gibson TW, Brisson BA, Sears W. Perioperative survival rates after surgey for diaphragmatic hernia in dogs and cats: 92 cases (1990–2002). *J Am Vet Med Assoc* 2005; 227: 105–109.

Hackner SG. Emergency management of traumatic pulmonary contusions. *Comp Cont Ed Pract Vet* 1995; 17: 677–686.

Hodges CC, Fossum TW, Evering W. Evaluation of thoracic duct healing after experimental laceration and transection. *Vet Surg* 1993; 22 (6): 431–435.

Killeen KL, Mirvis SE, Shanmuganathan K. Helical CT of diaphragmatic rupture caused by blunt trauma. *Am J Roentgenol* 1999; 173 (6): 1611–1616.

Lipscomb VJ, Hardie RJ, Dubielzig RR. Spontaneous pneumothorax caused by pulmonary blebs and bullae in 12 dogs. *J Am Anim Hosp Assoc* 2003; 39 (5): 435–445.

Lisciandro GR, Mann KA, Voges AK, Lagutchick MS. Accuracy of focused assessment with sonography for trauma (FAST) to detect pneumothorax in 134 dogs with blunt and penetrating thoracic trauma. Abstracts of the 12th international VECC Symposium. 2006. San Antonio, TX.

McAnulty JF. A simplified method for stabilization of flail chest injuries in small animals. *J Am Anim Hosp Assoc* 1995; 31 (2): 137–141.

Nchimi A, Szapiro D, Ghaye B. Helical CT of blunt diaphragmatic rupture. *Am J Roentgenol* 2005; 184 (1): 24–30.

Olsen D, Renberg W, Perrett J, et al. Clinical management of flail chest in dogs and cats: a retrospective study of 24 cases (1989–1999). *J Am Anim Hosp Assoc* 2002; 38: 315–320.

Powell LL, Rozanski EA, Tidwell AS, Rush JE. A retrospective analysis of pulmonary contusion secondary to motor vehicular accidents in 143 dogs: 1994–1997. *J Vet Emerg Crit Care* 1999; 9: 127–136.

Sherman SC. Reexpansion pulmonary edema: a case report and review of the current literature. *J Emerg Med* 2003; 24 (1): 23–27.

Suter PF. Trauma to the thorax and cervical airways. *Thoracic Radiology of the Dog and Cat.* Switzerland: PF Suter, 1984; 130–151.

Sweet DC, Waters DJ. Role of surgery in the management of dogs with pathologic conditions of the thorax – Part II. *Comp Cont Ed Pract Vet* 1991; 13: 1671–1676.

Trinkle JK, Furman RW, Hinshaw MA, et al. Pulmonary contusion-pathogenesis and effect of various resuscitative measures. *Ann Thorac Surg* 1973; 16: 568–573.

Wagner RB, Crawford WO, Schimpf PP. Classification of parenchymal injuries of the lung. *Radiology* 1988; 167: 77–82.

White RN, Burton CA. Surgical management of intrathoracic tracheal avulsion in cats: long-term results in 9 consecutive cases. *Vet Surg* 2000; 29: 430–435.

White RN, Oakley MR. Left principal bronchus rupture in a cat. *J Small Anim Pract* 2001; 42 (10): 495–498.

Witt AL, Mathews KA, Holmberg DL. Successful management of traumatic right atrial rupture. *J Vet Eemrg Crit Care* 2000; 10: 85–89.

Zierold D, Lee SL, Subramanian S, et al. Supplemental oxygen improves resolution of injury-induced pneumothorax. *J Pediatr Surg* 2000; 35: 998–1001.

TRAUMATIC BRAIN INJURY

Rebecca S. Syring

1. INCIDENCE AND ETIOLOGY OF TRAUMATIC BRAIN INJURY IN CATS AND DOGS

a. The overall incidence of head trauma is not well studied in veterinary patients. However, in a large multi-center study of 191 cats and 1099 dogs with traumatic injuries, 42% of cats and 26% of dogs exhibited clinical signs of head trauma (Kolata, 1980).

b. At a large urban veterinary teaching hospital emergency room, the medical records of 290 dogs and cats were found to be coded with a diagnosis of head trauma during a 2-year period (Syring et al., 2001). This compromised approximately 1% of the total emergency service admissions during that time frame.

c. There are limited studies reporting morbidity or mortality rates in dogs and cats with head trauma and none that compare the effects of treatment regimens on outcome; therefore, the treatment recommendations of head injured dogs and cats has largely been extrapolated from information reported in experimental studies and human medicine:

  i. In a study of 52 dogs and 70 cats with clinical signs of head trauma, 73% of dogs and 74% of cats survived to hospital discharge (Syring et al., 2001). Several animals in this study were discharged prior to resolution of signs and subsequently lost to follow-up; therefore, these numbers may overestimate a good outcome by as much as 4% in dogs and 26% in cats.

  ii. In a retrospective study of 38 dogs with head injury, an 18% mortality rate was reported in the first 48 hours of treatment (Platt et al., 2001).

d. Etiology:

  i. Traumatic brain injury occurs secondary to both blunt and penetrating trauma.

  ii. Common causes of blunt trauma include vehicular trauma, acceleration-deceleration injury such as falling from a height or hitting a wall, and crushing injury such as being stepped upon or having something fall onto the animal.

  iii. Common causes of penetrating trauma include bite wounds, gunshot wounds, and miscellaneous projectile injury.

2. PATHOPHYSIOLOGY OF TRAUMATIC BRAIN INJURY

a. Primary injury:

  i. The injury incurred at the time of trauma as a result of the mechanical forces imparted to the brain.

  ii. Primary injury is often characterized by shearing or compressive forces to brain tissue (neurons, glial cells, and the vasculature) resulting in localized or diffuse injury:

Manual of Trauma Management in the Dog and Cat, First Edition. Edited by Kenneth J. Drobatz, Matthew W. Beal and Rebecca S. Syring.
© 2011 John Wiley & Sons, Inc. Published 2011 by John Wiley & Sons, Inc.

1. Concussion: characterized by a transient loss of consciousness following traumatic brain injury. No underlying pathology can be detected in the brain following a simple concussion.

2. Contusion: characterized by brain parenchymal hemorrhage, edema, and inflammation. The clinical signs associated with contusion may vary from mild to severe.

3. Diffuse axonal injury:

a. A microscopic injury to axons in the white matter as a result of shearing forces, associated with acceleration/deceleration, and rapid rotation of the head, applied to the brain at the time of trauma.

b. This type of injury is largely undetectable by advanced imaging and may be characterized microscopically by swollen and disconnected axons with mild injury and tears in the white matter with intraparenchymal hemorrhage in more severe cases.

c. Early posttraumatic coma is often associated with severe diffuse axonal injury, whereas more focal injuries often result in a progressive deterioration in neurological status. Alterations in mentation despite normal imaging studies should increase the suspicion for diffuse axonal injury.

4. Hematomas:

a. Epidural, subdural, or subarachnoid hemorrhage or intraparenchymal hemorrhage can occur following trauma resulting in compression of surrounding neural tissue and/or impaired regional blood flow:

i. Epidural hematomas arise between the skull and the dura mater—epidural hemorrhage usually occurs as a result of disruption of the meningeal vasculature (Figure 7.1).

ii. Subdural hematomas arise between the dura mater and brain tissue.

iii. Subarachnoid hemorrhage refers to blood accumulation between the

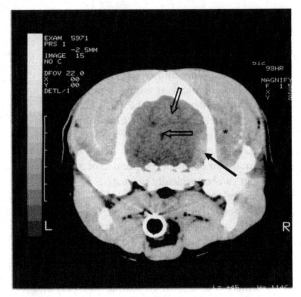

FIGURE 7.1 This computed tomography (CT) image was obtained from a young male dog who sustained blunt head injury secondary to vehicular trauma. This is a transverse image of the head at the level of the temporomandibular joint. A broad-based hyper-attenuating lesion is noted on the right lateral aspect of the brain (closed arrow), consistent with focal hemorrhage. The third ventricles are compressed and deviated toward the left (open arrows), as occurs with space occupying lesions. In addition, the hypo-attenuating signal in the temporalis muscle on the right (asterisk) likely represents edema. This dog was found to have an epidural hematoma that was evacuated at surgery and he recovered fully from the trauma. (Image used courtesy of Dr. Matthew W. Beal.)

arachnoid space and the pia mater. Traumatic subarachnoid hemorrhage is associated with a worse prognosis in humans.

iv. Both epidural and subdural hematomas can cause significant neurological deficits as a result of a global increase in intracranial pressure and focal hypoperfusion secondary to direct compression of brain parenchyma.

b. While focal hematomas have been traditionally considered uncommon in dogs and cats with head injury, more recent studies have reported an incidence of 10% in dogs with mild head injury (Platt et al., 2002) and in excess of 80%

in dogs and cats with severe head injury (Dewey et al., 1993).

5. Direct laceration of brain tissue as a result of compressed skull fractures or other penetrating injuries represents a very severe form of injury, resulting in physical disruption of neuronal tissue.

iii. There is often little that can be done medically to intervene and alter the course of primary injury, unless there is a skull fracture that can be surgically decompressed or a hematoma that can be surgically evacuated.

b. Secondary injury:

i. Secondary brain injury develops in the hours to days after the initial traumatic insult.

ii. As a result of the initial injury, damage to cell membranes and the surrounding brain tissues can perpetuate damage within the brain, which leads to a progressive brain injury and deterioration of clinical signs.

iii. Components of secondary brain injury:

1. Decreased cerebral oxygen delivery, as a result of decreased oxygen content in the blood or decreased cerebral blood flow, results in hypoxic or ischemic injury to the brain. This occurs either focally, as a result of vasospasm or focal injury, or globally, as a result of systemic hypotension or intracranial hypertension.

2. Tissue hypoxia and ischemia result in ATP depletion, leading to cell membrane pump failure. This leads to intracellular accumulation of sodium, water, and calcium, resulting in cerebral edema and ultimately cell death.

3. Glutamate and aspartate, two important excitatory amino acids, accumulate in the extracellular space as a result of cellular damage and decreased clearance by astrocytes. The presence of these amino acids extracellularly results in activation of a variety of neuronal receptors, exacerbation of cerebral edema, intracellular calcium accumulation, and increases the overall cerebral metabolic rate.

4. Intracellular calcium accumulation with cell membrane pump failure, liberation of free iron following hemorrhage, the potential for ischemia-reperfusion and the presence of high concentrations of lipid within the brain all contribute to the production of free radicals and oxidative injury, which further damages brain tissue.

5. Inflammatory mediators are produced in response to direct injury and secondary to hypoperfusion. These inflammatory mediators will cause an influx of inflammatory cells and activate the arachadonic acid and coagulation cascades, resulting in microvascular plugging, acceleration of oxidative injury, and microvascular thrombosis.

c. Early and aggressive management of the head injured animal should be aimed at minimizing the risk for development of progressive secondary brain injury:

i. Systemic derangements that can contribute to the risk for secondary brain injury include hypotension, hypoxia, hyperglycemia, hypoglycemia, hypercapnea, prolonged hypocapnea, hyperthermia, inflammation, and electrolyte or acid-base disturbances.

ii. Maintenance of cerebral oxygen delivery is probably the most important measure to limit secondary injury (see Chapter 3: Shock in the Trauma Patient, Figure 3.1).

iii. Cerebral oxygen delivery is dependent upon adequate cerebral blood flow (CBF) and adequate oxygen content in the circulation:

1. Maintenance of CBF:

a. CBF is a product of cerebral perfusion pressure (CPP) and cerebral vascular resistance.

b. In health, autoregulation of CBF ensures that blood flow to the brain is maintained over a wide range (50–150 mm Hg) of mean arterial blood pressure (MAP):

i. With head injury, autoregulation of blood flow may be impaired, resulting in a dependence upon MAP to maintain CBF. Approximately 30% of people with mild head injury and most people with severe head injury have impaired pressure autoregulation of blood flow (Bouma et al., 1992).

ii. When autoregulation of blood flow is impaired, CBF is directly related to arterial blood pressure. Hypotension and hypertension result in cerebral ischemia and hyperemia, respectively, in this scenario.

   c. Cerebral perfusion pressure (CPP):

   i. In health CPP = MAP – RAP, where MAP represents the mean arterial pressure and RAP represents the right atrial pressure.

   ii. When intracranial pressure is elevated above RAP, the following equation should be utilized: CPP = MAP – ICP.

   iii. Normal intracranial pressure is 5–12 mm Hg in cats and dogs.

   iv. Goal should be to maintain CPP at or above 50–70 mm Hg in order to maintain sufficient oxygen and nutrient delivery to the brain. While a CPP of 70 mm Hg is optimal, overly aggressive attempts to further increase CPP with fluids or vasopressors once the target range has been reached may increase the risk for acute lung injury (Brain Trauma Foundation, 2007).

   v. Since intracranial pressure is not measured in most veterinary patients, a normal MAP should be strived for in order to optimize CPP.

   2. Maintenance of adequate oxygen content is dependent upon hemoglobin saturation with oxygen (SaO_2), hemoglobin concentration, and dissolved oxygen concentration (PaO_2) (see Chapter 3: Shock in the Trauma Patient).

3. ASSESSMENT OF THE PATIENT WITH TRAUMATIC BRAIN INJURY

   a. Many patients with traumatic brain injury will have sustained additional injuries to other major body systems, such as the circulatory and respiratory systems, and/or injury to the contents of the abdomen or musculoskeletal system (see Chapter 1: Global Approach to the Trauma Patient).

   b. The initial assessment should focus on evaluation of the neurological, cardiovascular, and respiratory systems. Particular attention should be paid to the need for therapeutics to optimize systemic perfusion, maintain systemic blood pressure, and support adequate oxygenation and ventilation, as this may limit perpetuation of secondary brain injury (see Chapter 3: Shock in the Trauma Patient; Chapter 6: Trauma-Associated Thoracic Injury; Chapter 4: Monitoring of the Trauma Patient).

   c. Physical examination of the central nervous system:

   i. A limited neurological examination focusing upon level of consciousness, posture, pupil size, symmetry, and reactivity is sufficient for the primary survey prior to institution of stabilizing therapy. A more detailed examination, assessing all of the cranial nerves, gait, and postural reactions can be performed after patient stabilization.

   ii. Level of consciousness:

   1. Alterations in the level of consciousness to an animal following trauma may be indicative of injury to the brain. It is important to recognize that cardiovascular collapse, secondary to massive hemorrhage, or other reasons for shock, may also alter the level of consciousness. Therefore, level of consciousness should be reassessed following volume resuscitation and resolution of shock (see Chapter 3: Shock in the Trauma Patient).

   2. Classifying level of consciousness:

      a. Alert: a normal level of mentation

      b. Depressed: mentation is diminished from normal but aware of things occurring in the environment.

      c. Obtunded: markedly decreased level of consciousness, resulting in a general lack of awareness to things occurring in the environment, but the animal is able to respond to noise and touch.

      d. Stuporous: markedly decreased level of consciousness wherein animal is responsive only to noxious stimuli.

      e. Comatose: unresponsive to repeated noxious stimuli.

   iii. Posture:

   1. Opisthotonus: the presence of an extended (dorsiflexed) head and neck.

   2. Decerebrate (Decorticate) rigidity/ posturing:

      a. It is characterized by a decreased level of consciousness, opisthotonus, and extensor rigidity of all four legs.

b. Decerebrate posturing indicates a rostral brainstem lesion or any brain lesion resulting in brainstem compression and may be seen with significant intracranial hypertension and herniation. It is associated with a guarded prognosis.

c. It is important to differentiate decerebrate posturing from the Schiff-Sherrington posture:

    i. Schiff-Sherrington posture is associated with T3-L3 spinal lesions.

    ii. These animals will exhibit hypertonic front limbs and flaccid paresis of the hind limbs.

    iii. These animals will have a normal level of consciousness and cranial nerve examination so long as they are not hypovolemic nor have concurrent traumatic brain injury.

3. Decerebellate rigidity/posturing:

    a. It is characterized by extensor rigidity of the front limbs, opisthotonus, and the presence flexed hindlimbs at the coxofemoral joint with normal tone (Figure 7.2).

    b. These animals tend to be responsive unless concurrent injury is present elsewhere in the brain, as the cerebellum is not required for maintenance of consciousness.

    c. Decerebellate posturing is associated with cerebellar disease, such as cerebellar herniation as seen with intracranial hypertension.

iv. Pupils:

    1. Pupil symmetry:

      a. Differences in resting pupil size is termed anisocoria.

      b. An attempt should be made to discern which pupil is abnormal (i.e., is one pupil too dilated or is the other pupil too constricted). This will help to ascertain the reason for anisocoria.

    2. Pupil size:

      a. Miosis:

        i. Miosis usually indicates a forebrain injury, such as injury to the thalamus/hypothalamus where the sympathetic pathways originate.

        ii. Miosis also occurs with Horner's syndrome originating from extracranial injuries, such as a cervical spinal cord lesion or brachial plexus injury. Other signs of Horner's, such as ptosis, enophthalmos, or elevation of the third eyelid will often be present to help differentiate miosis related to Horner's syndrome from other injuries. In addition, neck pain and/or ataxia, paresis, or paralysis may be noted in the hindlimbs or all four limbs with cervical lesions, while decreased sensation and/or ability to move one front limb may be noted with brachial plexus injuries (see Chapter 9: Traumatic Spinal Injury and Chapter 8: Trauma-Associated Peripheral Nerve Injury).

        iii. Miosis also occurs with traumatic uveitis. Other signs of traumatic uveitis include blepharospasm, aqueous flare, and possibly hyphema in the anterior chamber (see Chapter 15: Trauma-Associated Ocular Injury).

        iv. Superficial corneal abrasions and ulcers may cause ciliary spasm resulting in miosis as well.

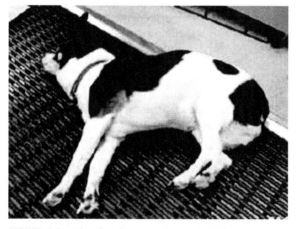

FIGURE 7.2 This dog demonstrates decerebellate posturing. Note the extended head and neck, increased tone in the front legs, and flexion of the hindlimbs at the coxofemoral joints. This dog was alert and aware of his surroundings.

b. Midrange:

    i. While seemingly normal, midrange pupils should always be assessed for responsiveness to light.

    ii. A midrange pupil that responds appropriately to light is normal.

    iii. A midrange pupil that is not responsive to light indicates a lesion in the brainstem (pons or medulla). It is important to note that the presence of a midrange unresponsive pupil is almost as grave as a fixed and dilated pupil.

c. Mydriasis:

    i. Mydriasis with weak or absent pupillary light response may indicate damage to the midbrain where the oculomotor nerve (cranial nerve III) originates:

        1. In this scenario, altered mentation should be noted, because of the close proximity to the reticular activating system that controls level of consciousness.

        2. If present without alterations in mentation, other reasons for a dilated unresponsive pupil should be considered, such as blindness secondary to retinal damage, cataracts, etc.

        3. Fixed and dilated pupils are associated with a poor prognosis and may be noted with direct trauma (such as focal hemorrhage) or secondary to herniation as a result of intracranial hypertension.

    ii. Pupillary dilation often occurs secondary to catecholamine release associated with critical injuries, even in the absence of head trauma. This is commonly seen in sick or stressed cats. In these animals, pupillary constriction should be present when a very bright light source is used to illuminate the eye.

3. Pupillary light response (PLR):

    a. In response to a bright light shined into one eye, both the ipsilateral (direct response) and contralateral eye (consensual response) should respond by constricting the pupil.

    b. Pupillary constriction is mediated by cranial nerve III (oculomotor nerve).

    c. An intact PLR requires that the following reflex arc be intact:

        i. The retina in that eye functions sufficiently to recognize the light.

        ii. Impulse travels up the optic nerve.

        iii. Crosses over at the optic chiasm to the contralateral side of the brain.

        iv. Travels up the contralateral optic tract.

        v. Optic tract ends at the contralateral pretectal nucleus in the midbrain.

        vi. Pretectal nucleus sends out axons to the Edinger–Westphal nucleus, which runs along both oculomotor (CN III) nerves.

        vii. Oculomotor nerve axons run back to the eyes, where they synapse with the ciliary ganglion that mediates constriction of the iris.

    d. Interpretation of an absent PLR:

        i. The PLR should always be assessed after hemodynamic resuscitation, as shock can impair PLR.

        ii. Unilateral optic nerve damage:

            1. The direct PLR is absent in the eye with optic nerve damage; the contralateral eye does not have a consensual PLR.

            2. The direct PLR is present in the contralateral eye (the unaffected eye) and a normal indirect PLR should be present.

        iii. Unilateral oculomotor nerve damage:

            1. The direct PLR is absent when light is shown in the affected eye but a normal indirect PLR is present.

            2. The direct PLR will be present in the unaffected eye but the indirect PLR will be absent.

4. When direct ocular injury or preexisting ocular pathology can be excluded (see Chapter 15: Trauma-Associated

Ocular Injury), interpretation of pupil size and reactivity can provide information regarding prognosis following head trauma:

a. The presence of an intact PLR, even when miosis is present, indicates that that the retina, optic nerve, optic chiasm, optic tract, and rostral brainstem functions normally. Miosis usually indicates a forebrain injury, such as injury to the thalamus/hypothalamus where the sympathetic pathways originate.

b. Transition of pupils from miosis toward mydriasis indicates a progressive injury to the brainstem. This is suggestive of either ongoing hemorrhage or development of intracranial hypertension, resulting in brainstem compression and possibly herniation.

c. Following resuscitation, the presence of bilateral mydriasis with an absent PLR is associated with a poor outcome (death or a persistent vegetative state) in 70–90% of humans with severe head injury. Conversely, only 30% of humans with severe head injury who exhibit bilateral reactive pupils following resuscitation have a poor outcome (Moppett, 2007).

5. Physiologic nystagmus (oculocephalic response):

a. Sometimes referred to as the "doll's eye" reflex.

b. Refers to the normal tracking motion of the eyes in response to movement of the head from side to side.

c. A normal response should consist of slow tracking of the eye away from the direction that the head is being moved, followed by fast tracking of the eye toward the direction that the head is being moved.

d. Absence of physiological nystagmus often signals a brainstem injury with damage to the vestibular nuclei (CN VIII) or the cranial nerves that control the extraocular muscles (CN III, IV, VI), all of which interconnect in the brainstem.

e. Care should be taken to move the entire body, rather than just moving the head and neck, when performing this test in animals if there is any concern that concurrent neck injury may be present.

d. Physical examination findings that may indicate the potential for traumatic brain injury:

i. Scleral hemorrhage.

ii. Aural hemorrhage: Aural hemorrhage is often indicative of injury to the petrosal bone and underlying neural tissue.

iii. Epistaxis.

iv. Proptosed eye/eyes: Proptosis is often associated with skull and brain injuries in cats and dogs with mesocephalic or dolichocephalic conformation because of the degree of force required to proptose the eye in animals with this facial conformation. Conversely, brachycephalic animals are more likely to sustain proptosis without significant underlying injuries (see Chapter 15: Trauma-Associated Ocular Injury).

v. Swollen head/face.

vi. Facial/oral fractures (see Chapter 16: Trauma-Associated Musculoskeletal Injury to the Head).

vii. Bradycardia and hypertension (The Cushing's Reflex):

1. This response is seen with intracranial hypertension that is causing decreased perfusion to the vasomotor center.

2. As intracranial pressure increases, blood flow is impaired to the brain.

3. The vasomotor center of the brain senses decreased perfusion and emits a sympathetic response.

4. This catecholamine surge results in massive peripheral vasoconstriction to improve cerebral perfusion.

5. Massive vasoconstriction results in hypertension.

6. The increased blood pressure is sensed at the baroreceptors, resulting in a reflex bradycardia.

7. Treatment of hypertension with concurrent bradycardia in a head injured animal should focus on lowering intracranial pressure (see below) and helping optimize MAP, rather than using pharmacologic agents to increase heart rate or lower blood pressure.

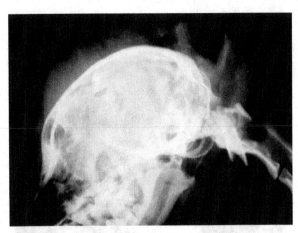

FIGURE 7.3 This lateral radiograph of the skull is from a dog that had been bitten on the head. On examination, a puncture wound was noted on the dorsal aspect of the head between the ears and discontinuity could be palpated over the skull. A large depressed skull fracture can be noted in the temporal bone.

4. DIAGNOSTIC IMAGING

  a. Skull radiographs (Figures 7.3 and 7.4a):

    i. Radiographs of the skull in head trauma patients are an insensitive diagnostic tool and rarely provide valuable information. They occasionally help detect depressed skull fractures (though many are missed with radiographs) and can help to provide information of concurrent maxillofacial and mandibular injuries.

    ii. Frequently, people and animals will have skull fractures but no evidence of underlying brain injury. More importantly, the radiographic absence of fractures does not rule out the presence of significant brain injury.

    iii. If a depressed skull fracture is noted on radiographs, broad-spectrum systemic antibiotics should be administered and surgical decompression should be considered.

  b. Advanced imaging:

    i. Advanced imaging will allow the clinician to rule in or out a significant mass lesion (epidural, subdural, or intraparenchymal hemorrhage), cerebral edema, herniation, or depressed skull fractures as contributing to the clinical signs.

    ii. Advanced imaging should be considered in any patient with moderate to severe head trauma on presentation, patients with lateralizing clinical signs, and in those patients who fail to improve or demonstrate deterioration during treatment.

    iii. Computed Tomography (CT scan) (Figure 7.4b):

      1. CT is superior to magnetic resonance imaging (MRI) for imaging of bone (to characterize fractures and dislocations) and for identifying hemorrhage or edema within the first 24 hours of injury.

      2. CT is more readily available, less expensive, performed more rapidly, and allows for better monitoring of the patient under anesthesia compared to MRI.

      3. CT findings that are associated with a worse prognosis in human patients with traumatic brain injuries include the presence of a midline shift, compression of the basal cisterns, and subarachnoid hemorrhage (Moppett, 2007).

      4. CT abnormalities were detected in 9 out of 10 dogs with clinical signs of mild head trauma (characterized as a modified Glasgow coma scale score of 15–18 on admission). The abnormalities detected in these dogs included skull fractures, hydrocephalus, parenchymal damage, hemorrhage, and an epidural hematoma (Platt et al., 2002).

    iv. Magnetic Resonance Imaging (MRI):

      1. MRI provides the most superior imaging detail of the neuroanatomy and is an excellent tool for detecting cerebral pathology.

      2. 48–72 hours after trauma, MRI becomes superior to CT for the detection of intracranial damage, such as maturing hematomas, axonal injury, and subtle neuronal injuries in humans (Lee and Newberg, 2005).

5. TREATMENT OF TRAUMATIC BRAIN INJURY

  a. Extracranial stabilization:

    i. Oxygenation:

      1. Oxygen supplementation should be considered for all patients with traumatic brain injury until you can prove that it is not needed, because of the risk for perpetuation of secondary brain injury when hypoxemia is present:

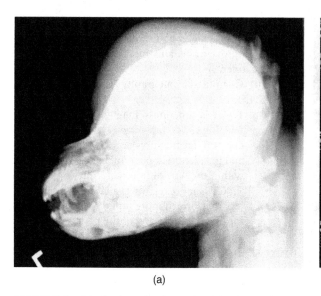

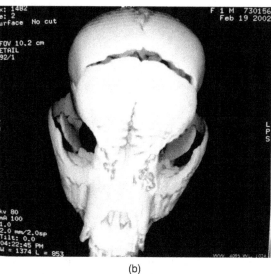

(a)   (b)

FIGURE 7.4 (a) This lateral radiograph of the skull is from a puppy who sustained head trauma after getting stuck in a recliner chair. Soft tissue swelling can be noted between the skull and skin over the dorsal aspect of the skull. A wide fracture is also noted over the temporal bone. (b) This puppy had a computed tomography (CT) scan of his brain. His brain was found to be normal on CT. Three-dimensional reconstruction of the CT scan in a bone window demonstrates the extent of the nondisplaced fracture along the suture line.

1. Oxygen can be supplemented non-invasively by face mask/flow-by or by placement into an oxygen cage. As many animals with head injury have decreased levels of consciousness, flow-by oxygen with a face mask is often well tolerated and will allow greater access to that animal than if it were in an oxygen cage.

2. Oxygen can also be supplied by more invasive routes, such as nasal insufflation or even intubation when necessary. Be aware that nasal insufflation should be avoided if it causes irritation and sneezing, as this may increase intracranial pressure.

2. Oxygen supplementation is absolutely required in any animal with a $PaO_2 < 60$ mm Hg, or an $SpO_2 < 92\%$.

3. Optimal goals of oxygen supplementation should be to maintain $PaO_2 > 80$ mm Hg, or an $SpO_2 > 96\%$.

ii. Ventilation:

1. Maintenance of ventilation is important in animals with head injury:

a. Hypoventilation will increase $PaCO_2$, which causes a respiratory acidosis.

b. In response to changes in pH, central chemoreceptors in the brain will alter cerebral blood flow, a process known as chemical autoregulation:

i. In the presence of acute acidosis (hypoventilation), cerebral vasculature will dilate and increase cerebral blood flow. This could increase intracranial pressure or result in cerebral hyperemia.

ii. In the presence of acute alkalosis (hyperventilation), cerebral vasculature will constrict and decrease cerebral blood flow. This could decrease intracranial pressure or worsen cerebral ischemia.

2. While monitoring of physical examination parameters such as respiratory rate and depth of thoracic excursions may aid in detection of hypoventilation, measurement of arterial PCO_2 is the optimal method to monitor ventilation.

3. Optimally, $PaCO_2$ should be maintained between 30 and 40 mm Hg. If $PaCO_2$ exceeds 45 mm Hg, methods to increase ventilation should be considered:

   a. Hypoventilation could be a result of direct trauma to the brain or could result from any of the following: thoracic pain (i.e., rib fractures), severe pulmonary (i.e., pulmonary contusion), pleural space disease, excessive sedation, or upper airway obstruction (i.e., swelling, hemorrhage, etc.).

   b. Correcting the underlying cause may improve ventilation:

      i. Analgesics should be given if thoracic pain is suspected.

      ii. Thoracocentesis could be considered if pneumothorax or pleural effusion is suspected.

      iii. Reversal of sedatives may be needed.

      iv. Tracheostomy to by-pass an upper airway obstruction may be required.

   c. Alternatively, intubation and manual/mechanical ventilation may be required until the underlying disorder can be corrected or when a quick fix is not obvious.

  iii. Perfusion:

   1. Optimization of systemic perfusion is key to the successful management of the head injured patient. Fluid therapy is usually the first line of therapy in order to improve cerebral perfusion pressure (CPP) in head injured patients. Restriction of intravenous fluids, for fear that they might increase intracranial pressure, is absolutely contraindicated.

   2. Intravenous fluids:

      a. There is no solid evidence in human medicine that any one type of fluid is superior to another for resuscitation of the patient with head trauma. Rather than focusing on the type of fluid to be used for resuscitation, the focus should be on optimizing perfusion rapidly such that cerebral perfusion pressure (CPP) is restored such that cerebral oxygen delivery is maintained (Brain Trauma Foundation, 2007).

      b. Isotonic crystalloids:

         i. Examples: 0.9% NaCl and balanced electrolyte solutions, such as Normosol-R (Hospira Inc., Lake Forest, IL).

         ii. Because 0.9% NaCl has a higher sodium concentration than the balanced electrolyte solutions, some prefer its use in head-injured patients, as water will be retained in the vasculature proportional to the amount of sodium in the solution. This may help to reduce brain water concentrations.

         iii. Isotonic crystalloids should be dosed to restore euvolemia as quickly as possible, correct dehydration over 12 hours, and provide for maintenance needs and ongoing losses (see Chapter 3: Shock in the Trauma Patient).

      c. Hypertonic crystalloids:

         i. Hypertonic saline, at concentrations of 7.0–7.8%, has several attractive properties for use in head trauma patients:

            1. Because of its hypertonicity, a much smaller volume of fluid is needed for restoration of euvolemia compared to isotonic solutions. This means that CPP may be restored more quickly with this type of fluid.

            2. Hypertonic saline solutions may help to decrease cerebral edema, similar to mannitol, by increasing the osmotic pressure in the vasculature, which will pull fluid from the interstitial and intracellular spaces. Hypertonic saline may be superior to mannitol when hypovolemia is present, as mannitol will ultimately cause an osmotic diuresis and can worsen hypovolemia.

            3. Hypertonic saline has been shown to minimize vasospasm, promote local vasodilation, and limit endothelial cell swelling.

These effects may promote micro-circulatory blood flow in the injured brain, thus improving local oxygen and nutrient delivery to maintain aerobic metabolism.

4. Hypertonic saline has been shown to have neurochemical effects that may help to decrease excitotoxicity and intracellular accumulation of calcium:

    a. With head injury and progressive secondary injury, massive neuronal depolarization and cell membrane pump failure related to ATP depletion occurs.

    b. As a result, glutamate, an excitatory amino acid that is primarily located within the intracellular space, leaks and accumulates extracellularly.

    c. Cell membrane pump failure results in decreased extracellular sodium, which promotes intracellular calcium accumulation. Both of these processes promote cell death.

    d. Administration of hypertonic saline helps to increase extracellular sodium concentrations and restores concentration gradients such that calcium is returned to the extracellular space and glutamate to the intracellular space, thus limiting secondary injury and neuronal death.

5. Hypertonic saline solutions may decrease inflammation, a perpetuator of secondary brain injury, by limiting leukocyte adhesion and migration. Decreasing inflammation may also limit oxidative injury and activation of the coagulation cascade.

  ii. See Chapter 3: Shock in the Trauma Patient for a more detailed discussion of the dosing of hypertonic saline solutions.

  d. Colloids:

    i. Artificial colloids, such as hydroxyethyl starches or dextran-70, can be considered in the head-injured patient for more rapid resuscitation (because of the smaller volume required for resuscitation), prolonged duration of volume expansion, and its potential to limit cerebral edema formation. There is no evidence that artificial colloids are superior to isotonic crystalloids in head injured patients (see Chapter 3: Shock in the Trauma Patient).

    ii. Human serum albumin:

      1. A post hoc analysis of a recent study in critically ill humans revealed that resuscitation with 4% human serum albumin significantly increased mortality (33.2%) compared to resuscitation with 0.9% NaCl (20.4%) in patients with traumatic brain injury (SAFE Study Investigators, 2007).

      2. It is not known why albumin was associated with increased mortality rates in this patient population.

  iv. Blood pressure:

    1. Systolic blood pressure should be maintained above 90 mm Hg:

      a. Systolic blood pressure can be monitored directly with an indwelling arterial catheter or noninvasively via oscillometry or Doppler ultrasonography (see Chapter 4: Monitoring of the Trauma Patient).

      b. It is commonly believed that the blood pressure obtained via Doppler ultrasonography represents the systolic blood pressure.

      c. If blood pressure cannot be maintained above 90 mm Hg despite repletion of volume deficits with intravenous fluids, then vasopressors (i.e., dopamine, norepinephrine, etc.) should be considered. It is absolutely critical that adequate volume expansion be ensured prior to pressor administration.

  b. Intracranial stabilization:

    i. Therapies to decrease intracranial pressure:

      1. Decrease brain volume:

a. Osmotic agents:
  i. Mannitol:
    1. Mannitol has two main mechanisms of action, as a rheologic agent and as an osmotic diuretic, both of which are beneficial to patients with traumatic brain injury:
      a. Immediately after intravenous administration, mannitol increases plasma volume, which reduces the hematocrit and blood viscosity. Decreased viscosity improves cerebral blood flow and oxygen delivery. This effect is short-lived and noted within the first few minutes of administration.
      b. Within 15–20 minutes of administration, mannitol exerts its mechanism of action by drawing fluid into the intravascular space from cells and interstitium as a result of its hyperosmolarity. This helps to reduce cerebral edema.
    2. The osmotic effect of mannitol is proportional to the dose administered, and it is thought that higher doses cause a greater effect:
      a. The recommended dose of mannitol ranges from 0.25 to 1.4 g/kg given as an intravenous infusion over 15–20 minutes. The author prefers doses of 1.0–1.4 g/kg but will use lower doses when concerns for volume depletion are present. An effect should be noted within 20–40 minutes of administration.
      b. A positive response to mannitol might include resolution of the cushing's reflex, improved mentation, posture, or return of PLR or pupil size toward normal. Lack of a response or a negative response to mannitol should preclude its continued use.
    c. Mannitol should not be given as a constant rate infusion over several hours nor should it be diluted, as this will limit its efficacy by reducing the osmotic gradient generated between the vascular and the brain tissue.
    d. Mannitol, in concentrations above 15%, readily crystallizes. Therefore, the bottle should be closely inspected prior to administration and an in-line 0.22 micron filter can be used to reduce the risk for infusion of crystals. Keeping bottles warmed (35–40°C) in a water bath or incubator may help to prevent crystal formation.
    e. Mannitol is also purported to have free radical scavenging properties, which may help to reduce oxidative injury in the brain. Evidence regarding mannitol's ability to scavenge free radicals in head injury is lacking.
    3. The most profound side effect of mannitol administration is the development of an osmotic diuresis, which causes free water loss:
      a. Mannitol should be given on an "as needed" basis, rather than being written as an automatic treatment order. No more than 3 doses of mannitol should be given in a 24-hour period. In the author's experience, most animals will need only one or two doses of mannitol.
      b. Placement of a urinary catheter may be necessary in recumbent animals and quantification of urine output should be performed in order to keep up with ongoing losses.
      c. Serum sodium concentrations should be monitored, at least once daily, during mannitol administration to assess for

hypernatremia and the need for alteration in fluid therapy.

4. Mannitol should be used with caution in animals with concurrent hypovolemia, as it will cause an osmotic diuresis, which will worsen hypovolemia and therefore compromise cerebral perfusion pressure. The patient should be fully volume expanded before considering use of mannitol. If an agent is needed to lower intracranial pressure before the animal is fully volume expanded, then hypertonic saline should be considered.

5. Some people advocate the use of furosemide (0.5–1.0 mg/kg IV) prior to mannitol. The reasoning behind this recommendation is that furosemide can induce a transient vasodilation, which may blunt the initial rise in ICP due to intravascular volume expansion that mannitol may cause prior to the onset of an osmotic diuresis. In addition, the two agents together cause a synergistic diuretic effect. With that being said, the risk for volume depletion is greater when furosemide is administered with mannitol and therefore its routine use is not recommended.

6. The potential risk that mannitol may increase intracranial bleeding probably does NOT outweigh global benefit to the brain.

ii. Hypertonic saline (7.0–7.8%):

1. In the presence of hypovolemia, hypertonic saline should be considered when an osmotic agent is desired to decrease intracranial pressure. This fluid will help to volume expand the animal and reduce cerebral edema.

2. A dose of 3–5 mL/kg has been recommended for use in dogs (2–3 mL/kg for cats) for volume expansion. Lower doses may be acceptable when using this fluid to lower intracranial pressure. This fluid should be administered no faster than 1 mL/kg/minute and the author usually gives the dose over 8–10 minutes.

3. A lower concentration of hypertonic saline (3%) has been investigated as a continuous infusion in children (0.1–1.0 mL/kg infusion) with refractory intracranial hypertension with some success (Adelson, 2003).

b. Corticosteroids:

i. There is no evidence available in veterinary medicine to support or refute the use of corticosteroids in head-injured animals. Therefore, one must look to human clinical medicine for guidelines.

ii. The Brain Trauma Foundation issued their strongest recommendation against the use of corticosteroids in human patients with traumatic brain injury. They concluded that there is no evidence in human medicine that the use of corticosteroids improves outcome or lowers intracranial pressure. (Brain Trauma Foundation, 2007).

iii. A prospective clinical trial involving over 10,000 human patients with moderate to severe traumatic brain injury demonstrated that high-dose methylprednisolone (2 g/person IV followed by 0.4 mg/h for 48 hours) was associated with an increased mortality rate. The reason for increase in mortality rate among those patients who received corticosteroids was unclear, but was not related to increased rate of infections nor gastrointestinal bleeding (Roberts et al., 2004).

iv. Not only is there a general lack of evidence that corticosteroids are useful in head injury, the following well-documented untoward side effects in veterinary patients, precludes their use in animals with head trauma:

1. Insulin resistance promoting hyperglycemia

2. Gastrointestinal bleeding

3. Perpetuation of a catabolic state

4. Decreased wound healing

5. Immunosuppression

c. Others:

  i. 21-Aminosteroids (Lazaroids; i.e., Tirilazad mesylate):

    1. Initial experimental evidence demonstrated that 21-aminosteroids were more effective than glucocorticoids in traumatic brain injury and that they did not possess the same untoward side effects of glucocorticoids (Hall, 1992).

    2. Two human clinical studies in head trauma failed to show a beneficial effect on outcome (Kassal, 1996; Marshall et al., 1998).

    3. These products have never been made available for commercial use and it does not appear that there are any plans for their marketing in the near future.

  ii. DMSO, desferoxamine, allupurinol, and other agents have been used in the management of head injury for their free-radical scavenging properties. There are no clinical studies, in animals or people, to support or refute their use.

2. Decrease brain blood volume:

a. Elevate head and neck (Figure 7.5):

  i. Elevation of the head and neck 15–30° above the posterior half of the body can be used to facilitate venous outflow from the brain. This may help to decrease blood volume in the brain and thereby decrease intracranial pressure.

  ii. Care should be taken to avoid kinking of the neck, which may occlude the jugular vein, not only defeating the purpose of the maneuver, but also having the potential to increase intracranial pressure.

  iii. Elevation of the head and neck to an angle greater than 30° is not recommended, as this can impede

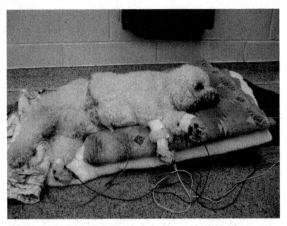

FIGURE 7.5 A dog with head trauma and altered mentation is placed with his head and neck elevated to a 15–30° angle. Note that a board was placed underneath the blankets that the dog was laying upon and the board was elevated, so that the degree of elevation occurred in a uniform plane. This dog is attached to a continuous ECG and has an indwelling urinary catheter connected to a closed collection system in place to allow for the dog better monitoring.

arterial inflow into the brain, thereby impairing cerebral oxygen delivery and worsening secondary injury.

  iv. Elevation of the head and neck should be performed after volume resuscitation in hypovolemic patients.

b. Hyperventilation:

  i. Mild hyperventilation ($PaCO_2$ 30–35 mm Hg) can be used to temporarily lower intracranial pressure. As $PaCO_2$ decreases, the resulting alkalosis will cause vasoconstriction of the cerebral vasculature, which may help to reduce intracranial pressure through a decrease in the brain blood volume.

  ii. Excessive or prolonged hyperventilation to $PaCO_2$ concentrations below 30 mm Hg may be harmful, as vasoconstriction may potentiate cerebral ischemia and worsen secondary injury:

    1. The Brain Trauma Foundation recommends that hyperventilation not be used in the first 24 hours following traumatic brain

injury in humans because of the global reduction in cerebral blood flow often noted during this time frame. (Brain Trauma Foundation, 2007).

   iii. The effect that hyperventilation has on the cerebral vasculature is transient in nature. Once the pH change has been buffered in the brain, the effect will be negated. Therefore, the therapeutic use of hyperventilation should be limited to short periods of time (i.e., < 1 hour) when acute decompensation is life-threatening.

ii. Therapies to decrease cerebral metabolic rate (CMR):

  1. Seizure prophylaxis:

   a. Seizure activity increases cerebral metabolic rate directly by neuronal activation and indirectly by increasing body temperature.

   b. Early posttraumatic seizures (within 7 days of injury) have been noted in 4–25% of people following head injury (Tempkin et al., 1991) prompting the frequent use prophylactic anticonvulsant therapy in humans. The incidence of early posttraumatic seizures in veterinary patients has not been documented.

   c. While prophylactic anticonvulsant therapy is not recommended in dogs and cats, if seizures are noted in the traumatized patient, they should be treated aggressively:

    i. Valium or midazolam (0.25–0.50 mg/kg IV) can be used to stop any ongoing seizure activity.

    ii. Rapid intravenous loading with an anticonvulsant should be performed. The author recommends 4 mg/kg of Phenobarbital IV every 30 minutes to 2 hours for a total of 4 doses to achieve therapeutic concentrations within 2–8 hours. During loading, any break through seizures should be treated with valium or midazolam.

  2. Sedation and analgesia:

   a. Pain and fear can result in agitation, increased motor activity, and vocalization.

These can increase body temperature and may contribute to increases in intracranial pressure.

   b. While sedatives may alter the neurological examination by decreasing level of consciousness, it is thought that the beneficial effects of sedation outweigh this fact.

   c. Care should be taken to avoid drugs that may cause refractory hypotension (i.e., acepromazine) or may increase cerebral metabolic rate (i.e., ketamine).

   d. While concern exists that opioids cause respiratory depression, which could result in hypercarbia and increased intracranial pressure, dogs and cats are much less sensitive to the respiratory depressant effects compared to humans. Pure opioid agonists (i.e., hydromorphone, fentanyl) should be used in head-trauma patients and the dose should be titrated to effect. The use of partial agonist/antagonists (i.e., Butorphanol or Buprenorphine) should be used with caution as these agents are more difficult to reverse with naloxone should respiratory depression be a problem.

   e. See Chapter 5: Analgesia and Anesthesia for the Trauma Patient.

  3. Body temperature:

   a. Increases in body temperature will result in increased cerebral metabolic rate. Care should be taken to avoid hyperthermia.

   b. Prophylactic hypothermia (32–33°C; 90–92°F) has been investigated in human medicine as a way to reduce cerebral metabolic rate and therefore limit secondary neurologic injury.

   c. While controlled hypothermia has not been investigated in veterinary patients, the author suggests that aggressive rewarming (i.e., forced air or circulating water blankets) should be avoided in animals who are cardiovascularly stable for risk that hyperthermia may result if the rewarming device is not removed in a timely fashion.

6. MONITORING THE PATIENT WITH TRAUMATIC BRAIN INJURY

a. Physical parameters:

    i. Serial neurological examination:

        1. Cranial nerve examination (see Table 7.1)

        2. Serial recording of the Modified Glasgow Coma Scale (Table 7.2)

    ii. Serial re-evaluation of patient perfusion, blood pressure and oxygenation is important to limit the risk for secondary brain injury with the goals of maintaining systemic perfusion with a systolic blood pressure above 90 mm Hg and a PaO_2 above 80 mm Hg (SpO_2 above 96%).

b. A high level of nursing care is often needed for head-injured animals, with attention paid to the following:

    i. Frequent turning/repositioning of the patient (every 2–4 hours) and provision of well-padded bedding to avoid pressure sores.

    ii. Physical therapy (muscle massage, passive range of motion therapy, encouraging the animal to stand/ambulate) to prevent muscle atrophy and contraction.

    iii. The eyes should be lubricated with artificial tears if there is impaired ability to blink or completely close eyelids.

    iv. Manual evacuation of the bladder and bowels may be necessary in those animals that are unable to on their own. Placement of a urinary catheter connected to a closed collection system may be helpful.

    v. Nutrition should be instituted within 72 hours of injury, with the goal of providing the daily resting energy requirement. If the animal is not alert enough to chew/swallow, a feeding tube or parenteral nutrition should be used:

        1. Nasoesophageal, esophageal, or gastric tubes can be used in animals that have a sufficient level of consciousness to limit the risk for aspiration pneumonia.

        2. Animals with markedly decreased levels of consciousness should be fed via a tube inserted beyond the stomach (nasojejunal) or via parenteral nutrition.

c. Intracranial pressure measurement:

    i. Intracranial pressure (ICP) is defined as the pressure that is exerted on the intracranial contents by the skull:

        1. The intracranial volume consists of the sum of the brain, blood, and cerebrospinal fluid volume within the brain as defined by the Monro-Kelli doctrine.

        2. Sudden increases in any of these three components can result in increased ICP when intracranial compliance is exceeded.

    ii. Intracranial compliance describes the adaptations in intracranial volume in response to an increase in any component of intracranial volume to maintain intracranial pressure. For instance, if intracranial blood volume increased secondary to hematoma formation, a compensatory decrease in cerebrospinal fluid volume may occur to maintain ICP.

    iii. In health, the normal ICP is 5–12 mm Hg in dogs and cats.

    iv. Therapy should be directed toward lowering intracranial pressure below 20 mm Hg.

    v. Intracranial pressure catheters can be positioned into the epidural space, intraparenchymal, or into the ventricle. Epidural and intraparenchymal catheters are less invasive than an intraventicular catheter:

        1. Intraparenchymal fiberoptic monitoring devices can be used in cats and dogs, but they are expensive and fragile.

        2. An epidural water-filled monitoring system has been validated in normal cats. This system is affordable, making the risk for damage to equipment negligible (Dewey et al., 1997).

    vi. While intracranial pressure monitoring is not routine in veterinary medicine, its measurement is feasible in head injured animals when a high level of care can be provided.

d. Jugular vein oxygen saturation:

    i. Jugular venous bulb oxygen saturation provides an indirect measure of global cerebral oxygen utilization:

        1. When cerebral oxygen demand exceeds its supply, the oxygen extraction ratio increases resulting in decreased venous oxygen saturation in blood returning from the brain.

        2. Cerebral oxygen supply can be decreased by decreased cerebral blood flow or decreased arterial oxygen content:

            a. Decreased cerebral blood flow can result from intracranial hypertension,

TABLE 7.1
CRANIAL NERVE EXAMINATION

Cranial Nerve	Function	How to Test Nerve Function	Normal Response	Signs Associated with Nerve Dysfunction
I Olfactory	Smell	1. Assess for response to different odors	1. Ability to smell	1. Inability to notice or track a scent
II Optic	Vision	1. Visual placing or tracking 2. Menace response (sensory) 3. Pupillary light response (sensory)	1. Places foot onto table without any tactile stimulus 2. Closing of eye 3. Constriction of pupil	1. Impaired visual placing/tracking but normal tactile placing 2. Absent menace response in affected eye 3. Absence of both a direct PLR in the affected eye and a consensual PLR in the contralateral eye
III Oculomotor	1. Pupillary constriction 2. Movement of the globe 3. Elevation of eyelid	1. Pupillary light response (motor) 2. Physiological nystagmus	1. Pupillary constriction 2. Normal tracking of eye from side to side as head is turned	1. Mydriasis 2. Loss of medial tracking when head is turned from side to side 3. Ventrolateral strabismus 4. Ptosis
IV Trochlear	1. Innervates dorsal oblique eye muscle		1. Movement of globe (dorsal oblique muscle)	1. Dorsolateral (rotational) strabismus
V Trigeminal	1. Facial sensation 2. Motor to muscles of mastication	1. Palpebral response (sensory) 2. Corneal reflex (sensory) 3. Open jaw	1. Closing of eye in response to touching the medial/lateral canthus of the eye 2. Closing of eye when cornea is touched 3. Fully closing of jaw when opened	Motor 1. Holds mouth open (no obstruction to closing lower jaw) Sensory 1. No blink in response to tactile stimulus around eye/cornea 2. No recognition or response to upper/lower lip stimulation or stimulation of the mucosa of the nostril
VI Abducens	1. Innervates lateral rectus eye muscle 2. Globe retraction	1. Physiologic nystagmus 2. Corneal reflex	1. Movement of globe laterally (lateral rectus) 2. Globe retraction	1. Medial strabismus 2. Loss of globe retraction

TABLE 7.1
(CONTINUED)

Cranial Nerve	Function	How to Test Nerve Function	Normal Response	Signs Associated with Nerve Dysfunction
VII Facial	1. Motor to muscles of facial expression 2. Sensation to palate, tongue	1. Palpebral, corneal, and menace response (motor)	1. Blinking of eye	Motor 1. Unable to blink eye 2. Decreased tear production 3. Facial asymmetry (ear droop, widened palpebral fissure)
VIII Vestibulo-cochlear	1. Hearing 2. Equilibrium	1. Response to auditory stimuli 2. Checking for resting or positional nystagmus	1. Recognition of noise 2. No nystagmus or head tilt	1. No recognition of noise 2. Head tilt, nystagmus, ataxia
IX Glossopha-ryngeal	Motor to the pharyngeal and palatal muscles	Touching the caudal oropharynx	Elevation of the pharynx and contraction of pharyngeal muscles	Dysphagia, lack of gag response.
X Vagus	–	–	–	–
XI Accessory Spinal	1. Assists with cranial movement of the forelimb	Palpation of muscles		Atrophy of the, trapezius, sternocephalic and brachyocephalic muscles
XII Hypoglossal	Movement of the tongue	Visual inspection of tongue; pull on tongue for retraction		Difficulty prehending and swallowing food; deviation of tongue; lack of tongue retraction

systemic hypotension, vasospasm, hypo-volemia, and hyperventilation.

b. Decreased arterial oxygen content can result from anemia, hypoxemia, and dyshemoglobinemias.

3. Cerebral oxygen demand can be increased by increases in cerebral metabolic rate. Common causes of increased cerebral metabolic rate include seizures, hyperthermia, head injury, and some anesthetic agents, such as ketamine.

ii. Measurement of jugular venous bulb oxygen saturation:

1. In people, the catheter should be inserted into the internal jugular vein in a cephalad direction to a level just below the base of the skull. When inserted into the internal jugular vein in people, the blood obtained from consists almost exclusively (97%) of venous return from the brain, with small contribution from the skull, cranial musculature, and meninges:

a. In human medicine, the *internal* jugular vein is routinely catheterized because it is much larger than the external jugular vein. In veterinary medicine, we routinely catheterize the *external* jugular vein because it is much larger and accessible. It is not known which of these two veins carries the majority of

TABLE 7.2
THE MODIFIED GLASGOW COMA SCALE SCORING SYSTEM

Modified Glasgow Coma Scale	Score
Motor activity (choose one)	
Normal gait, normal spinal reflexes	6
Hemiparesis, tetraparesis, decerebrate activity	5
Recumbent, intermittent extensor rigidity	4
Recumbent, constant extensor rigidity	3
Recumbent, constant extensor rigidity with opisthotonus	2
Recumbent, hypotonia of muscles, depressed or absent spinal reflexes	1
Brain stem reflexes (choose one)	
Normal pupillary light reflexes and oculocephalic reflexes	6
Slow pupillary light reflexes and normal to reduced oculocephalic reflexes	5
Bilateral unresponsive miosis with normal to reduced oculocephalic reflexes	4
Pinpoint pupils with reduced to absent oculocephalic reflexes	3
Unilateral unresponsive mydriasis with reduced to absent oculocephalic reflexes	2
Bilateral unresponsive mydriasis with reduced to absent oculocephalic reflexes	1
Level of consciousness (choose one)	
Occasional periods of alertness and responsive to the environment	6
Depression or delirium, capable of responding but response may be inappropriate	5
Semicomatose, responsive to visual stimuli	4
Semicomatose, responsive to auditory stimuli	3
Semicomatose, responsive only to repeated noxious stimuli	2
Comatose, unresponsive to repeated noxious stimuli	1
Total Score	

The value is assigned in each of three categories (motor activity, brainstem reflexes, and level of consciousness) to describe the animal's current neurologic status. The sum of the values from each of these three categories is the animal's coma scale score.
Suggested prognosis: Total score: 3–8: Grave; 9–14: Guarded; 15–18: Good.

venous return from the brain in cats and dogs.

b. Dogs and cats have significantly more musculature overlying the skull than people. It is not known what effect the additional musculature over the skull in cats and dogs has on jugular bulb venous oximetry, but it is possible that a smaller percentage of this blood will be from the brain.

c. Placement of such a monitoring device may be contraindicated in patients with increased intracranial pressure, as even transient occlusion of the jugular vein could result in rapid elevations in intracranial pressure, which could be fatal.

2. All air should be quickly expelled from the sampling syringe and the syringe should be capped to the environment to prevent alterations in oxygen saturation. Environmental contamination will errantly increase the oxygen saturation within the sample.

3. Samples should be processed within 10 minutes of collection at room temperature or can be processed within 4 hours if maintained on ice.

iii. Interpretation of jugular venous bulb oxygen saturation:

1. Normal jugular venous oxygen saturation is 55–75%—this is lower than is considered normal for systemic mixed venous oxygen saturation.

2. This measurement has a high specificity (i.e., when this value is low you can be assured that cerebral ischemia is present) but it is not very sensitive (i.e., focal regions of cerebral ischemia may be present despite normal values).

3. Jugular venous oxygen saturations below 50% warrant institution of therapies to increase oxygen supply (by increasing cerebral blood flow or arterial oxygen content) or decreasing cerebral metabolic rate (such as sedation, seizure management, or controlled hypothermia).

4. In the absence of intracranial pressure monitoring in veterinary medicine, monitoring of jugular venous oxygen saturation may provide a relatively noninvasive technique to assess the efficacy of various treatments (i.e., mannitol administration, volume resuscitation, hyperventilation, etc) in improving cerebral oxygen balance.

e. Transcranial Doppler ultrasonography:

i. Transcranial Doppler ultrasonography provides a noninvasive measure of cerebral blood flow velocity utilizing a conventional ultrasound machine equipped with pulsed Doppler.

ii. Arterial blood flow is often interrogated at the basilar artery, located on dorsal midline near the base of the skull or the middle cerebral artery, located near the ear and zygomatic arch on the lateral aspect of the skull.

iii. The information obtained can provide an indirect, noninvasive estimation of cerebral perfusion pressure as well as intracranial pressure.

iv. This technology has been evaluated in four dogs with naturally occurring traumatic brain injury. This technology may prove to be a clinically useful noninvasive tool for estimation of intracranial pressure status in veterinary patients; however, further research is needed. (Fletcher et al., 2005)

2. PROGNOSIS

a. Coma scoring systems:

i. In human medicine, the Glasgow Coma Scale (GCS) has been used to prognosticate outcome:

1. This scoring system allocates points for each of the following three categories: eye opening response, verbal responses, and motor responses. Higher scores correspond to improved neurological function, with a maximum possible score of 15.

2. A cumulative score below 9 during the first 24 hours is associated with a poor outcome, whether that be death, a persistent vegetative state, or severe neurological disability.

ii. The Small Animal Coma Scale was developed for use in veterinary medicine (Shores, 1983):

1. This scoring system allocates points for each of the following three categories: motor activity, brainstem reflexes, and level of consciousness. Higher scores correspond to improved neurological function, with a maximum possible score of 18. This same scoring system has more recently been referred to as the Modified Glasgow Coma Scale (Table 7.2).

2. This scoring system is yet to be prospectively validated in a large number of cats and dogs with traumatic brain injury.

3. A small retrospective study of 38 dogs with head injury found a linear association between the admission Modified Glasgow Coma Scale score and outcome, with higher scores having a greater probability of survival. A Modified Glasgow Coma Scale score of 8 at admission was associated with 50% probability of survival at 48 hours. In this study, gender, body weight, and the presence of skull fractures were not useful in predicting outcome (Platt et al., 2001).

b. Biochemical disturbances:

i. The degree and duration of hyperglycemia has been associated with severity of injury and neurological outcome in adult and pediatric head trauma. Hyperglycemia has been documented in cats and dogs following head trauma, and the degree of hyperglycemia on hospital admission was associated with severity of neurological injury (Syring et al., 2001).

BIBLIOGRAPHY

Adelson PD, Bratton SL, Carney NA, et al. Guidelines for the acute medical management of severe traumatic brain injury in infants, children, and adolescents. *Pediatr Crit Care Med* 2003; 4 (3 Suppl): S72–S75.

Alderson P, Roberts I. Corticosteroids for acute traumatic brain injury. *Cochrane Database of Systematic Reviews* 2005, Issue 1. Art. No.: CD000196. DOI: 10.1002/14651858.CD000196.pub2.

Bouma GJ, Muizelaar JP, Bandoh K, Marmarou A. Blood pressure and intracranial pressure-volume dynamics in severe head injury: relationship with cerebral blood flow. *J Neurosurg* 1992; 77: 15–19.

Brain Trauma Foundation. Guidelines for the management of severe head injury. *J Neurotrauma* 2007; 24: S1–S106.

Dewey CW. Emergency management of the head trauma patient. *Vet Clin North Am Small Anim Pract* 2000; 30: 207–225.

Dewey CW, Downs MO, Aron DN, Mahaffey EA. Acute traumatic intracranial haemorrhage in dogs and cats. *Vet Comp Orthop Traumatol* 1993; 6: 153–159.

Dewey CW, Bailey CS, Haskins SC, et al. Evaluation of an epidural intracranial pressure monitoring system in cats. *J Vet Emerg Crit Care* 1997; 7: 20–33.

Fletcher DJ, Seiler G, Mikszewski J, Drobatz K. Transcranial color coded duplex sonography as an indicator of severity in traumatic brain injury – a pilot study. *J Vet Emerg Crit Care* 2005; 15: S4.

Hall ED. The neuroprotective pharmacology of methylprednisolone. *J Neurosurg* 1992; 76: 13–22.

Kassell NF, Haley EC. Randomized, double-blind, vehicle-controlled trial of tirilazad mesylate in patients with aneurysmal subarachnoid hemorrhage: a cooperative study in Europe, Australia, and New Zealand. *J Neurosurg* 1996; 84: 221–228.

Kolata RJ. Trauma in dogs and cats: an overview. *Vet Clin North Am Small Anim Pract* 1980; 10: 515–522.

Lee B, Newberg A. Neuroimaging in traumatic brain imaging. *NeuroRx* 2005; 2: 372–383.

Marshall LF, Maas AL, Marshall SB, et al. A multicenter trial on the efficacy of using tirilazad mesylate in cases of head injury. *J Neurosurg* 1998; 89: 519–525.

Moppett IK. Traumatic brain injury: assessment, resuscitation, and early management. *Br Med J* 2007; 99: 18–31.

Platt SR, Radaelli ST, McDonnell JJ, et al. The prognostic value of the modified Glasgow Coma Scale in head trauma in dogs. *J Vet Intern Med* 2001; 15: 581–584.

Platt SR, Radaelli ST, McDonnell JJ, et al. Computed tomography after mild head trauma in dogs. *Vet Rec* 2002; 151: 24.

Roberts I, Yates D, Sandercock P, et al. Effect of intravenous corticosteroids on death within 14 days in 10,008 adults with clinically significant head injury (MRC CRASH trial): randomized placebo controlled trial. *Lancet* 2004; 364: 1321–1328.

SAFE Study Investigators. Saline or albumin for fluid resuscitation in patients with traumatic brain injury. *N Engl J Med* 2007; 357: 874–884.

Schnell RM, Cole DJ. Cerebral monitoring: jugular venous oximetry. *Anesth Analg* 2000; 90: 559–566.

Shores A. Craniocerebral trauma. In: Kirk RW, ed. *Current Veterinary Therapy X*. Philadelphia, PA: WB Saunders, 1983; 847–854.

Smith DH, Meaney DF, Shull WH. Diffuse axonal injury in head trauma. *J Head Trauma Rehab* 2003; 18: 307–316.

Syring RS, Otto CM, Drobatz KJ. Hyperglycemia in dogs and cats with head trauma: 122 cases (1997–1999). *J Am Vet Med Assoc* 2001; 218: 1124–1129.

Tempkin NR, Dikmen SS, Winn HR. Posttraumatic seizures. In: Eisenberg HM, Aldrich EF, eds. *Management of Head Injury*. Philadelphia, PA: WB Saunders, 1991; 425–435.

Wakai A, Roberts I, Schierhout G. Mannitol for acute traumatic brain injury. *Cochrane Database of Systematic Reviews* 2007, Issue 1. Art. No.: CD001049. DOI: 10.1002/14651858.CD001049.pub4.

TRAUMA-ASSOCIATED PERIPHERAL NERVE INJURY

Jessica Snyder

1. GLOBAL APPROACH TO PERIPHERAL NERVE TRAUMA

a. Peripheral nerves can be classified as cranial nerves, brachial plexus or thoracic limb nerves, or lumbar intumescence or pelvic limb nerves.

b. The peripheral nerve has three layers of supporting connective tissue. Individual axons are surrounded by the endoneurium. Bundles, or fascicles, of nerve fibers are then surrounded by the perineurium. The entire nerve is encased in the epineurium.

c. Trauma to the peripheral nerves can cause either temporary signs resulting from a localized conduction block as a result of bruising of the nerve (neuropraxia), or more severe and potentially permanent signs if structural disruption, stretching, or crushing of the axons with retention of the connective tissue scaffold (axonotmesis) or complete transection of the axons and the connective tissue support (neurotmesis) occurs.

d. Traumatic nerve injury in dogs and cats is most commonly associated with fractures of the pelvis, femur, or humerus; bite wounds; lacerations; gunshot wounds; and iatrogenic causes such as orthopedic surgery and injection-associated injury.

e. Peripheral nerve and muscle can also be injured if blood or oxygen supply is interrupted to the limb (in situations of thrombosis or thromboembolism, arterial bleeding, or with excessively tight bandages or tourniquets causing ischemia), or if hemorrhage

or edema at the site of injury causes an increased compartment pressure.

f. Treatment generally consists of stabilizing other systemic injuries and providing supportive care to prevent further injury to tissues around the injured nerve(s) while providing supportive measures and time for the nerve to heal, although in some instances decompressive surgery or surgical anastomosis is appropriate. The prognosis for return to function in cases of complete nerve transection is very poor without prompt repair:

  i. Prophylactic antibiotic therapy is indicated for nerve injury associated with contaminated wounds.

g. Peripheral nerve repair may be primary or secondary:

  i. Primary nerve repair involves immediate nerve anastomosis.

  ii. Secondary nerve repair involves suturing nerve stumps to the surrounding soft tissue to prevent retraction of the nerve for later surgical repair.

  iii. Even with aggressive attempts to repair transected nerves, complications are common and include neuroma formation and inadequate nerve regeneration.

  iv. Nerve grafts may be attempted when end-to-end anastomosis is not possible.

h. The rate of axonal regrowth is 1–4 mm per day:

  i. The time period expected for return of

Manual of Trauma Management in the Dog and Cat, First Edition. Edited by Kenneth J. Drobatz, Matthew W. Beal and Rebecca S. Syring.
© 2011 John Wiley & Sons, Inc. Published 2011 by John Wiley & Sons, Inc.

function of most traumatic peripheral nerve injuries is within 6 months.

ii. Beyond this time, it is unlikely that there will be return of function.

iii. The most important prognostic indicator is the presence of deep pain sensation.

2. CRANIAL NERVES

a. Cranial nerve injury can occur after any blunt or penetrating head trauma.

b. The cranial nerves (from cranial to caudal as they exit the skull) include the olfactory, optic, oculomotor, trochlear, trigeminal, abducent, facial, vestibulocochlear, glossopharyngeal, accessory, and hypoglossal nerves:

    i. Optic nerve injury:

        1. Optic nerve dysfunction may be seen with traumatic proptosis of the globe.

        2. Optic nerve dysfunction manifests as ipsilateral blindness, mydriasis, and absent direct pupillary light response. The contralateral pupil will lack a consensual response from the affected side.

        3. When the unaffected eye is illuminated, both a direct and consensual (in the affected eye) pupillary light response should be present. If the oculomotor nerve is also damaged, then a consensual response in the affected eye will be absent.

        4. With enucleation, the contralateral optic nerve can be damaged if excessive traction is placed on the optic nerve of the eye being enucleated, causing traction on the optic chiasm and therefore affecting the opposite optic nerve (see Chapter 15: Trauma-Associated Ocular Injury).

    ii. Trigeminal nerve injury:

        1. Bilateral motor trigeminal nerve injury may be seen with temporomandibular joint subluxation (see Chapter 16: Trauma-Associated Musculoskeletal Injuries of the Head):

            a. These animals are unable to close their jaw, but facial sensation generally remains intact.

            b. Many affected animals will begin to show improvement within 4 weeks following injury.

        2. Unilateral trigeminal nerve injury may occur secondary to bite wounds, lacera-

tions, or other trauma to the face at the base of the ear (see Chapter 21: Trauma-Associated Aural Injury):

        a. Unilateral trigeminal injury manifests as ipsilateral masticatory muscle atrophy.

iii. Facial nerve paralysis, Horner's syndrome, and vestibulocochlear nerve dysfunction can be iatrogenic following bulla osteotomy. Hypoglossal nerve paralysis has also been infrequently reported following ventral bulla osteotomy:

    1. Permanent facial nerve paralysis has been reported in 23% of dogs and 28% of cats following total ear canal ablation and ventral bulla osteotomy (Sharp, 1990; Bacon et al., 2003).

    2. With blunt head trauma, fracture of the petrosal temporal bone can affect the vestibulocochlear nerve and cause peripheral or central vestibular signs (ataxia, head tilt, nystagmus) and ipsilateral facial nerve paralysis (see Chapter 21: Trauma-Associated Aural Injury and Chapter 7: Traumatic Brain Injury).

    3. Ipsilateral facial nerve paralysis (an inability to close the ipsilateral eyelid or retract the ipsilateral lip) may be seen with lacerations to the face.

    4. Horner's syndrome can also be seen with injury to the soft tissue of the neck (puncture wounds) and chest, and with skull fractures and retrobulbar contusions (Figures 8.1 and 8.2).

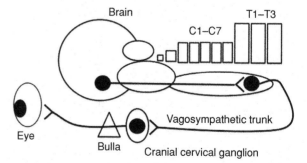

FIGURE 8.1 Pathway detailing the sympathetic innervation to the eye. With an injury at any point along this three neuron pathway, a Horner's syndrome, characterized by miosis, ptosis, enophthalmos, and third eyelid protrusion, will result.

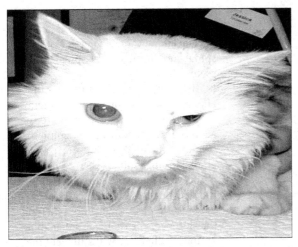

FIGURE 8.2   Cat with Horner's syndrome following cervical trauma.

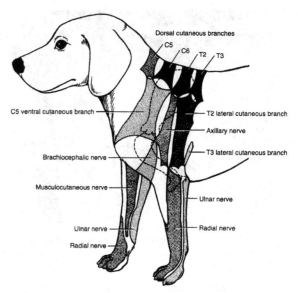

FIGURE 8.3   Nerve locations and zones of cutaneous sensation of the thoracic limb. (Reprinted with permission: deLahunta A and Glass EN, 2008. Veterinary Neuroanatomy and Clinical Neurology, W.B. Saunders, Philadelphia, PA)

iv. Traumatic laryngeal paralysis while common in humans is less so in the case of dogs and cats, as their larynx is more protected. Nonetheless, laryngeal paralysis can be seen in dogs and cats following choke chain injuries and penetrating bite wounds or foreign bodies damaging the recurrent laryngeal nerve. Laryngeal paralysis secondary to endotracheal intubation and prosthetic tracheal ring placement for the treatment of tracheal collapse has been reported in dogs. Symptoms of laryngeal paralysis include inspiratory (+/− expiratory) dyspnea, voice change, and respiratory stridor.

v. Hypoglossal nerve injury:

1. See (iii) regarding complications of bulla osteotomy. Hypoglossal nerve paralysis has also been reported in dogs following traumatic atlantooccipital luxation.

c. Diagnostic tools for assessing cranial nerve dysfunction include thorough neurological examination and otoscopic examination (to look for the presence of blood in the ear canal indicating possible petrosal bone injury), oral examination (possibly including assessment of proper abduction of the arytenoid cartilage on inspiration), and skull radiography and/or computed tomography. Animals with any evidence of injury to the cranial nerves following trauma should be assessed for the presence of concurrent traumatic brain injury (see Chapter 7: Traumatic Brain Injury).

3. PERIPHERAL NERVES OF THE THORACIC LIMB

a. The nerves of the brachial plexus, from cranial to caudal as they exit the C6 to T2 spinal cord segments, are the suprascapular, subscapular, axillary, radial, median, and ulnar nerves. Refer to Figure 8.3 for nerve locations and zones of cutaneous sensation.

b. Brachial plexus avulsion:

i. Brachial plexus avulsion is the most common traumatic peripheral nerve injury of the thoracic limb and is a common sequela to vehicular trauma, when the thoracic limb is sheared away from the body. Avulsion of the nerve roots is common, potentially because there is less surrounding connective tissue over the nerve roots.

ii. The ventral nerve roots, and the nerve roots of C8 and T1, are most commonly affected.

iii. For clinical signs to be apparent, two or more adjacent nerve roots must be affected.

iv. Complete brachial plexus avulsion:

1. All of the roots from the spinal cord segments C6 to T2 are affected.

2. The limb is paralyzed and flaccid. The withdrawal reflex, extensor carpi

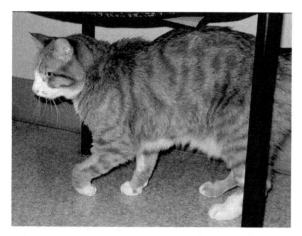

FIGURE 8.4 Cat with brachial plexus avulsion following vehicular trauma.

radialis reflex, and biceps reflex cannot be elicited.

3. The presence or absence of sensation is the most important prognostic indicator.

v. Caudal brachial plexus avulsion:

1. The nerve roots from the C6 and C7 spinal cord are not affected, and shoulder and elbow function may be spared.

2. These animals will often hold the limb off of the ground and flex the elbow, and sensation may be lost over craniolateral antebrachium and dorsum of the paw due to damage of the nerve responsible for this zone of cutaneous sensation. (Figure 8.4).

3. There may be an ipsilateral Horner's syndrome (a partial Horner's syndrome with miosis of the pupil should not be confused with intracranial trauma):

a. Horner's syndrome represents an interruption of sympathetic innervation to the eye and is characterized by enophthalmos, ptosis, miosis, and third eyelid protrusion.

b. The pathway is a three neuron pathway that begins in the hypothalamus, travels down the brainstem and cervical spinal cord to exit at the T1–T3 spinal cord segments, then travels cranially with the vagosympathetic trunk to synapse at the cranial cervical ganglion, and finally courses by the tympanic bulla to the eye (Figure 8.1).

4. These animals may also have loss of the ipsilateral cutaneous trunci reflex:

a. The lateral thoracic nerve exits the spinal cord at the C7–T1 spinal cord segments.

b. Normally, this nerve provides the efferent response (bilateral contraction of the cutaneous trunci muscle) to the afferent local stimulus of pinching the skin over the ipsilateral thoracic and cranial lumbar spine.

c. Because the contralateral lateral thoracic nerve is intact in cases of caudal brachial plexus avulsion, pinching the skin over the thoracolumbar spine on the affected side will still yield the appropriate contralateral response.

vi. Cranial brachial plexus avulsions are uncommon, but carry a better prognosis as these animals retain the ability to bear weight on the limb. There may be ipsilateral paralysis of the diaphragm with involvement of the C5, 6, and 7 nerve roots.

vii. Diagnostic testing for suspected brachial plexus avulsion includes a thorough neurological examination, cervical radiography to rule out simultaneous vertebral facture or luxation, and possibly advanced imaging to definitively rule out concomitant traumatic intervertebral disk disease, vertebral fracture or luxation, or compressive hematoma:

1. Magnetic resonance imaging (MRI) allows for visualization of the nerve roots. These lesions cannot be evaluated as well with computed tomography (CT).

2. Electrodiagnostic examination (electromyography, motor evoked responses [H wave, F wave, magnetic motor evoked potentials], and cord dorsum potentials) may offer additional information. Electromyography and nerve conduction studies should be delayed at least 5–7 days from the onset of the clinical signs to allow for abnormalities to become apparent.

viii. Treatment for brachial plexus avulsion includes physical therapy (passive range of motion exercises and massage, to prevent muscle contracture) and protecting the limb from self-mutilation and from dragging on the ground. Most cases of neuropraxia will improve within 4–6 weeks. If there is no improvement within 4–6 months, then it is not likely that there will be return of function, and amputation may be necessary.

ix. Prognosis is guarded. Recovery rates to an acceptable level of function range from 20 to 28% in the veterinary literature (Dewey, 2003; Shores, 1993; Wheeler et al., 1986).

c. Radial nerve paralysis (uncommon):

i. Radial nerve injury should be suspected if the extensor carpi radialis reflex is absent. The radial nerve is the major weight-bearing nerve of the thoracic limb. With radial nerve injury, the limb will buckle and knuckle when weight is applied, and the limb is often carried with the elbow flexed. There may be a decreased or absent response to stimulation of the cranial antebrachium and dorsal surface of the foot (Figure 8.3).

ii. More diffuse injury, such as brachial plexus avulsion, should be suspected with sensory abnormalities of the medial or caudal limb, if a Horner's syndrome is present, or if the ipsilateral cutaneous trunci response is absent.

iii. The radial nerve may be injured with fractures of the distal humerus, although this is uncommon (see Chapter 18: Trauma-Associated Musculoskeletal Injury to the Appendicular Skeleton).

iv. Specific treatment for radial nerve paralysis may include primary nerve repair, physical therapy, carpal arthrodesis, and muscle relocation:

   1. Amputation can be considered if the injury results in significant discomfort or disability or if the limb is becoming traumatized secondary to dragging, pressure sores, or the animal is self-traumatizing the limb. If required, many cats and dogs do very well following limb amputation.

4. PERIPHERAL NERVES OF THE PELVIC LIMB

a. The nerves of the lumbosacral intumescence, from cranial to caudal as they exit the L4 to S3 spinal cord segments, are the femoral, obturator, cranial gluteal, caudal gluteal, sciatic, pudendal, and perineal nerves. Refer to Figure 8.5 for nerve locations and zones of cutaneous sensation.

b. Femoral nerve:

i. The femoral nerve exits the L4, 5, and 6 spinal cord segments. This correlates with the

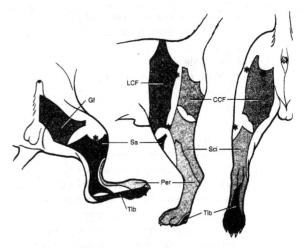

FIGURE 8.5 Nerve locations and zones of cutaneous sensation of the pelvic limb. (Reprinted with permission: deLahunta A and Glass EN, 2008. Veterinary Neuroanatomy and Clinical Neurology, W.B. Saunders, Philadelphia, PA)

level of the 3rd and 4th vertebral bodies in most animals. Mid-lumbar vertebral trauma and very rarely femoral fractures may be associated with femoral nerve dysfunction.

ii. Femoral nerve involvement should be suspected if the patellar reflex is depressed. Spinal cord intumescence injury rather than peripheral nerve disease should be suspected with bilateral pelvic limb involvement, decreased tail or anal tone, or paravertebral pain on spinal palpation.

iii. The femoral nerve innervates the major weight bearing muscles of the pelvic limb. Injury to this nerve causes an inability to fix the stifle in place when weight is placed on the limb, resulting in buckling of the leg.

c. Sciatic nerve:

i. The sciatic nerve exits the L6, L7, and S1 spinal cord segments. This correlates with the 4th, 5th, and 6th vertebral bodies in most animals.

ii. Sciatic nerve involvement should be suspected with a decreased or absent pelvic limb withdrawal response.

iii. Branches of the sciatic nerve include the peroneal nerve and the tibial nerve:

   1. Peroneal injury causes a tendency to knuckle the dorsal surface of the paw because of an inability to flex the tarsus.

2. Tibial nerve injury causes a plantigrade stance because of an inability to extend the tarsus.

iv. Clinical signs:

1. With sciatic nerve injuries, animals are able to bear weight on the limb, but they walk with a plantigrade stance and often knuckle on the paw.

v. Etiology:

1. Approximately 11% of pelvic fractures in cats and dogs are associated with peripheral nerve injury, most commonly involving the sciatic nerve (Jacobson and Schrader, 1987). Sciatic nerve injury may be associated with fractures of the sacral wing, acetabulum, ischium, ileum, and sacroiliac luxations (see Chapter 19: Trauma-Associated Musculoskeletal Injury to the Pelvis, Sacrum, and Tail).

2. Iatrogenic injury to the sciatic nerve has been reported in dogs and cats following sacroiliac luxation repair, intramedullary pinning of femoral fractures, cemented hip prosthesis, tibial plateau leveling osteotomy, and perineal herniorrhaphy. Treatment for these injuries involves removal of implants, connective tissue, or suture entrapping the nerve, and reconstructive nerve surgery. The prognosis is guarded, with 13/27 (48%) animals with iatrogenic sciatic nerve injury recovering completely and 7/27 (26%) animals showing no improvement (Forterre et al., 2007).

3. Sciatic nerve injury may also be seen with intramuscular injections, gunshot wounds, bites, and lacerations of the caudal thigh.

vi. Treatment:

1. Therapy for sciatic nerve injury includes surgical correction of pelvic fractures (if appropriate) and allowing appropriate time for manifestations of injury to resolve.

2. Animals that knuckle on the paw may be fitted with an orthopedic boot (ankle foot orthosis) to protect the dorsum of the paw from abrasions and also to improve locomotion.

3. Sciatic nerve paralysis may be treated with talocrural joint fusion and muscle transfer.

4. Peroneal nerve paralysis may be treated with relocation of the long digital flexor muscle.

d. Pudendal nerve:

i. The pudendal nerve exits the spinal cord at the nerve roots S1–3.

ii. Clinical signs of injury:

1. Decreased tail and anal tone.

2. Fecal incontinence (dropping stool).

3. Flaccid, easily expressed bladder ("lower motor neuron bladder") characterized by leaking or dripping urine.

iii. Etiology:

1. Pudendal nerve injury may occur secondary to sacral fracture and sacrococcygeal luxation (tail pull injury) in cats and dogs (see Chapter 19: Trauma-Associated Musculoskeletal Injury to the Pelvis, Sacrum, and Tail).

2. It has been reported that 20% of cats with pelvic fractures also have sacral fractures (Smeak and Olmstead, 1985).

3. Sacrococcygeal luxation is more common in cats than in dogs, and the presence of anal tone and intact perineal sensation are important prognostic indicators.

4. Cats that fail to regain urinary incontinence within one month have a poor prognosis (Smeak and Olmstead, 1985).

iv. Diagnosis of sacral fractures and sacrocaudal fracture/luxation is often made by survey radiography:

1. MRI or CT can be used to rule out associated injuries of the lumbosacral spinal cord.

2. CT may be indicated if fracture is suspected but not observed on conventional survey radiographs, as this modality is more sensitive for bone disease.

3. Treatment for sacral fractures involves stabilization and, if appropriate, dorsal laminectomy for nerve root decompression. (see Chapter 19: Trauma-Associated Musculoskeletal Injury to the Pelvis, Sacrum, and Tail).

4. Treatment for sacrococcygeal luxation involves tail amputation (in cases of intractable pain, mutilation, or necrosis) or appropriate time for clinical signs to abate (see Chapter 19: Trauma-Associated

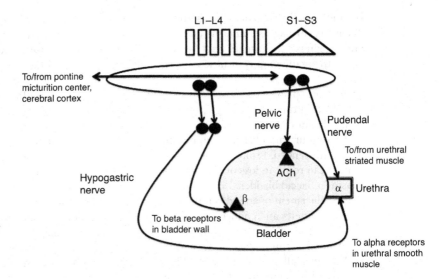

L1–L4   S1–S3

To/from pontine
micturition center,
cerebral cortex

Pelvic
nerve

Pudendal
nerve

To/from urethral
striated muscle

ACh

Hypogastric
nerve

β   α   Urethra

To beta receptors
in bladder wall   Bladder

To alpha receptors
in urethral smooth
muscle

FIGURE 8.6   The neuroanatomy of micturition, detailing the pathways of the sympathetic, pelvic, and pudendal nerves.

Musculoskeletal Injury to the Pelvis, Sacrum, and Tail).

5. URINARY SYSTEM DYSFUNCTION

a. Neurological dysfunction of the urinary bladder commonly occurs following spinal trauma (see Chapter 9: Traumatic Spinal Injury).

b. Anatomy of the pelvic, pudendal, and hypogastric nerves (Figure 8.6):

  i. The hypogastric nerve originates in the cranial lumbar spinal cord and sends nerve fibers to the caudal mesenteric ganglia. The hypogastric nerve then passes through the pelvic plexus to the detrusor muscle.

  ii. The pudendal nerve originates in the S1, 2, and 3 spinal cord segments and travels to the external urethral sphincter and urethral striated muscle.

  iii. The pelvic nerve originates in the S1, 2, and 3 spinal cord segments and travels through the pelvic plexus and then to the detrusor muscle.

c. The innervation to the urinary bladder is complex (Figure 8.6):

  i. Parasympathetic innervation is provided via the pelvic nerve, which stimulates cholinergic (muscarinic) receptors in the urinary bladder and causes detrusor muscle contraction in the bladder wall.

  ii. Sympathetic innervation is provided via the hypogastric nerve, which activates β adrenergic receptors in the bladder wall, causing bladder wall relaxation, and also activates α adrenergic receptors in urethral smooth muscle, causing urethral contraction.

  iii. Somatic innervation is provided via the pudendal nerve, which causes urethral skeletal muscle contraction.

  iv. The brain stem micturition center, with forebrain influence, mediates the spinal reflex arcs involved in micturition.

d. Failure to completely empty the bladder can be caused by a lack of detrusor contractile function, anatomic or functional urethral obstruction, or both. Anatomic obstructive disorders (in the trauma patient, consider urethral rupture or tear and obstruction by hematoma formation) are more common and should always be ruled out, especially if no other neurologic deficits are present (see Chapter 11: Trauma-Associated Urinary Tract Injury):

  i. An upper motor neuron bladder is large, firm, and difficult to express. The urethral sphincter tone may be increased. This type of bladder is seen with spinal lesions cranial to L5–7:

    1. Diagnostic evaluation:

      a. See Chapter 9: Traumatic Spinal Injury for diagnostic approach to spinal cord disease.

b. Additionally, consider CBC, serum chemistry, urinalysis and urine culture, and imaging of the urinary tract (survey or contrast radiography or ultrasonography).

2. Therapeutic plan:

a. Address primary neurologic, metabolic, or obstructive disease.

b. Prevent urinary bladder from becoming overdistended. Prolonged overdistention can result in loss of bladder tone, causing a flaccid bladder:

    i. Placement of an indwelling urinary catheter and connection to a closed collection system is recommended to empty the bladder and to keep it small. Alternatively, the bladder can be intermittently catheterized or manually expressed.

    ii. Manual bladder expression, because of the risk of iatrogenic bladder rupture, should be performed with caution in the trauma patient.

    iii. Aseptic technique is crucial when performing bladder catheterization or maintaining an indwelling urinary catheter. In the case of an indwelling urinary catheter, the urine and/or the catheter tip should be cultured when the catheter is removed. Urine culture should be performed 24–48 hours following catheter removal.

c. Treat urinary tract infection, if present. Monitor for the development of urinary tract infection.

d. Decrease the urethral resistance with a muscle relaxant, such as diazepam (0.2–0.5 mg/kg IV or PO prior to expression), or an alpha adrenergic blocker, such as phenoxybenzamine (0.2–0.5 mg/kg PO SID—BID) or prazosin (DOGS: 1 mg/15 kg body weight PO SID—TID; CATS: 0.25 mg/cat PO SID—BID):

    i. Blood pressure should be monitored in the animal receiving phenoxybenzamine and prazosin. The effects on the bladder may not be seen for 2–3 days with phenoxybenzamine while the onset of action may be quicker for prazosin.

    ii. Phenoxybenzamine should be used with caution in cases of cardiac disease, renal disease, or diabetes mellitus.

    iii. In the case of cats, owners should be cautioned of the risk of hepatic necrosis with oral diazepam (an extremely rare but serious complication). Diazepam may also cause marked sedation as a side effect.

ii. A lower motor neuron bladder is flaccid, distended, and easily expressed. This type of bladder is seen with spinal lesions caudal to L5–L7. Bladder atony may also result from chronic distention secondary to urinary retention (seen in animals that are stressed, painful, or receiving anticholinergic agents, opioids, or tricyclic antidepressants; or post urethral obstruction):

    1. Diagnostic evaluation: see diagnostic approach to upper motor neuron bladder above.

    2. Therapeutic plan: see therapeutic plan for upper motor neuron bladder above:

        a. Consider Bethanecol (a cholinergic agonist) at 5–20 mg/dog or 1.5–5 mg/cat PO TID:

            i. Bethanecol is contraindicated in cases of gastrointestinal or urinary obstruction.

            ii. Bethanecol may increase urethral resistance, and should be administrated with phenoxybenzamine (0.2–0.5 mg/kg PO every 12–24 hours) or diazepam (0.1–0.5 mg/kg PO every 12–24 hours) if this occurs.

            iii. Side effects may include vomiting, diarrhea, and inappetence.

        b. Other agents used less frequently to increase bladder contraction include the following:

            i. Metoclopramide 0.2–0.4 mg/kg IM, PO, SQ every 6 hours.

            ii. Cisapride 0.1–1 mg/kg PO every 8–12 hours. (Cisapride is no longer commercially available and must be obtained through a compounding pharmacy.)

BIBLIOGRAPHY

Anderson A, Coughlan AR. Sacral fractures in dogs and cats: a classification scheme and review of 51 cases. *J Small Anim Pract* 1997; 38: 404–409.

Bacon NJ, Gilbert RL, Bostock DE, et al. Total ear canal ablation in the cat: Indications, morbidity, and long-term survival. *J Small Anim Pract* 2003; 44: 430–434.

Bailey CS. Patterns of cutaneous anesthesia associated with brachial plexus avulsions in the dog. *J Am Vet Med Assoc* 1984; 185: 889–899.

Bennett D, Vaughan LC. The use of muscle relocation techniques in the treatment of peripheral nerve injuries in dogs and cats. *J Small Anim Pract* 1976; 17: 99–108.

Chrisman CL. Peripheral neuropathies. In: Bojrab MJ, ed. *Disease Mechanisms in Small Animal Surgery*. Philadelphia, PA: Lippincott, Williams, and Williams, 1993; 1158–1174.

Cottrill NB. Differential diagnosis of anisocoria. In: Bonagura JD, ed. *Kirk's Current Veterinary Therapy XIII*. Philadelphia, PA: WB Saunders, 2000; 1045–1050.

Cuddon PA. Electrophysiology in neuromuscular disease. *Vet Clin North Am Small Anim Pract* 2002; 32: 31–62.

deLahunta A, Glass E. *Veterinary Neuroanatomy and Clinical Neurology*. 3rd edition. Philadelphia, PA: WB Saunders, 2009.

Dewey CW. Disorders of the peripheral nervous system: mononeuropathies and polyneuropathies. In: Dewey CW, ed. *A Practical Guide to Canine and Feline Neurology*. Ames: Iowa State Press, 2003; 367–412.

Dewey CW. Functional and dysfunctional neuroanatomy: the key to lesion localization. In: Dewey CW, ed. *A Practical Guide to Canine and Feline Neurology*. Ames: Iowa State Press, 2003; 3–30.

Dewey CW. Neurology and neuropharmacology of normal and abnormal urination. In: Dewey CW, ed. *A Practical Guide to Canine and Feline Neurology*. Ames: Iowa State Press, 2003; 357–366.

Evans HE, ed. *Miller's Anatomy of the Dog*. 3rd edition. Philadelphia, PA: WB Saunders, 1993.

Forterre F, Tomek A, Rytz U, et al. Iatrogenic sciatic nerve injury in 18 dogs and 9 cats (1997–2006). *Vet Surg* 2007; 36: 464–471.

Gibson KL, Daniloff JK. Peripheral nerve repair. *Comp Cont Educ* 1989; 11: 938–944.

Holt D, Brockman D. Diagnosis and management of laryngeal disease in the dog and cat. *Vet Clin North Am: Small Anim Pract* 1994; 24: 855–871.

Jacobson A, Schrader SC. Peripheral nerve injury associated with fracture or fracture-dislocation of the pelvis in dogs and cats: 34 cases (1978–1982). *J Am Vet Med Assoc* 1987; 190: 569–572.

Kern TJ, Erb HN. Facial neuropathy in dogs and cats: 95 cases (1975–1985). *J Am Vet Med Assoc* 1987; 191: 1604–1609.

Kern TJ, Aromando MC, Erb HN. Horner's syndrome in dogs and cats: 100 cases (1975–1985). *J Am Vet Med Assoc* 1989; 195: 369–373.

Lane IF. Diagnosis and management of urinary retention. *Vet Clin North Am Small Anim Pract* 2000; 30: 25–57.

Lesser AS. The use of a tendon transfer for the treatment of traumatic sciatic nerve paralysis in the dog. *Vet Surg* 1978; 7: 85–89.

Moissonnier P, Vigneron O, and Duchossoy Y. The use of the cutaneous saphenous nerve as a source of nerve graft material in the dog (the use of the CSN as a graft). *Vet Comp Orthop Traumatol* 2001; 14: 84–89.

Rodkey WG, Sharp NJH. Surgery of the peripheral nervous system. In: Slatter D, ed. *Textbook of Small Animal Surgery*. Philadephia, PA: WB Saunders, 2003; 1218–1226.

Sharp NJH. Chronic otitis externa and otitis media treated by total ear canal ablation and ventral bulla osteotomy in thirteen dogs. *Vet Surg* 1990; 19: 162–166.

Sharp NJH, Wheeler SJ. Postoperative care. In: Sharp NJH, Wheeler SJ, eds. *Small Animal Spinal Disorders: Diagnosis and Surgery*. London: Mosby-Wolfe, 2005; 339–362.

Shores A. Traumatic and neoplastic diseases of the brachial plexus. In: Bojrab MJ, ed. *Disease Mechanisms in Small Animal Surgery*. Philadelphia, PA: Lippincott, Williams & Williams, 1993; 1175–1182.

Smeak DD, Olmstead ML. Fracture/luxations of the sacrococcygeal area in the cat. *Vet Surg* 1985; 14: 319–326.

Wheeler SJ, Clayton Jones DG, Wright JA. The diagnosis of brachial plexus disorders in dogs: A review of twenty-two cases. *J Small Anim Pract* 1986; 27: 147–157.

TRAUMATIC SPINAL INJURY

Daniel Fletcher

1. GENERAL APPROACH TO THE SPINAL TRAUMA PATIENT

a. Spinal trauma can result in a wide range of injuries, including spinal cord contusion, vertebral fracture or luxation, and traumatic intervertebral disk herniation. Common causes of spinal trauma include motor vehicle accidents, falls, projectile injuries, trauma from falling objects, and bite wounds.

b. Patients with spinal trauma commonly have polytrauma, necessitating rapid and thorough assessment of major organ systems and survey for evidence of other life-threatening injuries.

c. Once life-threatening injuries to the other major body systems have been identified and addressed, evaluation for possible spinal cord injury can be undertaken. It should be noted that neurologic deficits should be interpreted cautiously in the patient in whom perfusion has not been adequately restored, as these neurologic deficits may improve or correct with restoration of perfusion:

    i. An initial, brief evaluation of spinal cord function should include testing for the presence of superficial and deep pain sensation in all 4 limbs as well as presence of segmental reflexes. The results of this survey yield an initial neuroanatomic localization of the injury and assessment of injury severity.

    ii. Gentle palpation of the spine can yield evidence of spinal instability, malalignment, crepitus or pain, but the absence of such findings does not rule out the presence of spinal instability. All trauma patients with evidence of spinal cord dysfunction should be immobilized to reduce the risk of further traumatic injury to the spinal cord. The patient should be securely taped to a rigid board that is at least as long as the entire spine and wide enough to support all 4 limbs. Minimally, 2″ white tape or Elasticon should be used to secure the patient to the board over the shoulder and over the hip. See Figure 9.1 for an example. Additional tape should be used if needed.

    iii. Imaging, potentially including radiography, myelography, computed tomography, and/or magnetic resonance imaging should be employed for definitive diagnosis.

d. Initial management of the spinal trauma patient should include immobilization of unstable fractures as discussed above, pain management (see Chapter 5: Anesthesia and Analgesia for the Trauma Patient), correction of perfusion deficits (see Chapter 3: Shock in the Trauma Patient), and medical therapies aimed at reduction of secondary spinal cord injury.

e. Consideration of the basics of the pathophysiology of spinal cord injury is important when developing an appropriate diagnostic and therapeutic plan:

Manual of Trauma Management in the Dog and Cat, First Edition. Edited by Kenneth J. Drobatz, Matthew W. Beal and Rebecca S. Syring.
© 2011 John Wiley & Sons, Inc. Published 2011 by John Wiley & Sons, Inc.

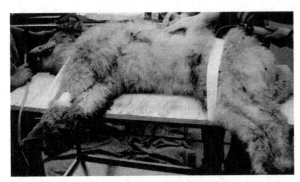

FIGURE 9.1 A dog with a T13 compression fracture taped to a back board. The rigid board should be at least as long as the entire spinal column, and the dog should be secured with at least two tape strips over the shoulders and hips.

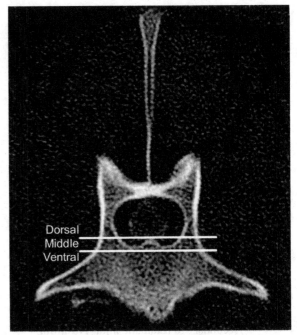

FIGURE 9.2 The dorsal, middle and ventral spinal compartments illustrated on a transverse Computed Tomography image of a canine lumbar vertebra.

i. Injury to the spinal cord can be divided into two main components: primary injury and secondary injury:

    1. Primary injury is damage to the vertebrae, spinal cord, and supporting structures that occurs as a direct result of the trauma.

    2. Secondary injury consists of a large number of biochemical processes that occur as a result of the primary injury, and that perpetuates spinal cord damage in the hours to days after the primary injury occurs.

ii. There are a number of different types of primary injury, including spinal luxation and vertebral fracture, traumatic intervertebral disk herniation, spinal cord contusion, and extra-axial hemorrhage:

    1. The types and severity of spinal luxations and vertebral fractures are dependent upon the structures affected. A three compartment model of the vertebra has been proposed to describe the stability of these types of injuries (see Figure 9.2):

        a. The dorsal compartment includes the articular processes, laminae, pedicles, and spinous processes.

        b. The middle compartment contains the dorsal longitudinal ligament, the dorsal aspect of the vertebral body, and the dorsal portion of the annulus fibrosis.

        c. The ventral compartment contains the ventral longitudinal ligament, the lateral and ventral aspects of the annulus fibrosis, the nucleus pulposus, and the remaining portions of the vertebral body.

    2. Damage to any two of the three compartments results in spinal instability.

    3. In addition, the type and severity of the force applied to the spine will determine the type of fracture or luxation that results:

        a. Vertebral lamina, facet, or pedicle fractures result from extension of the spine. Because disruption of the annulus is common, these fractures are unstable upon extension of the spine, but remain stable in flexion.

        b. Vertebral body fractures may occur secondary to shearing or compressive forces on the spine. They are generally unstable. In addition, bone fragments may be found within the vertebral canal, causing compression of the spinal cord.

        c. Vertebral compression fractures are generally caused by pure flexion forces. Spinal instability is uncommon with vertebral compression fractures because of the high likelihood of maintenance of dorsal ligamentous stabilizing structures.

d. Spinal luxation in the absence of vertebral fracture results from flexion with or without rotation of the spine. The instability resulting from these types of injuries is due to compromise of both the dorsal and ventral ligamentous structures.

e. Spinal luxation in the presence of vertebral fracture results from rotational forces with or without the presence of flexion forces. These injuries are also unstable due to the compromise of dorsal and ventral ligamentous structures.

4. Traumatic intervertebral disk herniation typically occurs in dogs with Hansen's Type I intervertebral disk disease. Chondroid degeneration of the dorsal annulus fibrosus predisposes the annulus to rupture secondary to traumatic injury, resulting in herniation of the nucleus pulposus into the vertebral canal. This type of degenerative disk disease is most common in chondrodystrophic dogs, but can be present in any breed. Although it is much less common, cats can also develop chondroid degeneration of the intervertebral disk, predisposing them to traumatic herniation.

5. Spinal cord contusion (hemorrhage into the spinal cord parenchyma) is rarely reported in the veterinary literature as an independent finding after spinal trauma. However, contusions likely commonly occur secondary to vertebral fracture, spinal luxation, or traumatic intervertebral disk herniation. Contusions form as a result of disruption of parenchymal blood vessels within the spinal cord. They may also develop secondary to traumatic motion of the spinal cord within the vertebral canal, resulting in coup and contrecoup lesions, similar to cerebral contusions that develop after head trauma.

6. Extra-axial hemorrhage results in accumulation of blood and hematoma formation. These accumulations can occur in the subdural or epidural spaces and can result in significant spinal cord compression and neurologic dysfunction. Although epidural and subdural spinal hematomas have been reported secondary to trauma in humans, they are rare. Several case reports in the veterinary literature describe the development of epidural hematomas secondary to intervertebral disk herniation, but there are no published reports of these types of injury secondary to trauma.

iii. Secondary injury to the spinal cord occurs in the hours to days after the primary injury. A series of vascular and biochemical events ultimately lead to progressive spinal cord damage:

1. In healthy animals, blood flow to the spinal cord is maintained in the face of fluctuations in systemic blood pressure through local spinal cord autoregulatory mechanisms. Traumatic injury to the spinal cord results in a deficit of these autoregulatory mechanisms, and systemic hypotension, which is common in patients with trauma, leads to decreased spinal cord blood flow, ultimately leading to spinal cord ischemia and necrosis.

2. Damage to neuronal membranes, release of excitatory neurotransmitters such as glutamate, and activation of voltage-gated calcium channels lead to an influx of calcium into the neuron. This results in triggering of the inflammatory cascade via phospholipase A2 activation, depletion of ATP via binding of calcium to phosphates, mitochondrial dysfunction, and neuronal cell swelling, perpetuating neuronal dysfunction and destruction.

3. Free radical production in the spinal cord is favored after injury by the presence of increased intracellular calcium, ischemia-reperfusion phenomena, the presence of iron and copper due to hemorrhage, and the high lipid content of CNS tissues. The cycle of oxidative damage leads to perpetuation of neuronal injury.

4. Extracellular concentrations of excitatory neurotransmitters such as glutamate and aspartate are increased after trauma due to release by damaged neurons as well as decreased clearance by ischemic astrocytes. These excitatory neurotransmitters activate a number of neuronal receptors, causing influx of sodium and calcium, as well as causing cellular swelling.

5. Traumatic spinal cord injury results in production of inflammatory mediators. These mediators contribute to secondary injury by inducing NO production, triggering influx of inflammatory cells, and activating the arachidonic acid cascade. Several of these inflammatory mediators are potent activators of coagulation, resulting in microvascular thrombosis and further spinal cord ischemia.

6. Spinal shock is the transient development of lower motor signs caudal to the level of an acute spinal cord injury. This is likely due to the loss of descending excitatory input to lower motor neurons, resulting in hyperpolarization of these neurons and decreased excitability. In time, these lower motor neurons again become excitable due to their inherent plasticity in order to adapt to the decreased input received from descending tracts. In dogs and cats, the initial flaccid paralysis usually lasts for no more than 12 hours, and spastic paralysis develops within 24–48 hours. This is in contrast to humans, in whom flaccid paralysis can last for days to weeks after an acute injury.

2. DIAGNOSTIC EVALUATION

a. Neurologic examination:

  i. An initial brief neurologic examination should be done to obtain a neuroanatomical diagnosis and determine if an unstable fracture is present:

    1. Nonambulatory animals should be evaluated on presentation in the position in which they arrive. Until the presence of an unstable injury has been ruled out, all patients should be treated as if the spine is unstable.

    2. The initial neurologic examination should consist of the following:

      a. Cranial nerve examination and evaluation of mentation.

      b. Presence of segmental reflexes in all four limbs.

      c. Presence of superficial pain sensation in all four limbs.

      d. If superficial pain sensation is absent, presence of deep pain sensation in affected limbs.

      e. Gentle spinal palpation to identify areas of instability, pain, crepitus, or malalignment.

      f. Panniculus reflex to provide additional localizing information in animals with thoracolumbar trauma.

      g. Presence of Schiff-Sherrington posture, which indicates thoracolumbar injury in the T2–L4 region. This consists of extensor rigidity in the thoracic limbs in addition to paraplegia:

        i. It is important to note that this finding is useful in the context of neurolocalization, but should not be considered a prognostic indicator. It may be present in animals with spinal cord lesions of varying severity.

        ii. It is crucial to differentiate Schiff-Sherrington posture from decerebrate rigidity, characterized by extensor rigidity of all four limbs, or a decerebellate posture, with rigid extension of the thoracic limbs and relaxed or flexed pelvic limbs but no paraplegia. Decerebrate rigidity indicates a rostral brainstem lesion and carries a guarded prognosis, while decerebellate posture suggests a cerebellar lesion, and both also commonly accompany cranial nerve deficits (see Chapter 7: Traumatic Brain Injury).

  h. Evaluations requiring more manipulation of the patient should be done only if unstable injuries of the spine have been deemed unlikely. These evaluations include the following:

    i. Evaluation of the ability of the animal to ambulate.

    ii. Presence of voluntary motor function in all four limbs.

    iii. Orthopedic evaluation to determine if musculoskeletal injury could be responsible.

  ii. Severe spinal trauma should be suspected in all patients with normal mentation and without cranial nerve deficits but which are unable to ambulate and have no evidence of musculoskeletal injury to explain their ambulation deficits. Significant spinal cord injury may be present even if the animal was noted to ambulate immediately post injury.

iii. Patients with cervical injuries often have neck pain with minimal or no neurologic deficits. The clinician's index of suspicion for cervical injury should be increased in patients with no cranial nerve deficits and normal mentation with or without neurologic deficits who resist movement of the neck or have neck pain.

iv. Brachial plexus injury should be suspected in any animal with absence of withdrawal reflex in one thoracic limb, Horner's syndrome (ptosis, miosis and enophthalmus) in the ipsilateral eye, and ipsilateral loss of the panniculus reflex (see Chapter 8: Trauma-Associated Peripheral Nerve Injury).

b. Imaging:

i. Spinal radiographs are generally indicated in animals with suspected vertebral injury. Screening lateral radiographs of the entire spine can usually be obtained safely, and can provide valuable diagnostic information in animals with multiple spinal injuries:

1. Sedation for spinal radiographs should be used with caution, as relaxation of the paraspinal musculature can lead to increased spinal instability and further spinal cord trauma. Because positioning of the patient can be crucial to obtaining spinal radiographs of good diagnostic quality, radiographs with poor patient positioning should be interpreted cautiously.

2. Patients that are stressed and attempting to move should be immobilized by taping them to a back board. Lateral radiographs can be taken with the patient immobilized in this way. Ventrodorsal radiographs should only be taken with the use of a horizontal beam technique with the patient stabilized in lateral recumbency (see Figure 9.3).

3. Radiography has been shown to have relatively low sensitivity for vertebral fractures (72%) and subluxations (77.5%) in canine trauma patients, as well as low negative predictive values for the presence of fracture fragments within the vertebral canal (51%). This suggests that spinal radiographs alone

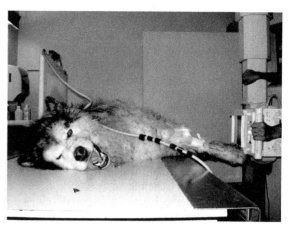

FIGURE 9.3   A ventrodorsal spinal radiograph being taken of a dog with a T3 compression fracture using a horizontal beam technique.

should not be used to definitively rule out the presence of spinal luxation or vertebral fracture.

4. Intervertebral disk herniations are also difficult to diagnose on spinal radiographs. Narrowing of an affected disk space has been shown to be the most useful radiographic sign of intervertebral disk herniation, but has low sensitivity (64–69%) and positive predictive value (63–71%) for diagnosis of herniation.

ii. In order to definitively diagnose the location and extent of spinal injury, advanced imaging techniques such as myelography, computed tomography, and/or magnetic resonance imaging are often required:

1. These advanced imaging modalities require general anesthesia, which relax the stabilizing paraspinal muscles and increase the risk of additional spinal cord injury. Care must be taken to minimize movement of the spinal column during these procedures.

2. Positioning of patients for contrast injection during myelography can cause an increased risk of spinal trauma. In addition, although compressive lesions are readily diagnosed with myelography, little information about other spinal cord insults, such as hemorrhage, is obtained.

3. Magnetic resonance imaging is superior for evaluation of spinal cord hemorrhage and edema, as well as damage to supporting soft tissue structures such as the epaxial musculature and ligaments. However, several studies in human medicine have shown that significant spinal fractures can be overlooked on magnetic resonance images.

4. Computed tomography (CT) has been shown to be an extremely sensitive diagnostic test for acute bony lesions in human polytrauma, with sensitivity of up to 100% in several studies. In addition, contrast-enhanced CT provides information on the presence of spinal cord edema and hemorrhage. This combination of characteristics makes it the preferred imaging modality for human patients with polytrauma including the spinal column.

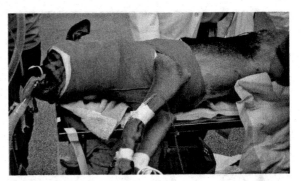

FIGURE 9.4   A dog with a cervical spinal injury in a fiberglass cast.

3. TREATMENT OF SPINAL INJURY

a. Treatment of primary spinal injury due to trauma may include surgical and medical intervention. Specific therapy targeted at the underlying primary injury must be tailored to each patient:

   i. Vertebral fractures and spinal luxations may be treated nonsurgically, or with surgical decompression, reduction, and/or fixation:

   1. There is considerable debate in the veterinary literature regarding indications for surgical vs. nonsurgical management of vertebral fractures and spinal luxations. Ultimately, it is often the personal opinion of the surgeon and the choice of the owner that determines which patients are surgical candidates. However, several general indications are widely agreed upon to be indications for surgical management:

   a. Patients with minimal voluntary motor function or complete paralysis.

   b. Patients with clinical or radiographic evidence of highly unstable fractures.

   c. Patients with obvious progression of neurologic signs despite appropriate nonsurgical management.

   2. There are various surgical options for stabilization and internal fixation, including the use of bone plates, screws, Steinmann pins, and polymethylmethacrylate (PMMA) cement. These are challenging procedures requiring advanced training, and are an indication for referral to a board certified surgeon or neurosurgeon. Advantages of surgical management include accelerated stabilization of the spine and more rapid return to function, but these procedures are expensive, may result in worsening of spinal cord injury due to instability of the extraspinal muscles during anesthesia and surgical manipulation, and carry the risk of implant failure or complications, such as infection and wound dehiscence.

   3. Nonsurgical management of vertebral fracture and spinal luxation involves external coaptation and strict cage rest for 6–8 weeks to allow healing. Splints can be fashioned from fiberglass, thermoplastics, plaster, metal rods, or other materials that can be fashioned to conform to the patient's body shape (see Figures 9.4 and 9.5). Immobilization of the entire spine must be achieved. The splint is held in place using bandage material, taking care to provide the required spinal stability without compromising the ability of the patient to ventilate. The bandage should be evaluated daily for evidence of soiling, abrasions, pressure sores, or other complications, and replaced promptly if problems are noted. Nonsurgical management is generally less expensive, does not require specialized equipment, and allows owners to provide care at home, but requires fastidious and labor-intensive nursing care, long recovery periods, and a greater likelihood of persistent neurologic deficits. Client education is of paramount importance, especially with large breed

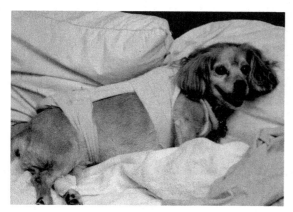

FIGURE 9.5 A dog with a thoracolumbar spinal injury in an orthoplast splint and bandage.

dogs in which nursing care often requires the efforts of multiple people.

ii. Traumatic intervertebral disk herniations may also be treated either surgically or nonsurgically. In general, patients with loss of voluntary motor function or rapidly progressing neurologic deficits should be considered for surgical management. Depending upon the site of the herniation, dorsal laminectomy, hemilaminectomy, or a ventral slot procedure may be indicated to relieve the spinal cord compression. Less severely affected patients, such as ambulatory patients with ataxia, or nonambulatory patients with improving motor function, may respond to medical management, consisting of strict cage rest for 6–8 weeks to allow resolution of spinal cord inflammation.

iii. Spinal cord contusion rarely occurs as a sole entity, and is usually the result of a compressive lesion or spinal instability. Treatment involves addressing the concurrent primary injury via surgical or nonsurgical management and medical therapy to reduce secondary injury.

iv. Treatment of traumatic extra-axial hematomas in people consists of surgical evacuation to relieve the spinal cord compression. These are rarely diagnosed in veterinary medicine secondary to trauma, but surgical decompression is recommended in these cases.

b. Secondary injury, which develops immediately after the traumatic event and continues in the hours to days postinjury, is responsible for much of the progression of neurologic dysfunction noted after a traumatic event. Many therapies to amelio-

rate secondary injury have been proposed in the clinical and experimental literature:

i. Maintenance of systemic blood pressure and blood oxygen content is of paramount importance in reducing secondary spinal cord injury. As described above, spinal cord blood flow autoregulatory mechanisms are commonly compromised by trauma. Patients sustaining spinal trauma frequently have respiratory, cardiovascular, or head trauma as well as significant hemorrhage, all of which can lead to decreased systemic blood pressure and oxygen delivery. In the face of impaired autoregulation, the damaged spinal cord is at high risk of ischemic injury. Aggressive fluid resuscitation should be implemented to maintain adequate perfusion:

1. Isotonic crystalloids (e.g., Normosol-R, Lactated Ringer's solution, 0.9% saline, Plasmalyte-A) at an initial dose of 20–30 mL/kg over 15–20 minutes are an excellent choice in the trauma patient. This dose can be repeated as needed to achieve and maintain normotension.

2. Hypertonic crystalloids (e.g., 7.2% hypertonic saline, HTS) at a dose of 4 mL/kg, or synthetic colloids at a dose of 5 mL/kg over 15–20 minutes are also good resuscitation fluids in well-hydrated trauma patients. These solutions will achieve a volume expansion effect in excess of the administered dose by pulling fluid from the extravascular space. In addition, HTS can improve cardiac contractility, reduce endothelial cell swelling, decrease inflammation, and protect the blood-brain/spinal cord barrier.

3. Packed red blood cells (pRBCs) at a dose of 10–15 mL/kg, or a polymerized hemoglobin solution (e.g., Oxyglobin) at a dose of 10–30 mL/kg at up to 10 mL/kg/h in the dog, 5–15 mL/kg in the cat at up to 5 mL/kg/h, can be used in patients with anemia secondary to blood loss to provide additional oxygen-carrying capacity in addition to intravascular volume. Note that Oxyglobin is not labeled for use in cats, and that cats are generally more susceptible to volume overload and development of pulmonary edema or

pleural effusion. Cats with underlying heart disease are at significantly increased risk of complications, and all cats administered Oxyglobin should be closely monitored for signs of increased respiratory rate and effort. The decision to transfuse a patient with anemia should be based on clinical signs of an inability to compensate for decreased oxygen-carrying capacity (e.g., tachycardia and hypotension unresponsive to volume replacement) (see Chapter 3: Shock in the Trauma Patient).

4. In patients unresponsive to fluid therapy, vasopressor agents should be used to maintain adequate systemic blood pressure. The decision to begin vasopressor therapy is ideally made with the benefit of an objective measurement of cardiac preload, such as central venous pressure (CVP) measurement. For guidelines, see Chapter 3: Shock in the Trauma Patient and Chapter 4: Monitoring of the Trauma Patient. Patients with inappropriate vasodilation may benefit from dopamine infusion (5–12 ug/kg/min) or norepinpehrine (1–10 ug/kg/min). Patients with decreased cardiac contractility may respond to dopamine or dobutamine (1–20 ug/kg/min) infusion. Although uncommon, seizures can occur in cats with dobutamine infusions, especially at doses greater than 5 ug/kg/min. In most cases, seizures resolve with discontinuation of the infusion and treatment with diazepam (0.5 mg/kg intravenously).

ii. Oxygen supplementation is indicated in all patients sustaining traumatic injury until definitive evidence of adequate pulmonary function and ventilation is obtained. Decreased oxygen delivery to the traumatized spinal cord due to hypoxemia can significantly contribute to secondary injury. Options for oxygen supplementation include flow by delivery via mask or nasal prongs (maximum $FiO_2 \sim 40\%$), unilateral or bilateral nasal cannulae (maximum $FiO_2 \sim 60\%$), oxygen tents or hoods, and oxygen cages. Blood oxygenation can be assessed via pulse oximetry (minimum acceptable $SpO_2 = 94\%$) or arterial blood gas analysis (minimum acceptable $PaO_2 = 100$ mm Hg).

iii. The use of corticosteroids to ameliorate secondary injury after spinal cord trauma is highly controversial in both human and veterinary medicine. There is evidence from the experimental and clinical literature of both benefit and harm from the use of these drugs in patients with spinal cord injury. The decision to treat with these drugs should be made with a thorough understanding of the evidence for both benefit and harm:

1. Methylprednisolone sodium succinate (MPSS) has been extensively studied in both experimental studies and clinical trials as a therapy to address secondary injury. Mechanisms by which MPSS has been proposed to offer a neuroprotective effect in patients with spinal cord injury include improvement of local blood flow, free-radical scavenging, and anti-inflammatory activity. The experimental evidence strongly suggests that the free radical scavenging property of MPSS is the most important protective effect in patients with spinal cord injury. Although the anti-inflammatory effects of other common corticosteroids (e.g., dexamethasone, prednisone) are likely to reduce the discomfort associated with spinal trauma, they do not possess the free-radical scavenging of MPSS and are unlikely to have any significant neuroprotective effect.

2. Clinical evidence for the beneficial effect of MPSS in spinal cord injury comes primarily from the National Acute Spinal Cord Injury Study (NASCIS) trials. Only the NASCIS 2 trial was placebo controlled. There was a mild improvement in motor scores at 6 weeks for patients treated with MPSS (30 mg/kg bolus, followed by a constant rate infusion of 5.4 mg/kg/h for 48 hours) compared to the placebo group, but this effect was not present at 6 months or 1 year postinjury. Only in a post hoc, subgroup analysis were the authors able to show an improvement in motor scores at 6 weeks, 6 months, and 1 year in the group of patients treated with MPSS for 48 hours beginning 3–8 hours post injury. No difference in outcome between the treatment groups was noted at any of the time

points for patients treated less than 3 hours or greater than 8 hours after injury. There were no differences in mortality between the groups, but there was an increased incidence of severe pneumonia and a trend for an increased risk of sepsis in the groups treated with MPSS for 48 hours at the 6 week time point.

3. The results of the NASCIS 2 trial have been the subject of great controversy in human medicine, and although the use of high dose MPSS for patients with spinal cord injury continues to be considered standard of care, several surveys have shown a lack of confidence in this therapy among human neurosurgeons.

4. There have been no placebo-controlled trials evaluating the efficacy of MPSS in veterinary patients with spinal cord injury. Studies have shown significant side effects of corticosteroid treatment in spinal cord injured dogs, including gastrointestinal ulceration as well as prolonged hospital stays.

5. Given the clinical and experimental evidence, MPSS at an initial dose of 30 mg/kg followed by a CRI of 5.4 mg/kg/h or repeated boluses of 15 mg/kg every 6 hours for 24–48 hours may be considered as neuroprotective therapy in patients with spinal cord injury. However, given the prevalence of complications, the lack of clinical trials demonstrating efficacy in veterinary species, and the likelihood that the mild functional improvements noted in the one human clinical trial would not correlate to significant improvements in quality of life in veterinary species, it is the author's opinion that the risks of this treatment outweigh the potential benefits. There is no clinical or experimental evidence of a neuroprotective effect of other corticosteroids, such as dexamethasone or prednisone, but these drugs may be useful at an anti-inflammatory dose (initially, 1–2 mg/kg per day prednisone, 0.15–0.3 mg/kg per day dexamethasone, tapering over 1–2 weeks) to reduce discomfort associated with the injury.

iv. Polyethylene glycol (PEG) is a hydrophilic polymer that has been shown to rapidly seal defects in mechanically damaged nerve fibers, allowing them to begin conducting sensory and motor impulses. In addition, PEG seals damaged cells and prevents release of excitatory neurotransmitters and other cytotoxic substances leading to secondary injury. A clinical trial of intravenous PEG (two doses, 2 mL/kg of a 30% solution intravenously 4–6 hours apart) in dogs with acute intervertebral disk herniation within 72 hours of onset of clinical signs showed that treated dogs had improved outcomes compared to historical controls. Although these data are preliminary and this drug has not been evaluated in patients with other types of spinal trauma, PEG may provide a promising new therapy for acute spinal trauma.

4. PROGNOSIS

a. Prognosis for recovery of neurologic function after spinal trauma is difficult to predict. The type and severity of the primary injury and the degree to which secondary injury has progressed will contribute to outcome:

i. Patients with loss of deep pain perception at the time of presentation have a worse prognosis than those with intact deep pain sensation. Loss of deep pain perception is evidence of functional spinal cord transection, as it reflects function of small diameter tracts adjacent to spinal cord gray matter, deep within the cord. However, some patients with loss of deep pain perception can go on to recover neurologic function with treatment.

ii. Patients with spinal luxation and vertebral fracture may have a worse prognosis than those with traumatic disk herniation. In one study, only 2 of 17 (12%) dogs with vertebral fractures or spinal luxation and absence of deep pain sensation regained the ability to walk, while 69% of dogs with spontaneous intervertebral disk herniation and loss of deep pain perception did so. Further studies are required to determine if patients with traumatic intervertebral disk herniation have similar prognoses to those with nontraumatic intervertebral disk herniation.

iii. In dogs with cervical vertebral fractures, nonambulatory status and delay of greater than 5 days to referral for surgical stabilization have been associated with worse outcome. Cervical vertebral fracture stabilization is associated with a high perioperative mortality (36%), but dogs that survive this period have a good prognosis for neurologic recovery. Hypoventilation is a potential complication of cervical spinal injury, but dogs with surgically corrected disease that hypoventilate postoperatively had a good prognosis with positive pressure ventilation and aggressive supportive care in one retrospective study (Beal, 2001).

iv. Prognosis in cats with spinal injury is similar to dogs, but in one retrospective study, a high incidence of myelomalacia was noted at surgery and/or necropsy in cats with loss of deep pain perception after spinal trauma. Clinical signs of myelomalacia include progressive ascending or descending lower motor neuron signs (affecting muscles served by nerves arising from the affected areas) in combination with ascending analgesia (caudal to the most cranial aspect of the lesion). Respiratory failure commonly occurs within 2–4 days, and the condition is irreversible. This should not be confused with spinal shock, a transient development of lower motor signs caudal to the level of an acute spinal cord injury described above. The resulting flaccid paralysis can last for up to 12 hours after injury.

b. Prognosis is also dependent upon the extent of other, concurrent injuries. Frank discussions with the owner regarding the cumulative effect on prognosis of the multiple injuries commonly present in patients with polytrauma are extremely important early in the management of these patients.

BIBLIOGRAPHY

Bagley RS. Spinal fracture or luxation. *Vet Clin North Am Small Anim Pract* 2000; 30(1): 133–153, vi–vii.

Beal MW, Paglia DT, Griffin GM, Hughes D, King LG. Ventilatory failure, ventilator management, and outcome in dogs with cervical spinal disorders: 14 cases (1991–1999). *J Am Vet Med Assoc* 2001; 218(10): 1598–1602.

Boag A, Otto C, Drobatz K. Complications of methylprednisolone sodium succinate therapy in dachshunds with surgically treated intervertebral disc disease. *JVECC* 2001; 11(2): 105–110.

Bracken MB, Shepard MJ, Collins WF, *et al.* A randomized, controlled trial of methylprednisolone or naloxone in the treatment of acute spinal-cord injury. Results of the Second National Acute Spinal Cord Injury Study. *N Engl J Med* 1990; 322(20): 1405–1411.

Bruecker KA. Principles of vertebral fracture management. *Semin Vet Med Surg (Small Anim)* 1996; 11(4): 259–272.

Grasmueck S, Steffen F. Survival rates and outcomes in cats with thoracic and lumbar spinal cord injuries due to external trauma. *J Small Anim Pract* 2004; 45(6): 284–288.

Hall ED, Springer JE. Neuroprotection and acute spinal cord injury: a reappraisal. *NeuroRx* 2004; 1(1): 80–100.

Hawthorne JC, Blevins WE, Wallace LJ, Glickman N, Waters DJ. Cervical vertebral fractures in 56 dogs: a retrospective study. *J Am Anim Hosp Assoc* 1999; 35(2): 135–146.

Kinns J, Mai W, Seiler G, *et al.* Radiographic sensitivity and negative predictive value for acute canine spinal trauma. *Vet Radiol Ultrasound* 2006; 47(6): 563–570.

Laverty PH, Leskovar A, Breur GJ, *et al.* A preliminary study of intravenous surfactants in paraplegic dogs: polymer therapy in canine clinical SCI. *J Neurotrauma* 2004; 21(12): 1767–1777.

Olby N, Levine J, Harris T, Munana K, Skeen T, Sharp N. Long-term functional outcome of dogs with severe injuries of the thoracolumbar spinal cord: 87 cases (1996–2001). *J Am Vet Med Assoc* 2003; 222(6): 762–769.

Olby N. Current concepts in the management of acute spinal cord injury. *J Vet Intern Med* 1999; 13(5): 399–407.

Selcer RR, Bubb WJ, Walker TL. Management of vertebral column fractures in dogs and cats: 211 cases (1977–1985). *J Am Vet Med Assoc* 1991; 198(11): 1965–1968.

Smith PM, Jeffery ND. Spinal shock – Comparative aspects and clinical relevance. *J Vet Intern Med* 2005; 19(6): 788–793.

URINARY TRACT TRAUMA

Merilee F. Costello

1. INTRODUCTION

a. Trauma to the urinary tract is an important rule-out in any trauma patient.

b. Common causes of trauma to the urinary tract include the following:

  i. Blunt trauma:

    1. In animals with blunt pelvic trauma, 39% are reported to have concurrent trauma to the urinary tract (Mathews, 2004).

  ii. Penetrating trauma including gunshot wounds, bite wounds, or other penetrating objects.

  iii. Iatrogenic trauma:

    1. Urethral catheterization when relieving urethral obstruction.

    2. Surgical trauma:

      a. Cryptorchid orchiectomy

      b. Surgery to remove urethral calculi

      c. Inadvertent ligation and transaction of the ureters during ovariohysterectomy

c. Trauma to the urinary tract often goes undetected:

  i. Incidence of trauma to the urinary tract that is not identified in dogs and cats has been reported as 20–50% and 15.4%, respectively (Aumann et al., 1998):

    1. In these studies, in some cases, the diagnosis was not made until clinical signs of azotemia and electrolyte abnormalities occurred; other cases were diagnosed at necropsy.

  2. In cats, a palpable bladder was noted in 20% of the cats with a ruptured bladder.

2. UROPERITONEUM

a. The most common cause of uroperitoneum in dogs and cats is trauma to the abdomen or pelvis.

b. Uroperitoneum occurs secondary to traumatic injury and subsequent urine leakage from the urethra, bladder, ureter, or kidney:

  i. Other etiologies of uroperitoneum include the following:

    1. Bladder rupture due to neoplastic infiltration, most commonly transitional cell carcinoma

    2. Urethral calculi and urinary obstruction

    3. Traumatic urethral catheterization

    4. Cystocentesis

c. Pathophysiology:

  i. As urine accumulates in the peritoneal space, nitrogenous waste products, potassium, and hydrogen ion are reabsorbed into the bloodstream, resulting in severe azotemia, hyperkalemia, and metabolic acidosis respectively:

    1. The degree of reabsorption is partly dependent on the molecular size:

      a. Urea is a small molecule that rapidly equilibrates with the bloodstream, resulting in little difference in the BUN levels between the blood and the abdominal effusion.

b. Creatinine is a large molecule and does not diffuse as readily, thus, uroperitoneum will result in a significantly higher creatinine level in the abdominal effusion as compared to the blood. This diffusion characteristic enables the clinician to compare abdominal effusion creatinine concentration to that in the blood as a screening test for uroperitoneum in dogs and cats that have sustained trauma (see Diagnosis below). (Aumann et al., 1998).

c. Despite its small size and propensity to rapidly diffuse across the peritoneal membrane, comparison of abdominal fluid potassium concentration to that in the blood appears to be a useful screening test for uroperitoneum in dogs and cats (see Diagnosis below) (Aumann et al., 1998).

2. Hyperkalemia is the likely cause of death in most dogs and cats with untreated uroperitoneum. Hyperkalemia decreases resting membrane potential (making it less negative) and results in severe electrocardiographic abnormalities (see Diagnosis below) including bradycardia. If left untreated, asystole and (rarely) ventricular fibrillation will result. Consequently, the focus of treatment for dogs and cats with hyperkalemia must be on management of hyperkalemia (see Treatment below) and concurrent life-threatening injuries.

3. Metabolic acidosis is commonly seen in animals with uroperitoneum due to a failure to excrete hydrogen ion.

ii. The severity of azotemia has been directly correlated with the duration of uroperitoneum in dogs; however, this has not been documented in cats (Aumann et al., 1998).

d. Historical findings:

i. Dogs and cats with traumatic uroperitoneum most often have a history of exogenous trauma.

ii. One classic historical finding in dogs with uroperitoneum is a failed attempt to jump into the rear of a car/truck resulting in blunt caudal abdominal trauma.

e. Clinical signs and physical examination findings:

i. Clinical signs associated with uroperitoneum may vary depending on both the duration and the underlying etiology.

1. Anuria, dysuria:

a. It is important to note that the ability to urinate does not rule out traumatic rupture of the urinary tract.

b. Even with bladder disruption, bladder integrity may be intermittently maintained by blood clot formation.

2. Hematuria:

a. Hematuria is a common clinical sign in humans, dogs, and cats with traumatic injury to the urinary tract and subsequent uroperitoneum.

b. Hematuria can also occur secondary to damage to the bladder mucosa and kidneys without being associated with rupture and urine leakage.

c. Significant urinary trauma can also occur without concomitant hematuria, so its absence does not rule out injury.

3. Vomiting and anorexia may occur secondary to uremia.

4. Restlessness, panting, abdominal guarding, abdominal distention, and a hunched appearance may all be manifestations of uroperitoneum.

ii. Physical examination findings that can occur secondary to the systemic effects of uroperitoneum and the subsequent electrolyte changes, acid base abnormalities and uremia may include the following:

1. Neurological:

a. Altered levels of consciousness may occur secondary to abdominal pain, uremia, and poor cardiovascular function (hypovolemia, bradycardia, conduction disturbances) secondary to uroperitoneum and hyperkalemia.

2. Cardiovascular:

a. Animals with longstanding uroperitoneum, dehydration, hypovolemia, and hyperkalemia may demonstrate all of the "classic" manifestations of hypovolemia including pale mucous membranes, a prolonged CRT, and poor pulse quality;

however, bradycardia or a relative bradycardia (normal heart rate) is often present.

   b. Bradycardia:

      i. Few injuries in the traumatized patient result in relative bradycardia. The presence of a relative or inappropriate bradycardia should trigger a vigorous search for its cause:

         1. Uroperitoneum causes bradycardia secondary to hyperkalemia (see above).

         2. Traumatic brain injury causes bradycardia due to increased intracranial pressure (see Chapter 7: Traumatic Brain Injury).

      ii. Hypothermia may also contribute to the bradycardia seen in animals with uroperitoneum and hyperkalemia.

   c. Dehydration may result from decreased intake and loss of fluids into the peritoneal space.

   d. Dehydration may progress to hypovolemia (see Chapter 3: Shock in the Trauma Patient).

   e. Hypovolemia may also result secondary to concurrent injuries.

3. Respiratory:

   a. Uroperitoneum is frequently associated with significant metabolic acidosis.

   b. Respiratory compensation for metabolic acidosis may include an increase in minute ventilation that is clinically represented by larger tidal volume breaths and occasionally tachypnea.

4. Abdominal palpation:

   a. Pain on abdominal palpation results secondary to the chemical peritonitis induced by the interaction of urine with the peritoneal membrane.

   b. Abdominal distention and the presence of a fluid wave may be noted in long-standing uroperitoneum.

   c. Animals with uroperitoneum, secondary to bladder or proximal urethral disruption, may lack a palpable bladder on abdominal palpation. However, this is not always the case:

      i. A palpable bladder does not rule out bladder rupture.

      ii. In cats, a palpable bladder has been reported in 20% of cats with ruptured bladder (Aumann et al., 1998).

5. Hypothermia:

   a. Potential causes include uremia as well as poor peripheral perfusion.

6. A rectal examination may reveal crepitus or irregularity of the pelvis associated with fractures or dislocations (see Chapter 17: Musculoskeletal Trauma to the Pelvis, Sacrum, and Tail).

7. Examination of the perineal region and inguinal region may show swelling, edema, or bruising associated with urine leakage into the adjacent tissues:

   a. These changes are rarely apparent immediately, so frequent re-evaluation is necessary during the first 24–72 hours as fluids are administered and urine production increases.

8. If the patient has a concurrent urinary tract infection, urine leakage into the peritoneal space will result in a septic peritonitis:

   a. In these cases, clinical signs of septic/vasodilatory shock and hypoperfusion may predominate (see Chapter 3: Shock in the Trauma Patient).

f. Diagnosis of uroperitoneum and its clinical sequelae:

   i. Clinicopathologic abnormalities:

      1. An "emergency blood screen" consisting of PCV/TS/Blood Glucose/Venous or Arterial Blood Gas Analysis/Electrolytes/BUN/CREA/Lactate is a very useful tool to aid in the early identification of many of the clinicopathologic manifestations of uroperitoneum:

         a. PCV/TS:

            i. Hemoconcentraiton may result secondary to dehydration associated with decreased fluid intake, fluid shifts into the peritoneal space, and loss of fluids associated with vomiting.

            ii. Decreased total solids may occur due to loss of protein into the abdominal space associated with chemical peritonitis.

            iii. Concurrent abdominal injuries and injuries to other organ systems may also impact PCV/TS in the traumatized patient.

    b. Venous or arterial blood gas analysis:

      i. Metabolic acidosis is expected in animals with uroperitoneum, due to a failure to excrete hydrogen ion.

      ii. Metabolic acidosis secondary to increased production of lactate and hydrogen ion due to concurrent injuries is not unexpected in animals with uroperitoneum and abdominal trauma.

      iii. Respiratory alkalosis may be noted due to pain, stress, or concurrent thoracic injuries.

      iv. Mixed disturbances are expected.

    c. Electrolytes:

      i. Common electrolyte disturbances in dogs and cats with uroperitoneum include hyperkalemia, hyponatremia, and hypochloremia:

        1. See Hyperkalemia above.

        2. Hyponatremia and hypochloremia may result because urine is low in sodium and chloride and these electrolytes rapidly equilibrate across the peritoneal membrane. Additional chloride may be lost in vomitus (Aumann et al., 1998).

    d. BUN/CREA:

      i. Absorption of urea results in an elevation in the BUN.

      ii. Absorption of creatinine over time will result in an elevation of the CREA.

    e. Lactate:

      i. Hyperlactatemia in the traumatized patient most often results from a failure of delivery of oxygen to the tissues.

      ii. Dehydration and secondary hypovolemia may contribute to lactic acidosis in the dog or cat with uroperitoneum.

  ii. Electrocardiography (ECG):

    1. ECG abnormalities are common in the traumatized patient and result from shock, cardiac injury, hypoxemia, metabolic acidosis, hyperkalemia, or a combination of these.

    2. ECG abnormalities associated with hyperkalemia may manifest in animals with uroperitoneum (Dibartola et al., 2000):

      a. Mild hyperkalemia:

        i. Tenting or spiking of the "T" wave is seen with mild hyperkalemia due to rapid repolarization.

        ii. Shortening of the QT interval due to rapid repolarization.

      b. Moderate hyperkalemia:

        i. Prolongation of the PR interval due to delayed conduction through the AV node.

        ii. Widening of the QRS complex due to delayed conduction through the AV node.

        iii. Widening and flattening of the P wave may occur due to impaired conduction through the atria.

      c. Severe hyperkalemia:

        i. Absence of the P wave due to absence of atrial contraction

        ii. Bradycardia

        iii. Sinoventricular rhythm

        iv. QRS merges with the T wave to form a sine wave.

      d. Terminal arrhythmias:

        i. Asystole

        ii. Ventricular fibrillation

  iii. Fluid analysis:

    1. Abdominal fluid accumulation is expected in animals with uroperitoneum. Abdominal fluid may be suspected based on physical examination, survey radiography results (see below), or FAST Scan (see below). A suspicion of abdominal effusion should prompt routine (blind) or ultrasound-guided abdominocentesis.

    2. Abdominal fluid analysis is an excellent screening test for the presence of uroperitoneum through the comparison of abdominal fluid creatinine and potassium to blood creatinine and potassium respectively:

      a. Abdominal fluid and blood samples should be acquired within $1/2$ hour of each other.

b. Abdominal fluid and blood samples must be handled concurrently and analyzed using the same methodology.

c. A ratio of the creatinine concentration in the effusion to serum creatinine above 2:1 is diagnostic for uroperitoneum in dogs and cats (Aumann et al., 1998; Schmiedt et al., 2001).

d. A ratio of the potassium concentration in the effusion to serum potassium above 1.4:1 is diagnostic for uroperitoneum in dogs and above 1.9:1 in cats (Aumann et al., 1998; Schmiedt et al., 2001).

3. The authors always evaluate both, potassium and creatinine ratios, in an effort to minimize the likelihood of false positive or negative results.

4. Once a diagnosis of uroperitoneum is made based on evaluation of abdominal effusion, diagnostic imaging is utilized to identify the source of uroperitoneum in an individual patient.

5. Cytological evaluation of abdominal effusion from animals with uroperitoneum is expected to demonstrate an acute inflammatory response as well as evidence of some degree of hemorrhage. The degree of the inflammatory response will be influenced by the duration of uroperitoneum. Concurrent abdominal injuries may impact the cytological characteristics of the abdominal fluid.

iv. Diagnostic imaging:

1. Various diagnostic imaging techniques are useful in the evaluation of the traumatized patient.

2. Diagnostic imaging is critical prior to surgical intervention in dogs and cats with uroperitoneum to better localize the source of the uroperitoneum.

3. Survey radiography:

a. Important to evaluate for concurrent fractures commonly associated with urinary trauma:

i. 39–46% of dogs with pelvic fractures have trauma to urinary tract (Selcer, 1982).

ii. Only 0.5% of cats with pelvic injuries have urinary tract injury (Aumann et al., 1998).

b. Changes seen on survey radiographs may be supportive of damage to the urinary system, but they rarely provide a definitive diagnosis:

i. May show loss of abdominal detail secondary to peritoneal effusion.

ii. Abdominocentesis is indicated when there is a loss of abdominal detail noted radiographically.

iii. Absence of a urinary bladder on survey radiographs may be supportive of, but is not diagnostic for, a bladder rupture.

4. Positive contrast radiography:

a. Excretory urography (Table 10.1) s useful for the diagnosis of renal vascular, renal pelvis, ureteral, and bladder injuries.

b. Retrograde cystourethrography (Table 10.2) is useful for the diagnosis of urethral and bladder disruption.

c. Uroperitoneum most often results from bladder and/or urethral disruption. As a result, retrograde urethrocystography is most appropriate for localizing the site of urinary leakage. These studies should be coupled with excretory urography to image the kidneys and ureters when there is any physical examination, imaging, or clinicopathologic data suggesting retroperitoneal injury.

5. Abdominal ultrasound:

a. Abdominal ultrasound may show perirenal or retroperitoneal fluid in cases of renal laceration, ureteral disruption, or abdominal effusion in cases of bladder rupture.

b. Focused assessment with sonography for trauma (FAST) is a method of evaluating dogs that have undergone trauma to evaluate for injuries resulting in fluid accumulation within the peritoneal and retroperitoneal spaces. Using ultrasound, transverse and longitudinal

---

TABLE 10.1
EXCRETORY UROGRAPHY—TECHNIQUE

---

1. It is recommended that a 12–24 hour fast and cleansing of the colon (laxatives, enemas) be performed prior to the contrast study
   a. This can be contraindicated in trauma patients due to the risk of dehydration, volume depletion, or further injury (particularly in cases with pelvic trauma)
2. Survey radiographs prior to injection of contrast will evaluate the GI tract and serve as baseline images.
3. Rapidly inject a bolus of water-soluble contrast media with iodine content equivalent to 600–800 mg iodine/kg body weight is used.
   a. Non-ionic contrast may be substituted but has not been shown to decrease contrast-induced renal failure.
4. Radiographs
5. Lateral and ventrodorsal radiographs are taken immediately and at 5, 10, 20, and 40 minutes postinjection
6. Complications may include vomiting, arrhythmias, weakness, collapse, hypotension, anaphylactic reaction to contrast agent, contrast-induced renal failure
7. Contrast agents available for our patients include
   a. Iohexal (Omnipaque, GE Healthcare), 300 mg iodine/mL
   b. Meglumine diatrizoate (Hypaque 60 Ionic,Mallinckrodt), 282 mg iodine/ml
   c. Sodium diatrizoate (RenoCal-76 Ionic, Bracco Diagnostics, Inc.) 370 mg iodine/mL

---

views are examined in each of these four locations (Boysen et al., 2004):

   i.   Just caudal to the xiphoid process

   ii.   The midline over the bladder;

   iii.   Over the most gravity-dependent area of the right flank

   iv.   Over the most gravity-dependent area of the left flank

   c. Abdominocentesis is indicated when fluid is suspected based on FAST scan.

g General approach to stabilization of dogs and cats with uroperitoneum:

   i.   The initial management must be aimed at treating any life-threatening injuries:

      1. Pulmonary injuries should be addressed with oxygen support, thoracocentesis, or

---

TABLE 10.2
POSITIVE CONTRAST RETROGRADE URETHROCYSTOGRAPHY—TECHNIQUE

---

1. It is recommended that a 12–24 hour fast and cleansing of the colon (laxatives, enemas) be performed prior to the contrast study
   a. This can be contraindicated in trauma patients due to the risk of dehydration, volume depletion, or further injury (particularly in cases with pelvic trauma)
2. Survey radiographs prior to injection of contrast will evaluate the GI tract and serve as baseline images.
3. A urethral catheter is placed, and the bladder distended with a 20% solution of a water-soluble organic iodide component
4. Lateral and ventrodorsal radiographs are taken
5. The urethral catheter is removed to the distal urethra and gently inflated to prevent reflux of contrast medium. An additional 10–15 mL of contrast medium is injected in dogs, an additional 5–10 mL in cats.
   a. During the last 2–3 mL of contrast injection, a lateral radiograph is taken.
6. For radiographic evaluation of the urethra, lateral radiographs are generally sufficient, although ventrodorsal oblique views (left and right) may be helpful.

---

positive pressure ventilation when indicated (see Chapter 6: Trauma-associated Thoracic Injury).

2. Cardiovascular support should be provided with fluid therapy, antiarrhythmics as indicated (see Chapter 3: Shock in the Trauma Patient).

3. Neurologic status should be addressed, and head or spinal trauma treated as needed (see Chapter 9: Traumatic Spinal Injury).

4. Management of life-threatening hyperkalemia is critical to the initial stabilization of dogs and cats with uroperitoneum:

    a. Intravenous volume expansion (see below):

        i. Rapid intravascular volume expansion will result in rapid (within minutes) dilution of blood potassium concentration. Its effects can be evident immediately after administration.

        ii. 0.9% NaCl lacks potassium and is very appropriate to utilize in this situation. LRS or Normosol-R are also reasonable crystalloid volume expanding fluids.

    b. Calcium gluconate:

        i. Calcium will not affect blood potassium levels; however, it will help mitigate the cardiovascular manifestations of hyperkalemia.

        ii. Calcium gluconate decreases the threshold potential (making it less negative); thus restoring a favorable electrical gradient between resting and threshold potentials.

        iii. Calcium gluconate has a very rapid onset of action. Increases in heart rate and ECG conformation are evident within minutes of administration.

        iv. 0.5 mL/kg of 10% calcium gluconate is administered intravenously over 1–3 minutes. Rapid administration of calcium gluconate IV will worsen bradycardia.

c. Dextrose +/− insulin:

    i. Concurrent administration of short acting, rapid onset insulin (regular insulin) and dextrose will help drive potassium intracel-

lularly resulting in decreased blood potassium concentration. Onset time for this effect is 20–40 minutes.

    ii. Dextrose 0.25–0.5 g/kg IV:

        1. Dextrose administration will stimulate endogenous insulin release resulting in the effect described above in (i).

    iii. Insulin 0.25 unit regular insulin/kg:

        1. The patient must be placed on supplemental dextrose (2.5% in the IV fluids) for 6–8 hours after insulin administration to prevent hypoglycemia.

        2. An alternative protocol involves the administration of 0.25 U/kg of regular insulin and 0.5 g/kg of dextrose intravenously with reassessment of blood glucose in 1 hour (to monitor for hypoglycemia).

    d. Sodium bicarbonate:

        i. This is similar to the effect of insulin/dextrose therapy. Administration of sodium bicarbonate will buffer hydrogen ion and result in an intracellular movement of potassium.

        ii. Onset time for this effect is 20–40 minutes.

        iii. 1–3 mEq/kg IV over 30 minutes.

        iv. The author prefers to utilize bicarbonate therapy in concert with the aforementioned therapies for life-threatening hyperkalemia especially when the patient demonstrates severe academia (pH<7.1) in concert with hyperkalemia.

        v. Venous or arterial blood gas analysis should be performed one hour after administration of bicarbonate therapy.

    ii. Urinary diversion:

        1. Abdominal drainage is an important aspect of patient stabilization.

        2. Effective drainage from the abdomen can be accomplished via placement of an intra-abdominal drain. Two drains will maximize drainage. One drain should be placed in the cranial abdomen and the second drain placed in the caudal abdomen, both exiting paramedian. Multi-fenestrated or T-Fluted drains work most effectively for abdominal drainage and urinary diversion. Any drain exiting the abdominal cavity should be connected to a closed collection system to minimize the risk of ascending nosocomial infection.

    a. Closed suction drain:

      i. Jackson-Pratt (Jackson-Pratt, Cardinal Health, McGaw Park, IL)

      ii. Flat suction drain (Sil-Med Corp., Taunton, MA)

    b. Locking-loop drainage catheter placed using the Seldinger technique.

    c. Foley catheter (Rusch, Inc., Duluth, GA).

    d. 16 g 5.25in or 14g 5.25in over-the-needle catheter with side-holes created.

  iii. Definitive treatment will vary based on the source of the uroabdomen (see below for specific traumatic causes of uroabdomen).

h. Prognosis:

  i. Prognosis is variable depending on the underlying cause and any concurrent traumatic injuries to other body systems. See below for a complete anatomy-directed discussion of specific injuries that result in uroperitoneum.

3. RETROPERITONEAL INJURIES

a. Renal Injuries (Renal contusion, rupture, or avulsion):

  i. Injury to the kidney can be difficult to identify due to the location in the retroperitoneal space.

  ii. Urine leakage due to direct renal injury leads to uroretroperitoneum:

    1. If the integrity of the retroperitoneal space has also been damaged secondary to the trauma, urine leakage will also result in uroperitoneum.

  iii. Renal contusions can lead to impaired renal function and potentially result in transient or permanent renal azotemia depending on the severity and extent of the damage to the renal parenchyma.

  iv. Renal avulsions can lead to severe and frequently fatal hemorrhage if the vascular pedicle is severed, as the kidneys receive 25% of cardiac output (Figures 10.1 and 10.2).

  v. Clinical signs and physical examination findings:

    1. Clinical signs are often vague and nonspecific, and may include weakness, lethargy, vomiting, anorexia, hematuria, abdominal or paralumbar/back pain.

    2. In severe cases or in patients with underlying renal disease, uroretroperitoneum can lead to electrolyte and metabolic disturbances often associated with vomiting, lethargy, and anorexia.

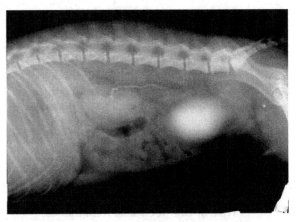

FIGURE 10.1 Lateral radiograph from an excretory urogram of a dog with a traumatic avulsion of the right kidney. Note that there is opacification of the left kidney, but no opacification of the right kidney.

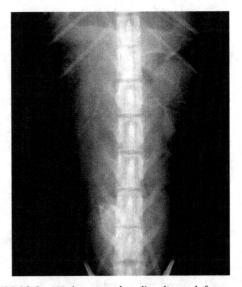

FIGURE 10.2 VD (or ventrodorsal) radiograph from an excretory urogram of a dog with a traumatic avulsion of the right kidney. Note that there is opacification of the left kidney, but no opacification of the right kidney.

3. Patients with hemorrhage into the retroperitoneal space may present with weakness, lethargy, or collapse:

   a. Physical examination in these patients will be consistent with hypovolemic shock including tachycardia, prolonged capillary refill time, pale mucous membranes, and weak peripheral pulse quality (see Chapter 3: Shock in the Trauma Patient).

vi. Clinicopathologic abnormalities:

   1. Renal contusions may be associated with renal azotemia in patients with underlying renal disease or bilateral renal trauma:

      a. Elevated BUN, creatinine, phosphorus with unconcentrated urine:

         i. Specific gravity <1.025 in dogs, <1.035 in cats

      b. Oliguria may result with severe renal injury.

   2. Urine leakage and subsequent uroretroperitoneum or uroperitoneum will result in a postrenal azotemia due to absorption of the urine and secondary increases in BUN, creatinine, phosphorus, and potassium:

      a. The onset of these clinical signs will vary with the severity of the urine leakage and accumulation.

      b. Only mild to moderate azotemia is expected when only unilateral renal injury is encountered, as acceptable GFR can be maintained by a single kidney.

   3. Comparison of retroperitoneal/peritoneal CREA and K^+ to blood CREA and K^+ will confirm uroretroperitonum/uroperitoneum, as discussed in the uroperitoneum section above.

   4. Renal avulsion and secondary hemorrhage will result in anemia and decreased total solids (see Chapter 3: Shock in the Trauma Patient and Chapter 4: Monitoring of the Trauma Patient).

   5. Additional clinicopathologic abnormalities are related to concurrent injuries.

vii. Diagnostic imaging:

   1. Survey radiographs:

      a. Fluid in the retroperitoneal space will lead to increased soft tissue density and loss of detail in the retroperitoneal space:

         i. While loss of retroperitoneal detail suggests fluids accumulation, it is not specific to the type of fluid and can occur with both, uroretroperitoneum as well as hemorrhage, into the retroperitoneal space.

      b. Retroperitoneal fluid frequently results in an inability to identify the border(s) of the kidneys (loss of retroperitoneal detail), ventral depression of the colon, and a diffuse "wispy" appearance to the retroperitoneal structures (see Chapter 3 Shock in the Trauma Patient, Figure 3.3).

   2. Excretory urography (see Table 10.1):

      a. This is indicated in cases of suspected renal or ureteral trauma based on physical examination, clinicopathologic changes, or survey radiographs.

      b. It is *imperative* that a patient be hemodynamically stable prior to contrast administration:

         i. If renal perfusion is poor, the decrease in GFR will result in poor renal opacification secondary to limited contrast uptake and a nondiagnostic study.

         ii. Contrast material has been shown to cause renal injury in human patients, so adequate renal perfusion is necessary to minimize this risk.

      c. Renal tear or laceration will result in leakage of contrast material into the renal subcapsular space, retroperitoneal space, or peritoneal space.

      d. Avulsion of the kidney and disruption of the vascular pedicle may result in a kidney that is not visualized or does not opacify during the nephrogram phase after intravenous contrast administration (Figures 10.1 and 10.2).

   3. Computed tomography (CT):

      a. Although not commonly utilized in the veterinary abdominal trauma patient, CT is a widely accepted and highly sensitive method for identification and classification of renal injuries in humans.

4. Ultrasonography:

   a. Abnormalities may include perirenal fluid, retroperitoneal effusion, peritoneal effusion, thrombus associated with renal artery, hypoperfusion of the affected kidney, or displacement of the kidney (Millward, 2009)

   b. Ultrasound guidance may be used to aid in the acquisition of retroperitoneal fluid for cytologic and chemical analysis.

viii. Treatment:

   1. Treatment for renal contusion and subsequent azotemia consists of supportive measures and therapy for renal failure:

      a. Intravenous fluid therapy to ensure adequate intravascular volume:

         i. Central venous pressure monitoring is a useful technique for ensuring adequate volume expansion from hypovolemic states. A CVP of 8–10 cmH_2O in dogs or 6–8 cmH_2O in cats is consistent with adequate volume expansion in the absence of primary myocaridal disease.

         ii. Management of oliguria (if present) consisting of ongoing maintenance of volume expansion coupled with the use of loop diuretics and osmotic diuretics to promote a polyuric state.

         iii. Peritoneal dialysis or hemodialysis may be indicated if anuria unresponsive to supportive measures occurs.

   2. In cases of uncontrollable hemorrhage due to renal pedicle avulsion, emergency exploratory laparotomy is indicated:

      a. Intravenous fluid therapy and blood component therapy should be administered with a goal of appropriate hemodynamic stabilization prior to induction of anesthesia:

         i. In cases of severe ongoing hemorrhage, hypotensive resuscitation may be indicated to avoid further exacerbating blood loss (see Chapter 3: Shock in the Trauma Patient).

      b. In the majority of cases, clamping of the vascular pedicle and a ureteronephrectomy performed by an experienced surgeon is required for control of hemorrhage.

      c. Selective coil embolization of a branch of the renal artery may be a technique that could spare renal function, when compared to ureteronephrectomy in cases with severe hemorrhage from the kidney.

   3. Animals that have sustained rupture of the kidney or renal pelvis with subsequent leakage of urine into the retroperitoneal space must be evaluated surgically:

      a. Repair of the lesion may spare the kidney. Renal parenchymal tears may be sutured using a horizontal mattress pattern.

      b. Ureteronephrectomy is considered a salvage procedure.

  b. Ureteral rupture:

    i. Ureteral rupture is a less common injury to the urinary tract in dogs and cats that have experienced blunt abdominal trauma.

    ii. Pathophysiology:

       1. There are multiple theories as to the mechanism by which abdominal trauma leads to ureteral rupture including the following:

          a. Direct compression of the ureter by the 12th rib or a transverse process of the lumbar vertebrae.

          b. Stretching of the ureter between the kidney and the urinary bladder.

          c. Abrupt cranial movement of the kidney and subsequent rupture.

          d. In humans, uretral rupture is thought to occur as a result of two separate and successive events (Campbell et al., 1992):

             i. Stretching of the ureter occurs secondary to spinal hyperextension.

             ii. Then, there is rapid deceleration resulting in compression of the ureter against the vertebral column.

       2. Rupture of the ureter results in uroretroperitoneum, and can lead to a uroperitoneum secondary to traumatic disruption of the retroperitoneal space.

       3. Clinical signs are similar to those for other traumatic injuries to the upper urinary tract (see 3a Renal Injuries above) and

will vary with concurrent injuries to other organ systems.

4. In one study of traumatic ureteral rupture in dogs and cats, 70% of the patients presented with shock or injuries to multiple organ systems (Weisse et al., 2002).

iii. Clinicopathologic abnormalities:

1. Urine leakage and subsequent uroretroperitoneum or uroperitoneum will result in a postrenal azotemia due to absorption of the urine and secondary increases in BUN, creatinine, phosphorus, and potassium:

    a. The onset of these clinical signs will vary with the severity of the urine leakage and accumulation.

    b. Only mild to moderate azotemia is expected when only unilateral renal injury is encountered, as acceptable GFR can be maintained by a single kidney.

2. Comparison of retroperitoneal/peritoneal effusion CREA and K^+ to blood CREA and K^+ will confirm uroretroperitonum/uroperitoneum, as discussed in the uroperitoneum section above.

3. Additional clinicopathologic abnormalities are related to concurrent injuries.

iv. Diagnostic imaging:

1. Survey radiographs show a loss of retroperitoneal (and possibly abdominal) detail, and abdominal ultrasonography may identify free fluid in the retroperitoneal and/or peritoneal space:

    a. This is consistent with ureteral damage, but it is not specific, as hemorrhage due to renal injury will also result in retroperitoneal fluid.

2. Definitive diagnosis best achieved with contrast studies:

    a. Excretory urography (see Table 10.1):

        i. As previously stated, it is *imperative* that a patient be hemodynamically stable, and a decrease in GFR will result in poor renal opacification and a nondiagnostic study.

        ii. Ureteral rupture results in extravasation of contrast material into the retroperitoneal space.

3. Ultrasonography:

    a. Abnormalities may include perirenal fluid, retroperitoneal, or peritoneal effusion.

    b. Ultrasound guidance may be used to aid in the acquisition of retroperitoneal fluid for cytologic and chemical analysis.

4. Other potential diagnostic modalities include antegrade pyelography, contrast-enhanced computed tomography (CT), and magnetic resonance imaging (MRI):

    a. Antegrade pyelography involves passing a needle through the renal parenchyma and into the renal pelvis, aspirating urine and injecting contrast directly into the renal pelvis:

        i. This is technically difficult unless there is pyelectasia present, which is not a common finding in animals with ureteral rupture.

    b. The sensitivity and specificity of these diagnostic modalities in the evaluation of ureteral trauma in veterinary trauma patients has not been evaluated.

v. Treatment:

1. Surgical intervention is mandatory for definitive treatment of ureteral rupture.

2. Numerous surgical options have been described, including ureteral repair, resection and anastomosis, reimplantation of the ureter into the bladder (ureteroneocystostomy), stenting across the defect with concurrent nephrostomy tube placement (to allow time for healing), and ureteronephrectomy:

    a. The choice of surgical procedures depends on the location and severity of the ureteral injury as well as the surgeon's preference.

    b. Surgical repair of the ureter is technically challenging and generally performed with an operating microscope. Ureteral stricture formation is a high risk, and the ureters are often repaired over a stent. Nephrostomy tube may be needed postoperatively for urinary diversion.

    c. Ureteronephrectomy is considered a salvage procedure and should only be used as a "last resort."

vi. Prognosis:

1. Ureteral rupture is a rare sequela to abdominal trauma in veterinary patients, so large studies evaluating outcome are not available.

2. Prognosis will vary depending on concurrent organ trauma.

3. A good prognosis has been reported in animals undergoing initial ureteronephrectomy after traumatic ureteral rupture; however, patients with underlying renal dysfunction may have persistent renal azotemia.

4. Although technically challenging and complicated, a kidney "sparing" procedure might offer the best option for definitive long-term preservation of renal function.

4. BLADDER INJURIES

a. Urinary bladder rupture:

i. Urinary bladder rupture is the most common cause of uroperitoneum in traumatized dogs and cats.

ii. In any patient with blunt abdominal trauma, there should be a high index of suspicion for bladder rupture, as these injuries can be overlooked:

1. In a study of trauma patients, in the first 12 hours after injury, the diagnosis of ruptured bladder was made in only 40% of the affected animals (Mathews, 2004):

a. In this same study, in 22.7% of patients, diagnosis of ruptured bladder was not made until necropsy.

iii. Pathophysiology:

1. Urinary bladder rupture can occur secondary to direct compressive force on the urinary bladder, exogenous penetrating injury (bite wounds, gunshot wounds, etc), or from penetration of the bladder by bone fragments due to concurrent orthopedic injuries.

2. Rupture of the urinary bladder leads to uroperitoneum and subsequent metabolic and electrolyte abnormalities:

a. Common electrolyte disturbances include hyperkalemia, hyponatremia, hypochloremia.

b. This occurs because urine is high in potassium and low in sodium and chloride, and these electrolytes rapidly equilibrate across the peritoneal membrane.

c. Azotemia.

iv. Clinical signs and physical examination findings:

1. Initial clinical signs are often vague and nonspecific:

a. May include lethargy, weakness, vomiting, diarrhea, dysuria, hematuria, or anuria.

b. Hematuria is a common clinical sign, but this is neither sensitive nor specific for bladder rupture.

c. Abdominal palpation:

i. Fluid wave

ii. Abdominal pain due to chemical peritonitis

iii. No palpable bladder:

1. This is not a definitive clinical sign—20% of cats with a ruptured bladder were noted to have a palpable bladder on physical examination (Aumann et al., 1998).

v. Clinicopathologic abnormalities:

1. Urine leakage and subsequent uroperitoneum will result in a postrenal azotemia due to resorption of urine and secondary increases in BUN, creatinine, phosphorus, and potassium:

a. The onset of these clinical signs will vary with the severity of the urine leakage and accumulation.

b. Severe azotemia and hyperkalemia is expected in long-standing uroperitoneum (>24 hours).

2. Comparison of peritoneal effusion CREA and K^+ to blood CREA and K^+ will confirm uroretroperitonum/uroperitoneum, as discussed in the uroperitoneum section above.

3. Hyponatremia and hypochloremia may also be noted.

4. Additional clinicopathologic abnormalities are related to concurrent injuries.

vi. Diagnosis:

1. Diagnostic imaging:

a. Survey radiographs:

  i. Loss of abdominal detail

  ii. Inability to visualize the bladder:

   1. It is important to note that this finding is supportive of bladder rupture but not diagnostic for this condition.

b. Ultrasonography:

  i. This is diagnostic for abdominal fluid accumulation; rarely diagnostic for ruptured bladder.

c. Analysis of creatinine and potassium in the abdominal effusion and comparison to concurrently derived blood levels is diagnostic for uroperitoneum as discussed in the uroperitoneum section above.

d. Contrast studies:

  i. Positive contrast urethrocystography (see Table 10.2):

   1. Ruptured bladder will result in extravasation of the contrast medium into the peritoneal space.

   2. May outline irregularities in the bladder wall or intraluminal blood clots.

   3. Fluoroscopy may be useful to help identify the anatomic site of leakage from the urinary bladder or urethra, as the study can be viewed in "real-time" while the contrast material is being injected.

  ii. Excretory urography is not required for the diagnosis of a ruptured bladder, so positive-contrast urethrocystography may be a safer diagnostic modality:

   1. Excretory urography can be associated with worsening of renal function in a hypovolemic or severely dehydrated trauma patient.

   2. Filling of the urinary bladder takes time and bladder distention is challenging.

   3. If there is *any* evidence of concurrent retroperitoneal injury, excretory urogram is indicated.

vii. Treatment:

   1. Emergency stabilization of dogs and cats with bladder disruption should proceed as described in Uroperitoneum above.

   2. Surgical intervention is indicated when the patient is euvolemic and free from clinical manifestations of electrolyte abnormalities (hyperkalemia):

    a. Complete abdominal exploration from xyphoid to pubis is indicated in animals with bladder rupture.

    b. Concurrent injuries are identified and managed.

    c. The bladder wall defect is identified and its edges debrided if necessary. The bladder wall is then closed using a simple continuous pattern of absorbable suture such as PDS. Suture size should be appropriate for the size of the patient.

    d. Placement of a urinary catheter to maintain bladder decompression for the first 24 hours is performed by some.

   3. Although there are reports of small bladder defects healing with urethral catheterization and time alone, surgery is advised in any case of uroperitoneum secondary to traumatic urinary bladder rupture.

viii. Prognosis:

   1. Prognosis for dogs with isolated bladder rupture that undergo surgical repair following appropriate medical stabilization is excellent.

   2. Definitive prognosis is often dictated by the severity of concurrent injuries.

5. URETHRAL INJURIES

  a. Urethral trauma/rupture:

   i. Urethral rupture is an infrequent complication of abdominal trauma in dogs and cats.

   ii. Pathophysiology:

    1. Trauma can occur to the urethra as a result of direct penetrating trauma from bite wounds, gunshot wounds, or secondary to fractures of the pubis and of penis.

    2. Urethral trauma can also occur secondary to blunt abdominal trauma.

    3. Trauma to the urethra is more common in male dogs due to the longer, more accessible urethra.

4. Subsequent urine leakage can lead to uroperitoneum in more proximal injuries, or significant swelling, inflammation and cellulitis of the intrapelvic and perineal tissues in more distal trauma.

5. There should be a higher index of suspicion of urethral injury in patients with pelvic fractures, particularly those involving the pubic bone.

iii. Diagnosis:

1. Definitive diagnosis is made with positive contrast urethrography (see Table 10.2):

a. Changes seen will be irregularities and contrast extravasation associated with the urethral wall.

iv. Treatment:

1. Minor urethral injuries (small lacerations, contusions) that present soon after the injury may be treated with conservative management:

a. Placement of a catheter into the bladder either via the urethra or through the body wall (cystostomy tube) to divert urine from the urethra:

i. Retrograde urethral catheterization should be attempted, but traversing the area that is torn or transected may be challenging.

ii. The catheter should remain in place for 7 days to allow for complete healing of the injured mucosa.

b. If retrograde catheterization is not possible, placement of a percutaneous or surgical cystostomy tube for urinary diversion is indicated:

i. Antegrade catheterization at the time of cystostomy tube placement should be attempted such that the urethra might heal over the catheter.

c. If retrograde catheterization is not possible and a cystostomy tube is in place, a retrograde urethrocystogram should be performed after 7–10 days to evaluate for urethral patency.

d. Fluoroscopy guided antegrade urethral catheterization is a newer technique that involves percutaneous catheterization of the bladder and advancement of a 0.035 in, standard stiffness, angled tip, hydrophilic guide wire in an antegrade fashion across the area of urethral disruption. Once through and through wire access is achieved (the guidewire enters the bladder percutaneously and exits through the normal urethral orifice), retrograde over-the-wire catheterization of the urinary bladder is possible followed by removal of the guide wire.

2. More severe injuries (such as urethral transection) or injuries associated with significant urine extravasation should be treated surgically:

a. Proximal urethral disruption may be accessible via the routine abdominal surgical approach (xiphoid to pubis).

b. Intrapelvic urethral disruption may require bilateral pubic and ischial flap osteotomy to gain access to the lesion for repair.

c. Surgical options include primary urethral anastomosis and permanent urethrostomy, and vary depending on the location and severity of the injury as well as the preference of the surgeon.

d. Surgery of the urethra will require temporary urinary diversion via cystostomy tube and/or or urinary catheterization.

v. Prognosis:

1. Urethral injuries are generally associated with a favorable outcome, but the presence of multiple traumatic injuries was associated with a worse outcome in one study (Anderson et al., 2006).

2. Potential complications associated with urethral trauma include stricture formation, necrosis and abscessation of perineal tissues, urethrocutaneous fistula formation, and urinary incontinence.

BIBLIOGRAPHY

Anderson RB, Aronson LR, Drobatz KJ, et al. Prognostic factors for successful outcome following urethral rupture in dogs and cats. *JAAHA* 2006; 42: 136–146.

Aumann M, Worth LT, Drobatz KJ. Uroperitoneum in cats: 26 cases (1986–1995). *JAAHA* 1998; 34: 315–324.

Booth HW. Managing traumatic urethral injuries. *Clin Tech Small Anim Pract* 2000; 15 (1): 35–39.

Boysen SR, Rozanski EA, Tidwell AS, et al. Evaluation of a focused assessment with sonography for trauma protocol to detect free abdominal fluid in dogs involved in motor vehicular accidents. *J Am Vet Med Assoc* 2004; 225: 1198–1204.

Campbell EW, Filderman PS, Jacobs SC. Ureteral injury due to blunt and penetrating trauma. *Urology* 1992; 40: 216–220.

Dibartola SP, Autran De Morais H. Disorders of Potassium. In: Dibartola SP, ed. *Fluid therapy in Small Animal Practice*. 2nd edition. Philadelphia, PA: WB Saunders Co., 2000

Mathews KA. Urinary perturbations of trauma. Proceed, *Int Vet Emerg and Crit Care Symp* 2004. San Antonio, TX.

Millward IR. Avulsion of the left renal artery following blunt abdominal trauma in a dog. *J Small Anim Pract* 2009; 50 (1): 38–43.

Schmiedt C, Tobias KM, Otto CM. Evaluation of abdominal fluid: Peripheral blood creatinine and potassium ratios for diagnosis of uroperitoneum in dogs. *JVECC* 2001; 11: 275–280.

Selcer BA. Urinary tract trauma associated with pelvic trauma. *JAAHA* 1982; 18: 785–793.

Weisse C, Aronson LR, Drobatz KJ. Traumatic rupture of the ureter: 10 cases. *JAAHA* 2002; 38: 188–192.

TRAUMA-ASSOCIATED ABDOMINAL PARENCHYMAL ORGAN INJURY

Andrew J. Brown, Charles S. McBrien, and Stephen J. Mehler

CHAPTER

11

1. **INTRODUCTION**

   a. Abdominal parenchymal organ injury occurs commonly in small animals secondary to trauma. Injury to the liver, spleen, or kidneys often results in acute hemorrhage. Signs can vary from mild and incidental to severe and fatal. Since the most common complication from abdominal parenchymal organ injury is hemorrhage, recognition of acute blood loss in the trauma patient is critical to a successful outcome.

2. **PHYSICAL EXAMINATION**

   a. A thorough physical examination is crucial to recognition of hypovolemia and identification of acute hemorrhage in the trauma patient.

   b. Initial evaluation of the trauma patient should focus on the major body systems.

   c. Animals with acute hemorrhage secondary to abdominal parenchymal organ injury will be presented with (or develop) signs consistent with hypovolemic shock (see Chapter 3: Shock in the Trauma Patient).

   d. Animals with shock will have a depressed mentation secondary to decreased oxygen delivery to the brain.

   e. A drop in arterial blood pressure will result in baroreceptor-mediated sympathetic nervous system activation. Animals with acute hemorrhage and hypovolemic shock will be tachycardic, tachypneic, have pale mucous membranes, prolonged capillary refill time, weak pulse quality, and cool extremities.

   f. Thorough auscultation of the animal's thorax should be performed to help rule out concurrent thoracic injury and incidental/preexisting cardiac disease.

   g. In the absence of respiratory compromise, dogs will be tachypneic but have normal respiratory effort. In contrast, cats with severe acute hypovolemic shock may be presented with open-mouthed breathing even in the absence of respiratory dysfunction. Resolution of the open-mouth breathing follows with correction of hypovolemia.

   h. Gentle abdominal palpation should be performed. Pain or tenderness on abdominal palpation may be detected although the absence of discomfort does not rule out significant organ injury.

   i. Thorough visualization and inspection of the animal may reveal abdominal bruising. Injury to the abdomen sufficient to result in cutaneous bruising is likely to also be extensive enough to cause abdominal parenchymal injury. The Cullen's sign is a blue/black bruising around the umbilicus that may occur following peritoneal hemorrhage. Inguinal bruising may be noted in animals with retroperitoneal hemorrhage.

   j. Ballotment of a fluid wave is an insensitive method of detecting free abdominal fluid and the absence of a fluid wave does not rule out abdominal hemorrhage

Manual of Trauma Management in the Dog and Cat, First Edition. Edited by Kenneth J. Drobatz, Matthew W. Beal and Rebecca S. Syring.
© 2011 John Wiley & Sons, Inc. Published 2011 by John Wiley & Sons, Inc.

k. Gross abdominal distension will only be seen if at least 40-mL/kg of fluid is within the peritoneum (Crowe and Devey, 1994). Potentially fatal hemorrhage from parenchymal injury can therefore occur even in the absence of abdominal distension.

l. Serial physical examinations should be performed to promptly identify deterioration in patient status and to note improvement with instituted therapy.

3. **EMERGENCY DIAGNOSTICS**

a. An emergency database can provide objective data to support a clinical diagnosis of hypovolemic shock secondary to acute hemorrhage.

b. An emergency database should consist of a packed cell volume (PCV), total protein by refractometry (TS), blood glucose (BG), and a blood smear.

c. When possible, a venous blood gas with electrolytes, lactate, blood urea nitrogen and creatinine will also provide valuable information.

d. PCV/TS:
  i. PCV/TS should be interpreted together.
  ii. Immediately following acute hemorrhage, the PCV/TS will be normal.
  iii. Following acute hemorrhage, TS will initially decrease without a proportional drop in PCV (e.g., TS < 5.5 and PCV of 45%). Fluid moves from the interstitium into the vasculature, diluting proteins and reducing the measured total solids. In dogs, splenic contraction secondary to the acute hypovolemia (and subsequent sympathetic stimulation) will increase the erythrocytes in the circulation allowing maintenance of normal PCV.
  iv. Over time and with continued bleeding, fluid therapy, and fluid retention by the kidneys, both the PCV and TS will be decreased.
  v. A baseline PCV/TS should be obtained at presentation, and values monitored frequently for changes and response to therapy.
  vi. It should be noted that animals can bleed to death with a normal PCV/TS in cases of very severe, acute hemorrhage. Consequently, transfusion therapy in patients with acute blood loss should be triggered by the documenta-

tion of blood loss, clinical signs of ongoing hypovolemic shock and, if present, a decreased PCV/TS.

e. Venous blood gas:
  i. A metabolic acidosis will be present with acute hemorrhage and hypovolemic shock.
  ii. The metabolic acidosis occurs as a result of lactate and hydrogen ion production during anaerobic metabolism secondary to decreased oxygen delivery to the tissue.
  iii. Lactate is measured on some blood gas analyzers. In addition, handheld lactatometers (Accutrend Lactate, Roche, Basel, Switzerland) are also available making it a quick, point-of-care monitoring tool requiring less than 0.5 mL of whole blood.
  iv. Normal serum lactate concentrations should be less than 1.0 mmol/L, though levels greater than 2.5 mmol/L are considered clinically significant. The normal range may vary slightly between instruments, institutions, and methodologies.
  v. Lactate concentration increases with increasing severity of hypovolemic shock.
  vi. Electrolyte concentrations are typically normal following acute blood loss from abdominal parenchymal injury. Hyponatremia may develop from hypotension-induced release of vasopressin and resorption of water at the distal nephron.

f. Coagulation assays:
  i. Abnormalities in coagulation are common following abdominal parenchymal organ injury and hemorrhage.
  ii. Trauma-induced tissue injury leading to exposure of tissue factor and activation of the coagulation cascade may result in a consumptive coagulopathy.
  iii. A *lethal triad* of hypothermia, acidosis, and coagulopathy may develop.
    1. Fluid resuscitation to correct hypovolemia will dilute clotting factor concentrations. This dilution will be more sustained following resuscitation with synthetic colloids.
    2. Synthetic colloids reduce factor VIII activity greater than through dilution alone (Stump et al., 1985), decrease plasma

levels of von Willebrand factor (de Jonge et al., 2001), and inhibit platelet function (Franz et al., 2001) and fibrin polymeration (Nielsen, 2005).

3. Coagulation times are prolonged with acidosis. Acidosis may occur secondary to an increase in lactate and hydrogen ion concentration, and following resuscitation with fluids containing a high concentration of chloride (e.g., 0.9% NaCl). A buffered crystalloid solution may therefore be a more appropriate resuscitation fluid than 0.9% NaCl in the patient with a traumatic hemoabdomen and hypovolemia.

4. Trauma patients are commonly hypothermic, which further worsens a coagulopathy. Hypothermia may result from environmental exposure or resuscitation with room-temperature fluids and cool blood products.

iv. Coagulation can be evaluated with laboratory or cage-side assays (e.g., iStat, Abbott Point of Care, East Windsor, NJ). Activated clotting times (ACT), activated partial thromboplastin time (aPTT), and prothrombin times (PT) are all readily available.

v. Coagulation assays should be performed if there is clinical evidence of bleeding or prior to performing an invasive procedure. Correction of a coagulopathy with fresh frozen plasma (15 mL/kg) should be confirmed through reevaluation of the coagulation assay.

g. Blood type:

i. Abdominal parenchymal organ injury commonly results in hemorrhage requiring transfusion with blood products.

ii. If time permits, blood typing for DEA 1.1 should be performed for all dogs:

1. Universal (DEA 1.1 negative) blood should be used if blood typing is not possible.

2. DEA 1.1 negative blood may be administered to all dogs.

3. DEA 1.1 positive blood should only be administered to DEA 1.1 positive dogs.

4. Dogs that have been previously transfused that require blood emergently should be administered DEA 1.1 negative blood. If the transfusion is less urgent, they will need to have their blood cross-matched to a donor unit.

iii. A blood type (A, B, AB) should be performed for *all* cats. Transfusion with incompatible blood can result in potentially fatal hemolytic transfusion reactions in cats. Due to the recent discovery of an additional high prevalence antigen (Mik) in cats, cross-matching should be performed before elective transfusions (Weinstein et al., 2007). The acute trauma patient may not afford the clinician this time.

h. Arterial blood pressure:

i. Objective data regarding hemodynamic status can be obtained with measurement of arterial blood pressure.

ii. If an animal is displaying clinical signs of hypovolemia, therapy (i.e., fluid resuscitation) should not be delayed pending the acquisition of an arterial blood pressure reading.

iii. Arterial blood pressure can provide useful information in patients with equivocal hemodynamic status and for assessing response to therapy. However, it should be recognized that significant hypovolemia may be present even in the face of a normal blood pressure.

iv. Continually monitoring arterial blood pressure can provide a valuable means of detecting patient decompensation

v. Arterial blood pressure can be measured with either direct (invasive) or indirect (e.g., Doppler) methods (see Chapter 4: Monitoring of the Trauma Patient).

i. Central venous pressure (CVP):

i. CVP represents the pressure in the intrathoracic vena cava and provides an assessment of preload.

ii. In the patient with traumatic hemoabdomen, CVP can be used to determine adequacy of resuscitation from a hypovolemic state.

iii. Monitoring CVP in the cardiovascularly stable trauma patient may aid in the detection of acute hypovolemia following recurrence of abdominal parenchymal organ hemorrhage.

iv. CVP is most commonly recorded following placement of a central venous catheter via the jugular vein.

v. Contraindications to central venous catheter placement via the jugular vein include hemostatic abnormalities (both hyper- and hypocoagulable states) and animals at risk of increased intracranial pressure.

vi. Normal central venous pressure is 0–5 cm H_2O (1 cm H_2O = 1.36 mm Hg).

vii. A low CVP (less than 0 cm H_2O) in a patient with abdominal parenchymal organ injury is consistent with hypovolemia.

viii. If a CVP reading is questionable, a small test bolus of 10–15 mL/kg of an isotonic crystalloid solution or a 3–4 mL/kg bolus of a synthetic colloid can be given over 5 minutes:

    1. If the patient has a low CVP due to hypovolemia, the CVP will either show no change or will have a transient rise toward normal, then rapidly decrease again.

    2. An increase of 2–4 cm H_2O with a return to baseline within 15 minutes is usually seen with euvolemia.

    3. A large increase (greater than 4 cm H_2O) and slow return to baseline (more than 30 minutes) is seen with hypervolemia

    4. A large increase (greater than 4 cm H_2O) and rapid return to baseline (within 15 minutes) is seen with reduced cardiac compliance.

ix. As a general rule, resuscitation to a CVP slightly above normal (5–8 cm H_2O) helps ensure adequate volume expansion.

j. Electrocardiogram:

i. Ventricular dysrhythmias are common following blunt trauma, and may require therapeutic intervention.

ii. In addition to concurrent myocardial contusion (also called blunt cardiac injury), pain, anxiety, and hemorrhage can all cause dysrhythmias (Bansal et al., 2005). These conditions are all common secondary to parenchymal organ injury; attention should therefore be paid to the potential for dysrhythmias to develop (see Chapter 6: Trauma-Associated Thoracic Injury).

k. Diagnostic Imaging:

i. Radiographs are not sensitive for detection of abdominal parenchymal organ injury:

    1. Fluid accumulation will result in a loss of peritoneal or retroperitoneal detail.

    2. Detail of soft tissue structures is dependent upon the amount of fat present.

    3. Comparison of detail and contrast of the intraperitoneal space with the retroperitoneal space is a convenient method of evaluation.

    4. A pneumoperitoneum (without abdominocentesis) suggests either a hollow viscus rupture or compromise to the body wall.

    5. Loss of detail in the retroperitoneal space is often described as "streaking" and occurs due to intermingling of fluid with retroperitoneal fat and structures. Loss of a visible renal silhouette and ventral depression of the colon on lateral radiographs suggest fluid in the retroperitoneal space.

ii. Abdominal ultrasound:

    1. FAST (focused assessment with sonography for trauma):

        a. May be performed within minutes of the patients' arrival by clinicians with little ultrasonographic training (Boysen et al., c11+bib+0002).

        b. The goal of the FAST is fluid detection.

        c. With the patient in lateral recumbency, four areas are examined in two planes:

            i. Subxiphoid.

            ii. Midline over the bladder

            iii. Gravity-dependent flank

            iv. Gravity-independent flank

        d. Fluid (when identified) may be obtained via ultrasound-guided paracentesis.

    2. Experienced ultrasonographers may detect abdominal parenchymal injury.

l. Abdominocentesis (Figure 11.1):

i. Abdominocentesis may be performed with or without (blind) ultrasound guidance.

ii. To avoid splenic injury, abdominocentesis is most commonly performed in left lateral recumbency.

iii. Using an aseptic technique, an over-the-needle catheter, butterfly catheter, or hypodermic needle is introduced 1–3 cm caudal to the umbilicus and just to the left of midline:

    1. Abdominocentesis can be performed using either an open or closed technique.

    2. The closed technique involves attachment of a syringe to the needle prior to

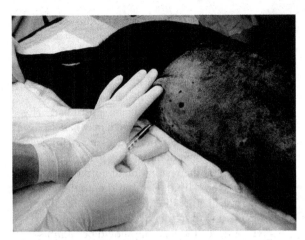

FIGURE 11.1   Abdominocentesis. Using an aseptic technique, an over-the-needle catheter, butterfly catheter, or hypodermic needle is introduced 1–3 cm caudal to the umbilicus and just to the left of midline and gentle negative pressure is applied with a syringe.

insertion, and fluid collected by aspiration of the syringe. This prevents air from entering the abdomen, which will be apparent as a pneumoperitoneum on radiographs (see above). The disadvantage of this technique is potential occlusion of the needle bevel by omentum.

3. An open technique relies on passive gravitational flow of fluid from the abdomen rather than syringe aspiration. A needle or catheter is inserted in the most gravity-dependent portion of the abdomen and fluid allowed to flow by gravity. With an open technique, there is a risk of air entering the abdomen causing a pneuomoperitoneum. This may be visualized radiographically and complicate their interpretation.

iv. Fluid may be collected and analyzed (PCV, TS, cytology, chemical analysis, and aliquots saved for bacterial culture as necessary).

v. A single negative abdominocentesis mandates a four-quadrant peritoneal tap when paired with high clinical suspicion of abdominal effusion:

    1. Abdominocentesis using a closed technique can be sequentially performed in each of four quadrants centered around the umbilicus.

    2. Alternatively, 2–4 separate open needles can be simultaneously inserted. A change in abdominal pressure between the needles may increase yield (Jandrey, 2008).

vi. False negative "blind taps" are reported in up to 80% of animals with effusion of less than 3 mL/kg.

vii. Presence of sanguineous fluid that does not clot indicates hemoperitoneum.

4. MEDICAL MANAGEMENT

    a. The primary therapeutic goal is restoration of normal cardiovascular function. This is achieved by attaining hemostasis and correcting hypovolemia.

    b. Fluid resuscitation will improve cardiac output, and subsequently restore tissue perfusion:

        i. There are multiple options for fluid resuscitation of the patient with parenchymal organ injury and hemoabdomen.

        ii. Resuscitation should be accomplished with multiple small volumes of parenteral fluid with frequent physical examination and close monitoring of end points of resuscitation.

        iii. *End points of resuscitation* used to help determine restoration of normovolemia include improvement in patient mentation, normalization of heart rate, increase in blood pressure, an increase in central venous pressure, resolution of lactic acidosis, and increased urine output.

        iv. Optimal choice of fluid therapy has not been determined in the trauma patient with acute hemorrhagic shock.

        v. Fluid choices include isotonic crystalloids, hypertonic saline, synthetic colloids, and blood products.

        vi. Each patient must be considered individually with careful attention paid to physical examination.

        vii. Consideration must be paid to respiratory function (including the suspicion of pulmonary contusion), underlying cardiac or renal disease, and ongoing hemorrhage.

        viii. "Hypotensive resuscitation" to a mean blood pressure of 60 mm Hg, or a systolic pressure of 80 mm Hg is a resuscitation technique that reduces ongoing hemorrhage yet permits perfusion of vital organs. By limiting the blood pressure, blood clots are not disrupted and excessive bleeding is reduced. Definitive hemostasis must be rapidly achieved by surgical exploration and/or correction of the coagulopathy, and this is followed by normotensive resuscitation (see Chapter 3: Shock in the Trauma Patient).

c. Isotonic crystalloids:

i.   Multiple small volume aliquots of an isotonic crystalloid solution is typically the first choice of fluid in the trauma patient with abdominal parenchymal injury.

ii.   Dogs that have signs consistent with mild hypoperfusion may only require 20–30 mL/kg of isotonic crystalloids, whereas a dog with evidence of severe hypoperfusion may require 70–90 mL/kg of isotonic crystalloids and the addition of colloids.

iii.   Hypovolemic cats may respond to a single 10–20 mL/kg bolus of an isotonic crystalloid solution, or may require a repeated isotonic crystalloid bolus and the addition of a colloid.

iv.   A buffered isotonic solution may be a more physiologic resuscitation fluid than normal saline. The high concentration of chloride in 0.9% NaCl may contribute to an existing metabolic acidosis. The use of 0.9% saline, however, will restore tissue perfusion and it is also compatible with blood and blood products.

v.   Caution should be exercised to avoid increasing hydrostatic pressure relative to colloid oncotic pressure, with the resultant increase in fluid flux out of the vasculature. This is especially true in the trauma patient that has respiratory compromise from pulmonary contusion.

vi.   Isotonic crystalloid therapy may prolong coagulation by dilution, worsening of acidosis (if using 0.9% NaCl) and hypothermia (if using room temperature fluids).

vii.   Only 25% of a crystalloid infusion will remain in the intravascular space after one hour.

d. Hypertonic saline:

i.   Hypertonic saline (typically, 7.2–7.5% NaCl) can provide rapid correction of hypotension in the trauma patient.

ii.   Infusion of a hypertonic crystalloid solution creates a large osmotic gradient that draws water from the interstitial and intracellular fluid compartments and results in rapid expansion of intravascular volume.

iii.   Its effects are diminished within 30 minutes but can be prolonged with the addition of a synthetic colloid.

iv.   Contraindications to hypertonic saline administration include dehydration, hyperosmolality, and uncontrolled hemorrhage.

v.   Trauma patients with abdominal parenchymal injury and hemoabdomen may benefit from the rapid correction of hypovolemia. However, ongoing intra-abdominal hemorrhage may worsen and the restoration of normovolemia may be short-lived. Caution should therefore be exercised before the use of hypertonic saline in a patient with traumatic abdominal injury.

vi.   A dose of 4–6 mL/kg should be administered at a rate no faster than 1 mL/kg/min. A dose of 2–3 mL/kg should be used in the cat.

e. Synthetic colloids:

i.   Synthetic colloids can be administered to the trauma patient to provide volume expansion following acute abdominal hemorrhage. Due to their particle size, colloids are retained in the intravascular space longer than crystalloids, and as result are more efficient at maintaining intravascular volume.

ii.   Loss of protein through hemorrhage, and dilution with interstitial fluids will decrease serum albumin, total solids (as measured by refractometry), and thus colloid oncotic pressure.

iii.   Hypovolemic patients with a total protein below than 4.5 g/dL may benefit from resuscitation with colloids.

iv.   A bolus of 5 mL/kg synthetic colloid may be required in the mildly hypovolemic trauma patient, whereas a dog with evidence of severe or refractory hypoperfusion may require up to 20 mL/kg (in small boluses with frequent reassessment). A bolus of 3–5 mL/kg is the initial dose range for a cat.

v.   Coagulation can be compromised at doses of synthetic colloids above 20 mL/kg per day.

vi.   Hemostasis is affected by dilution (to a greater degree than with crystalloids since colloids remain in the intravascular space longer), a reduction in factor VIII activity (greater than through dilution alone; Stump et al., 1985) a decrease in plasma levels of von Willebrand factor (de Jonge et al., 2001), and inhibition of platelet function (Franz et al., 2001) and fibrin polymerization (Nielsen, 2005).

f. Blood products:

i. Blood products may be needed in the patient with traumatic hemoabdomen to aid in the restoration of normovolemia, provide erythrocytes to optimize oxygen-carrying capacity and thus blood oxygen content, and to correct coagulopathy.

ii. Fresh frozen plasma should be administered if there is prolongation of routine coagulation assays (aPTT and PT) and there is either evidence of clinical bleeding or prior to an invasive procedure. A dose of 10–20 mL/kg should be administered followed by rechecking of the coagulation assays.

iii. Animals with severe acute blood loss may require packed red blood cells (PRBCs). Although no specific transfusion trigger exists, failure to achieve cardiovascular stability following crystalloid and colloid therapy (e.g., persistent tachycardia) and/or an acute drop in hematocrit to less than 20% would be indications for the provision of erythrocytes.

iv. Fresh whole blood may also be administered and has the benefit of providing coagulation factors, erythrocytes and will help restore normovolemia, all of which the trauma patient with an acute hemoabdomen will benefit from. Lack of immediate availability may limit the use of whole blood.

v. Autotransfusion is an autologous transfusion technique that utilizes the animal's intraperitoneal blood:

1. Blood should not be transfused if bacterial contamination has occurred (e.g., bowel rupture or penetrating injury).

2. Blood is collected from the abdomen using a peritoneal dialysis catheter, other multi-fenestrated catheter, over-the-needle catheter, or hypodermic needle.

3. The collection device is connected to a 60 mL syringe through an IV administration extension set with or without a three-way stopcock.

4. Blood may or may not be anticoagulated. A 60 mL syringe can be filled with 7 mL of ACD (acid-citrate-dextrose) or CPD (citrate-phosphate-dextrose) solution for small volume autotransfusion. Blood that

has been in contact with the peritoneum for longer than 45 minutes does not require anticoagulation as it is devoid of fibrinogen and platelets. Blood should be delivered back to the patient through a micropore (18–22 μm) filter (HemoNate Filter 18 Micron. Utah Medical Products, Inc. Midvale, UT).

5. For larger-volume autotransfusion, blood may be collected from the peritoneum as described in (2) above and then infused into a standard blood collection bag (Blood-Pack. Baxter Healthcare Corp. Deerfield, IL) (with anticoagulant) and then readministered through a standard blood administration set (Blood Set 80.5in. with 210 μm filter. Hospira Inc. Lake Forest, IL) followed by a micropore blood filter (HemoNate Filter 18 Micron. Utah Medical Products, Inc. Midvale, UT). This provides a "closed system" for autotransfusion and minimizes the likelihood of bacterial contamination during the collection process. (Figure 11.2)

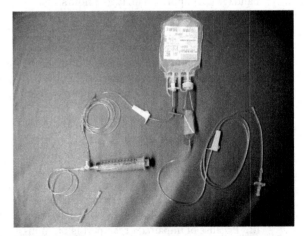

FIGURE 11.2 Autotransfusion. Blood is collected from the abdomen using a peritoneal dialysis catheter, other multi-fenestrated catheter, over-the-needle catheter, or hypodermic needle. The collection device is connected to a 60 mL syringe through an IV administration extension set with a three-way stopcock. Blood is aspirated and infused into a blood collection bag (with anticoagulant) and then delivered back to the patient through both a standard blood administration set and a micropore (18–22 μm) blood filter.

g. Abdominal counterpressure:

i. Abdominal counterpressure may aid in hemostasis by reducing vessel diameter to limit blood flow and by increasing intra-abdominal pressure to produce a tamponade effect on bleeding organs and vessels.

ii. Abdominal counterpressure can be rapidly achieved (with or without inclusion of the hindlimbs) using bandaging materials and tape. Preplacement of a urinary catheter should be considered prior to application.

iii. An increase in intra-abdominal pressure may lead to abdominal compartment syndrome, with resultant compromise to organ perfusion (e.g., renal) and hypoventilation. The duration of counterpressure should therefore be minimized to reduce the incidence of complications. The authors prefer to have the bandage removed within 6–8 hours.

iv. The counterpressure wrap should not be removed abruptly or severe hypotension may occur secondary to redistribution of blood and/or recurrent hemorrhage. Cut the wrap in a cranial to caudal direction and allow for hemodynamic equilibration to occur before making the next cut. The authors remove the bandage over approximately 2–4 hours.

h. Antibiotics are immediately indicated if there is a penetrating abdominal wound, or there are other lacerations, abrasions or wounds. In the absence of wounds, antibiotics are not indicated in blunt abdominal trauma. If possible, bacterial cultures should be obtained prior to the administration of antibiotics.

i. Analgesics (see Chapter 5: Analgesia and Anesthesia for the Trauma Patient):

i. Appropriate analgesia should be instituted as early as possible following presentation and adjusted according to response.

ii. Opioids provide good systemic analgesia with little effect on the cardiovascular system.

iii. Because of impaired organ perfusion, nonsteroidal anti-inflammatory drugs (NSAIDs) should be avoided in the early stages of patient stabilization.

j. Nursing care:

i. Animals with parenchymal organ injury require intensive nursing care.

ii. Close monitoring is essential (see below and Chapter 4: Monitoring of the Trauma Patient). All subjective and objective data should be frequently documented.

iii. Patient movement should be minimized to prevent disruption of clots with resultant hemodynamic decompensation. Radiographs and other diagnostic modalities should be delayed until stabilization has occurred.

iv. Placement of a urinary catheter should be considered. This will aid in the assessment of "ins and outs" as well as limiting the activity an animal has to do. For example, dislodgement of a clot whilst a dog is walked outside may lead to recurrence of abdominal hemorrhage.

k. Monitoring:

i. Patients with parenchymal organ injury should be closely monitored for response to therapy and to rapidly detect cardiovascular decompensation.

ii. Monitoring should focus on frequent and thorough physical examinations.

iii. Additional monitoring tools include blood pressure, central venous pressure, electrocardiogram, and measurement of lactate concentration.

iv. Further details on cardiovascular monitoring can be found in Chapter 4: Monitoring the Trauma Patient.

5. SURGICAL MANAGEMENT

a. Most animals with blunt abdominal parenchymal organ injury and hemoabdomen can be managed conservatively whilst others may require emergent surgery.

b. Following cardiovascular stabilization, animals with penetrating abdominal injury require immediate surgery:

i. Many animals with penetrating abdominal injuries have concurrent abdominal visceral damage, including bowel perforation.

c. In patients with blunt abdominal trauma, the inability to achieve cardiovascular stabilization after appropriate fluid resuscitation and/or restoration of oxygen delivery to the tissues is an indication for emergent surgery. This may become apparent shortly after presentation if improved hemodynamic parameters are unable to be achieved after appropriate fluid resuscitation (including the use of isotonic crystalloids, colloids, and blood products).

d. Similarly, a patient that responds appropriately to initial medical management (e.g., normalization of heart rate, mentation, and blood pressure) that subsequently decompensates secondary to further parenchymal bleeding requires emergent surgery.

e. Hypovolemia should be corrected prior to induction of anesthesia (if possible).

f. Vascular access should be adequate for the concurrent delivery of blood products, anesthetic, agents, crystalloid and colloid fluids, and for sampling arterial and venous blood. A minimum of two peripheral IV catheters should be placed.

g. Many anesthetic agents cause some degree of vasodilation. Rapid fluid administration may be necessary to compensate and to keep ventricular filling pressures appropriate.

h. The goals of surgery are to achieve hemostasis and to perform a full exploratory laparotomy to determine the extent of abdominal injury.

i. Fluids and blood products should be available to administer following cessation of hemorrhage.

j. A staged laparotomy may be considered in patients with exsanguinating penetrating abdominal injury.

k. Surgical approach to hemoabdomen:

   i. The patient is prepared for immediate surgery.

   ii. Anesthetic agents that are known to promote hypotension should be avoided.

   iii. The technique used to open the abdomen is critical:

     1. The midline skin is opened from xiphoid to pubis.

     2. The linea alba is identified and opened between the xiphoid and the umbilicus:

       a. At this point, the falciform fat is visible.

       b. The ventral surface of the falciform is not within the peritoneal cavity.

       c. This exposure is enough to allow the surgeon to get a hand into the abdomen:

         i. Locate the aorta and renal artery by tracing the artery from the hilus of the kidney.

         ii. Locate the opposite renal artery.

         iii. The next proximal major artery is the cranial mesenteric artery; proximal to that is the celiac artery.

         iv. The celiac artery is the major arterial blood supply to the liver, spleen,

all of the left limb and some of the right limb of the pancreas, stomach, and proximal duodenum.

d. Occlude the celiac artery with digital pressure. This procedure has been documented to prevent the devastating and often fatal hypotension that results when the tamponade effect of the abdominal distension is relieved.

e. The remaining linea is opened to the pubis.

f. Pack the abdomen with sterile laparotomy sponges:

   i. It is easy to lose sponges in the hemoabdomen patient. A sponge foreign body (gossipyboma) is an easily avoidable postoperative complication. It is prevented by counting sponges before opening and closing the abdomen. Radiopaque sponges are ideal; if there is any suspicion that a sponge was left in the abdomen, a radiograph is made to determine its location.

   ii. Packing the abdomen provides a tamponade effect that helps control hypotension.

   iii. Packing will help control venous hemorrhage.

   iv. Remove the celiac artery occlusion when the abdomen has been thoroughly packed off.

g. If the patient continues to hemorrhage despite celiac artery occlusion and abdominal sponge packing, the Pringle maneuver should be attempted:

   i. The hepatic artery, the portal vein, and the common bile duct are occluded using digital pressure.

   ii. After 10 minutes, the portal occlusion must be released for at least 1 minute every 10 minutes.

   iii. If the source of hemorrhage is found, it is repaired at this time and then a full exploratory is performed.

h. The three most common sources of hemorrhage from abdominal trauma are the spleen, liver, and kidney

i. Emergency surgery of the spleen:

i.   Anatomy of the splenic vasculature includes the splenic artery and splenic veins. The splenic artery is a direct branch of the celiac artery. Before the splenic artery branches and delivers oxygen rich blood to the spleen, it gives off the main blood supply to the left limb of the pancreas (pancreatic artery). The splenic artery also divides into smaller branches that bring arterial blood to the stomach in the form of the short gastric arteries (found in the gastrosplenic ligament) as well as the left gastroepiploic artery (main blood supply to the left portion of the greater curvature). Other branches of the splenic artery supply the greater omentum. Numerous small arteries form the hilar vessels of the spleen that are located along the majority of the base of the organ.

ii.   If a laceration is found it can be sutured primarily and splenectomy is avoided. Splenorrhaphy can be performed by primarily ligating any exposed and bleeding vessels. The capsule of the spleen is then sutured using simple interrupted, cruciate, or mattress suture patterns. Be sure to only grab the capsule with the fine needle as further punctures to the parenchyma will exacerbate bleeding.

iii.   For small lacerations, constant and firm pressure for 7 minutes with use of common hemostatic agents, such as Gelfoam (Pharmacia & Upjohn Company, Division of Pfizer Inc., New York, NY), are all that are needed in the patient with normal platelet number and function and that is not overtly coagulopathic.

iv.   Two general techniques exist for splenectomy.

v.   The first is mass ligation of the splenic artery and vein. For traumatic hemoabdomen patients, the splenic artery is identified, isolated, and ligated. The ligation should be distal to the left pancreatic artery but proximal to the branching of the splenic artery. One encircling ligature is placed and one transfixation suture is placed. A hemostat, second encircling suture, or vascular clip is applied distal to the last suture to prevent back bleeding when the artery is transected. The same is performed with the splenic vein distal to its entrance into the left gastric vein. It is important to remember that there are also small arteries and veins that will back bleed, within the gastrosplenic ligament and from the greater omentum that will likely need ligating. In some animals, the left limb of the pancreas will overlie the main splenic artery and vein beyond the point where they divide. Be careful that the left limb of the pancreas is identified before clamping or ligating these vessels.

vi.   The second technique for splenectomy is the hilar ligation technique. Although this technique takes longer and uses more suture material, there are fewer complications associated with the blood supply to the pancreas and stomach. For actively bleeding spleens, the major splenic artery and vein are located and temporary clamped with an appropriate vascular clamp (i.e., Satinsky forcep) or tourniquet. This will slow any parenchymal hemorrhage and enable better visualization along the hilus of the spleen. Each hilar artery and vein is identified, isolated, and ligated twice using an encircling ligature. After all ligations have been performed, the spleen is removed by cutting the hilar vessels distal to the last ligature.

vii.   Other commonly used instruments for splenectomy include, vascular clips, ligate-divide-stapler (LDS-2. US Surgical, A Division of Tyco Healthcare Group LP, Mansfield, MA), electrosurgery, radiosurgery, ultrasonic energy surgery, and other coagulation devices.

j. Emergency surgery of the liver:

i. Surgical anatomy includes the individual lobes of the liver, including; the left lateral, left medial, quadrate, right medial, right lateral, caudate process of the caudate lobe, and the papillary process of the caudate lobe. The arterial blood supply (20% of the nutrients and 50% of the oxygen delivery) to the liver is through the hepatic artery, a major branch of the celiac artery. The remaining 80% of the nutrient blood and 50% oxygen demand is from the portal vein (venous blood from the gastrointestinal tract, spleen, and pancreas). Venous return from the liver is through the hepatic veins, which are mostly intrahepatic, and enter directly into the vena cava. Each liver lobe, or set of lobes, also has a corresponding hepatic bile duct draining bile into the common bile duct.

ii. For small capsular and/or parenchymal lacerations, the techniques described above for splenic lacerations are implemented.

iii. For major liver lobe trauma, each major artery branch, hepatic vein branch, portal vein branch, and hepatic duct must be identified, isolated, and ligated. The Pringle maneuver (described above) will often need to be implemented to control hemorrhage during dissection of the hepatic veins off of the vena cava. Proper training in vascular surgery is often required for liver lobectomy or in cases with severe liver based hemorrhage. If the portal vein or vena cava are inadvertently ligated or damaged, the patient may be at risk for acute severe complications or death. In some cases, the diaphragm may need to be opened or the xyphoid and last two to three sternabrae transected on midline to increase exposure to the hepatic venous vasculature. In some cases, usually the left lateral and left medial liver lobes, the vascular pedi-

cle can be identified as a portion of it is extrahepatic. In these cases, a thoracic anastamosis/thoracoabdominal stapler (TA Premium 30, US Surgical, A Division of Tyco Healthcare Group LP, Mansfield, MA) may be used. The ideal cartridge to be used is a TA30 (referring to the 30 mm staggered staple line) V3 (referring to the three rows of staggered staples that are set), manufactured by the aforementioned company. Because of the short length of the staple line and short arm length of the staples, this device is only recommended for liver lobectomy when the vascular pedicle is free of surrounding liver parenchyma. Otherwise, the staples will fail to close appropriately around the large vessels and severe hemorrhage will ensue after transection.

k. Trauma to the kidney:

i. Surgical anatomy includes the renal artery and vein that are direct branches off of the aorta and to the caudal vena cava respectively. The kidneys and their vasculature are all located within the retroperitoneal space. The renal artery usually bifurcates into dorsal and ventral branches. Variations in number of both renal artery and veins exist in dogs and cats. The ureter begins as the continuation of the renal pelvis and ends at the ureterovesicular junction on the dorsal aspect of the bladder neck.

ii. Ureteronephrectomy is indicated in trauma cases with uncontrollable hemorrhage from the kidney, severe vascular damage to the kidney, or in cases with severe ureteral damage. In cases with minor capsular or parenchymal damage, similar techniques can be used as described above for splenic laceration repair. It is ideal to assess the function of the healthy kidney before removing the diseased kidney; however, in cases of uncontrollable hemorrhage or severe parenchymal damage, that may not be possible. The safest technique for dissecting out the vasculature of the kidney is to open the retroperitoneal space by incising the peritoneum covering the kidney. Blunt dissection continues laterally and dorsally around the kidney. The kidney is then gently rotated medially (toward midline) to expose the hilar vessels. In most cases, there will be evidence of retroperitoneal hemorrhage and swelling, the peritoneum overlying the kidney may be torn, or the kidney itself may be avulsed from its vascular supply. Once the renal artery and vein are identified, they should be isolated and ligated individually (artery first) using at least two ligations per vessel. Once the artery and vein have been transected, the ureter is gently retracted out of the retroperitoneal space, and its junction with the bladder is identified. The ureter is ligated once and transected at the level of its junction with the bladder.

l. If the source of hemorrhage is not identified, then the abdomen is systematically explored by slowly removing laparotomy sponges until bleeding is observed.

m. If the source of the hemorrhage is not identified or cannot be repaired, a staged laparotomy may be performed:

i. Laparotomy sponges are left in the abdomen and the abdomen is temporarily closed.

ii. The patient is stabilized and taken back to surgery in 24–48 hours to have the sponges removed and the abdomen is again fully explored.

iii. On re-exploration of the abdomen, warm, sterile saline is used to bathe the lap sponges and abdominal viscera before slowly removing the sponges. This helps prevent any major damage to the abdominal viscera from adhesions formed between the cotton-based sponges and the serosal surface of the organ. Another option is to use nonadhesive sterile drapes instead of cotton-based sponges as the primary contact layer.

n. In dogs and cats, the midline incision is closed in three layers:
   i. Rectus abdominus and its sheaths
   ii. Subcutaneous tissue
   iii. Skin

o. Although sometimes cost prohibitive, the use of CT angiography is a superb imaging modality for detecting the location of an abdominal parenchymal injury and an active bleed.

BIBLIOGRAPHY

Bansal MK, Maraj S, Chewaproug D. Myocardial contusion injury: redefining the diagnostic algorithm. *Emerg Med J* 2005; 22: 465–469.

Boysen SR, Rozanski EA, Tidwell AS, et al. Evaluation of a focused assessment with sonography for trauma protocol to detect free abdominal fluid in dogs involved in motor vehicle accidents. *J Am Vet Med Assoc* 2004; 225 (8): 1198–1204.

Brockman DJ, Mongil CM. Practical approach to hemoperitoneum in the dog and cat. *Vet Clin North Am Small Anim Pract* 2000; 30: 657.

Crowe DT, Devey JJ. Assessment and management of the hemorrhaging patient. *Vet Clin North Am Small Anim Pract* 1994; 24: 1095–1122.

Culp WTN, Silverstein DC. Abdominal trauma. In: Silverstein DC, Hopper K, eds. *Manual of Small Animal Emergency & Critical Care*. St. Louis: WB Saunders, 2008; 667–671.

de Jonge E, Levi M, Buller HR, et al. Decreased virculating levels of von willebrand factor after intravenous administration of a rapidly degradable hydroxyethyl starch (HES 200/0.5/6) in healthy human subjects. *Intensive Care Med* 2001; 27: 1825–1829.

Fossum TW. *Small Animal Surgery*. St. Louis, Missouri, 2007; 531–558, 624–631, 635–646.

Franz A, Braunilich P, Gamsjaer T, et al. The effects of hydroxyethyl starches of varying molecular weights on platelet function. *Anesth Analg* 2001; 92: 1402–1407.

Harari J. Abdominal trauma. In: Wingfield WE, Raffe MR, eds. *The Veterinary ICU Book*. Jackson: Teton NewMedia, 2002; 905–909.

Herold LV, Devey JJ, Kirby R. Clinical evaluation and management of hemoperitoneum in dogs. *J Vet Emerg Crit Care* 2008; 18: 40–53.

Jandrey KE. Abdominocentesis. In: Silverstein DC, Hopper K, eds. *Manual of Small Animal Emergency & Critical Care*. St. Louis: WB Saunders, 2008; 671–673.

Mongil CM, Drobatz KJ. Traumatic hemoperitoneum in 28 cases. *J Am Anim Hosp Assoc* 1995; 31: 217.

Nielsen VG. Colloids decrease clot propagation and strength: role of factor XIII-fibrin polymer and thrombin-fibrinogen interactions. *Acta Anaesthesiol Scand* 2005; 49: 1163–1171.

Stump DC, Strauss RG, Heniksen RA, et al. Effects of hydroxyethyl starch on blood coagulation, particularly factor VIII. *Transfusion* 1985; 25: 349–354.

Waddell LS, Brown AJ. Hemodynamic monitoring. In: Silverstein DC, Hopper K, eds. *Manual of Small Animal Emergency & Critical Care*. St. Louis: WB Saunders, 2008; 859–864.

Weinstein NM, Blais MC, Harris K, et al. A newly recognized blood group in domestic shorthair cats: the Mik red cell antigen. *J Vet Intern Med* 2007; 21: 287–292.

TRAUMA-ASSOCIATED BILIARY TRACT INJURY

Philipp D. Mayhew

1. INTRODUCTION

a. Traumatic injury to the extra-hepatic biliary tract (EHBT) is uncommon in dogs and rare in cats. When it occurs it can be difficult to diagnose and challenging to treat successfully.

b. Many patients will be systemically compromised and require intensive supportive therapy if a successful outcome is to be achieved.

c. To manage these cases appropriately, a thorough knowledge of EHBT anatomy, pathophysiology, and surgical principles is necessary.

2. ANATOMICAL CONSIDERATIONS

a. There are species variations in EHBT anatomy that can have important clinical ramifications. The basic anatomy of the canine biliary tract is depicted in Figure 12.1:

  i. Gall bladder: located in a fossa between the right medial and quadrate lobes of the liver.

  ii. Cystic duct: connects the gall bladder to the common bile duct and becomes the common bile duct at the point of entry of the first hepatic duct.

  iii. Hepatic ducts: drain bile from each liver lobe but convergence prior to entry into the common bile duct results in there being a wide variation in hepatic duct number in dogs and cats from as few as two to as many as seven.

  iv. Common bile duct (CBD): begins at the end of the cystic duct and accepts lobar bile drainage via a variable number of hepatic ducts:

    1. In its most distal aspect the CBD passes adjacent to pancreatic parenchyma before forming an intramural tunnel in the duodenal wall prior to its termination at the major duodenal papilla.

    2. Ductal morphology is different between dogs and cats:

      a. In dogs, the common bile duct and pancreatic duct enter the duodenum together, but not conjoined, at the major duodenal papilla, which is located approximately 3–6 cm aboral to the pylorus.

      b. In dogs, a minor duodenal papilla is located approximately 2–4 cm aboral to the major duodenal papilla and provides an entry point for the accessory pancreatic duct, which is the major channel for pancreatic secretions into the duodenum in dogs.

      c. In cats, the common bile duct and pancreatic duct are conjoined prior to their entry into the duodenum at the major duodenal papilla. Only ~20% of cats have a minor duodenal papilla, meaning that all pancreatic exocrine secretions must pass into the

Manual of Trauma Management in the Dog and Cat, First Edition. Edited by Kenneth J. Drobatz, Matthew W. Beal and Rebecca S. Syring.
© 2011 John Wiley & Sons, Inc. Published 2011 by John Wiley & Sons, Inc.

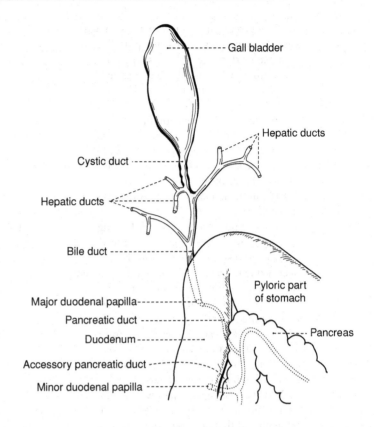

Gall bladder

Hepatic ducts

Cystic duct

Hepatic ducts

Bile duct

Pyloric part
of stomach

Major duodenal papilla

Pancreatic duct

Duodenum

Pancreas

Accessory pancreatic duct

Minor duodenal papilla

FIGURE 12.1 Anatomy of the canine extra-hepatic biliary tract. (Reprinted with permission: Miller's Anatomy of the Dog, Edition 3, Evans HE, 457, Copyright Elsevier (1993).)

gastrointestinal tract through the major duodenal papilla in the majority of cats.

v. Duodenum: the proximal part of the duodenum at the cranial duodenal flexure is a relatively immobile part of the small intestine due to its firm anchorage by the mesenteric root. This protects the complex anatomical arrangements of organs in the region (bile and pancreatic ducts, portal vein, hepatic artery) from traction injury but significantly limits manipulation of the area during surgery.

3. PATHOPHYSIOLOGY—CAUSE AND LOCATION OF BILIARY TRAUMA IN DOGS

a. Etiology of injury:

i. Blunt trauma:

1. Trauma to the EHBT can be the result of a number of different causes in dogs. The most frequent cause of injury is blunt abdominal trauma following a motor vehicle accident.

2. Blunt trauma sustained during a fall (high-rise syndrome) is a rare cause of EHBT injury.

3. It is most likely that a combination of the following factors combine to cause biliary tract injury: a short wide cystic duct that allows rapid filling of the common bile duct, a force applied to the gall bladder that leads to rapid emptying and a simultaneous shearing force that is applied to the common bile duct or hepatic ducts:

a. Blunt trauma-induced bile duct rupture has been described in cholecystectomized humans suggesting that rapid ductal filling is not always mandatory for injury to occur.

4. It is likely that during blunt trauma rapid cranial movement of the liver away from the relatively well fixed duodenum results in a traction force that can result in tearing or avulsion injuries of the common bile duct.

5. Concurrent injuries to other associated vascular structures such as the portal vein or hepatic artery are rarely seen possibly due to their increased elasticity or the likely fatal nature of these injuries leading to a lack of detection.

6. In humans, the most common cause of injury is during motor vehicle accidents when direct impact of the steering wheel against the abdomen occurs. It is likely that in dogs the shear force required to cause EHBT injury emanates from a direct blow to the abdomen.

7. It is also possible for injuries leading to perforation of the upper gastrointestinal tract to result in bile peritonitis. This occurs due to leakage of bile that has passed through the major duodenal papilla and then leaks out of an intestinal perforation.

ii. Penetrating wounds from gunshot, stab, or bite injuries can all lead to biliary tract injury:

1. Penetrating injury is a less common cause of EHBT trauma but has been recorded in both dogs and cats.

2. When assessing a patient with a gunshot wound to the abdomen, it should be remembered that the tissue within the trajectory of the projectile undergoes crush injury but that pathology is not limited to this tract:

a. The kinetic energy transferred to the body when the projectile hits its target leads to the formation of shock waves that radiate to other tissues as well as cavitation, which causes expansion of a tissue tract around the projectile. This causes expansion and then collapse as the projectile passes through. Negative pressure behind the projectile during cavitation increases tissue damage while drawing contamination into the wound.

b. The greater the velocity of the projectile, the greater the kinetic energy released and therefore the greater the likelihood of damage to tissues remote from the projectile's tract.

3. Stab wounds generally are low-velocity injuries that are more likely to cause direct laceration or perforation of tissues.

4. Dog bite wounds (see Chapter 20: Bite Wound Trauma):

a. Bite wounds rarely cause injury to the EHBT but have been reported to cause injury to the gall bladder as well as trauma to many other intra-abdominal organs.

b. Severe tissue injury results from crushing and shearing that often accompanies the violent shaking that occurs during an attack. Small dogs are particularly affected.

iii. Iatrogenic injury sustained during abdominal surgery is another unusual but reported cause:

1. Most likely to occur during surgical procedures.

2. Overzealous gall bladder expression can lead to rupture.

3. Postoperative leakage from a cholecystotomy, cholecystectomy, or choledochotomy incisions can also result in leakage and subsequent bile peritonitis.

4. In humans, the routine use of laparoscopic cholecystectomy for gall stone disease has made iatrogenic injury to the EHBT during this procedure the most frequently encountered cause of bile peritonitis. Such injuries may be seen more frequently in dogs and cats in the future with the increasing use of laparoscopic surgery in veterinary medicine.

b. Location of the injury:

i. There is a relationship between the cause and location of biliary tract rupture in dogs.

ii. The most likely site of leakage in dogs with bile peritonitis is the gall bladder due to the frequent occurrence of necrotizing cholecystitis, gall bladder infarction, and gall bladder mucocele.

iii. When leakage occurs as a result of trauma, however, the location of the perforation is almost always within the common bile duct or hepatic ducts, although leakage from the gall bladder has been rarely reported:

1. The most common lesions are tears or transections within the body of the common bile duct and less frequently within the cystic duct. Also common are avulsion injuries of the common bile duct from the duodenum or avulsions of hepatic ducts from the common bile duct.

2. This information is useful as it may allow a more focused and rapid identification of the site of leakage at surgery if trauma is known to be the cause.

4. PATHOPHYSIOLOGY—CAUSE AND LOCATION OF BILIARY TRAUMA IN CATS

a. Trauma to the extrahepatic biliary tract in cats is exceedingly rare and has only been reported in three cats.

b. Two cats had sustained injury from gunshots (Ludwig et al., 1997) and the third was hit by a car (Bacon and White, 2003).

c. In the two cats sustaining gunshot injury, perforation of the gall bladder was present in one cat and avulsion of the common bile duct from the duodenum was present in the other.

d. The cat that was hit by a car sustained a CBD avulsion injury.

5. PATHOPHYSIOLOGY—BILE PERITONITIS

a. The inevitable result of traumatic EHBT injury is spillage of bile into the abdominal cavity.

b. This can remain localized if surgical exploration occurs soon after the injury. More often, there is a delay in diagnosis leading to the establishment of generalized peritonitis. Severe systemic effects can result in high levels of morbidity and mortality in these patients.

c. Local effects:

   i. The release of bile salts into the peritoneum is principally responsible for the initial pathological changes that occur.

   ii. Bile salts cause inflammation, hemolysis, and necrosis of tissue. Their hyperosmolality leads to significant fluid shifts from the vascular space into the peritoneal cavity, which causes dehydration and eventually hypovolemic shock.

   iii. High proportions of one of the most toxic bile salts, taurocholic acid, in canine bile is thought to increase severity of lesions compared to humans.

   iv. The development of peritoneal inflammation and biliary effusion is likely to promote and sustain the growth of bacteria more readily once a bacterial source has been provided.

   v. In the absence of bacterial infection, biliary peritonitis causes a mild chemical peritonitis.

The establishment of septic effusion profoundly worsens pathology and subsequent prognosis:

   1. Multiple studies have demonstrated a significantly higher mortality in dogs with septic bile peritonitis compared to those with sterile effusion (Ludwig et al., 1997, Mehler 2004).

   2. Normal canine bile is sterile and therefore blunt trauma induced bile leakage is more likely to result initially in a sterile peritonitis. However, infection can result from ascending gastrointestinal contamination, intestinal translocation, or colonization by resident hepatic anaerobes.

   3. In penetrating injuries, bacterial infection can be introduced via direct inoculation.

d. Systemic effects:

   i. Biliary tract trauma with bile peritonitis can result in a partial or total absence of bile salts passing into the small intestine.

   ii. Bile salts perform an important role in binding bacterial endotoxins in the lower small intestine, thereby preventing their absorption into the portal circulation. Lack of this protective effect may predispose to sepsis, severe sepsis, and multiple organ failure.

   iii. Renal vascular compromise and fibrin deposition can result in acute renal failure.

   iv. Hypotension can result secondary to decreased cardiac output as a result of hypovolemia caused by third spacing of fluids and impaired myocardial contractility. This is exacerbated by systemic vasodilation as a result of the systemic inflammatory response that is occurring.

   v. Coagulation abnormalities can result from the failure of absorption of vitamin-K, a fat-soluble vitamin that in the absence of dietary fat emulsification by bile salts fails to become absorbed. Vitamin K is necessary for the carboxylation in the liver of the pro-coagulation factors II, VII, IX, and X to their active form.

6. CLINICAL SIGNS AND PHYSICAL EXAMINATION

a. In most cases, clinical signs of EHBT traumatic injury will be vague and nonspecific and may be overshadowed by the signs of concurrent injury sustained during trauma, which can lead to a delay in the diagnosis being made.

b. The most common clinical signs in dogs and cats with bile peritonitis are vomiting, anorexia, diarrhea, and weight loss, which may not be evident until several days after the traumatic incident.

c. Most patients with bile peritonitis will demonstrate abdominal pain and may exhibit abdominal distension secondary to the accumulation of biliary effusion.

d. Signs of systemic hypoperfusion may be present such as poor peripheral pulse quality, pale mucous membranes, tachycardia, and cold extremities.

e. Icterus is usually evident once the serum bilirubin concentration exceeds 1.5–2.0 mg/dL.

f. On physical examination, patients that sustain blunt trauma may show evidence of bruising, superficial abrasions, lacerations, or may have deeper wounds in the case of penetrating injury.

g. There may be evidence of concurrent orthopedic or neurological injury.

7. **DIAGNOSIS OF EHBT INJURY**

a. Injury to the EHBT can be clinically silent for substantial periods especially when the cause is blunt abdominal trauma. One study reported a mean delay between trauma and diagnosis of 14 days (Ludwig et al., 1997).

b. Any animal sustaining penetrating injury to the abdomen should undergo an abdominal exploratory procedure during which the biliary tract should be thoroughly evaluated.

c. The diagnosis of bile peritonitis is dependent upon laboratory and imaging findings, but ultimately the retrieval and analysis of fluid from the peritoneal cavity or exploratory laparotomy provide the definitive answer:

   i. Laboratory parameters:

      1. Frequently encountered laboratory abnormalities:

         a. Increased total bilirubin

         b. Increased alkaline phosphatase

         c. Increased alanine aminotransferase

         d. Hypoalbuminemia

         e. Leukocytosis ± band neutrophils

         f. Anemia

         g. Bilirubinuria (*Note*: bilirubinuria may be detected prior to onset of increases in serum bilirubin)

   ii. Diagnostic imaging:

      1. Plain radiography—Nonspecific findings such as loss of abdominal detail suggest peritonitis. In penetrating injuries, it may be possible to visualize retained projectiles. Most choleliths in cats and dogs are made of calcium salts (most frequently calcium bilirubinate in dogs and calcium carbonate in cats) and are radio-opaque. However, it should be noted that choleliths can be incidental findings that are not associated with the primary pathology, particularly in trauma.

      2. Ultrasonography—May facilitate the retrieval of fluid from the abdomen during simple or four quadrant abdominocentesis. Focused assessment with sonography for trauma (FAST)—a recently described technique uses ultrasound to rapidly evaluate the abdomen ultrasonographically for fluid accumulation posttrauma. Transverse and longitudinal views at four locations are obtained: just caudal to the xiphoid process, on the midline over the urinary bladder and left and right flank regions. This technique has been shown to be simple, rapid (median duration of 6 minutes) and sensitive even in inexperienced hands (see Chapter 3 Shock in the Trauma Patient).

      3. Computed tomography (CT) and magnetic resonance imagine (MRI)—No data are available on the use of CT and MRI in the diagnosis of EHBT trauma in veterinary patients. In humans, a technique known as magnetic resonance cholangiopancreatography can be used for evaluation of either obstructive or traumatic EHBT disease but is not currently available for dogs and cats.

   iii. Abdominal fluid retrieval (see Chapter 11 for figures of this procedure):

      1. Simple abdominocentesis—Obtaining a fluid sample from the abdominal cavity is often simple in these cases as a significant peritoneal effusion is usually present:

         a. With the dog or cat in left lateral recumbency, to avoid splenic injury, an area just caudal and lateral to the midline is clipped and scrubbed aseptically.

         b. A 20–22 gauge needle or over the needle catheter is introduced using sterile technique.

c. Aspiration is initiated as soon as the skin is penetrated:

i. If a fluid sample is retrieved it is placed in an EDTA tube for cytological analysis, a serum tube for analysis of bilirubin level and onto culture swabs for microbiological analysis.

d. To increase the likelihood of fluid retrieval, ultrasound guidance can be employed during abdominocentesis.

2. Four quadrant abdominocentesis—If simple abdominocentesis is unsuccessful locations 2–3 cm cranial and caudal and 2–3 cm lateral and medial to the umbilicus can be tapped to increase the likelihood for fluid retrieval.

3. Diagnostic peritoneal lavage (DPL)—If fluid retrieval fails with the aforementioned techniques but a suspicion for EHBT trauma remains high, DPL is recommended:

a. Technique:

i. Sedation and local anesthetic infusion is used.

ii. An over-the-needle catheter or preferably a specialized peritoneal dialysis catheter, are placed into the abdominal cavity through a small incision 2–3 cm caudal to the umbilicus.

iii. If fluid cannot be aspirated directly, 20 mL/kg of warm 0.9% NaCl can be instilled under strict aseptic technique.

iv. Fluid is allowed to distribute by abdominal massage and then retrieval is attempted. Only a small sample may be retrieved.

b. Advantages of this technique include the ability to sometimes retrieve fluid from patients when other modalities have failed and the ability to obtain fluid from a larger area of the peritoneal cavity.

c. One disadvantage of this technique is the inability to accurately quantify bilirubin due to dilutional effects of the fluid instilled. For cytological evaluation, the dilutional effect of DPL can be ameliorated through centrifugation of the retrieved DPL fluid prior to cytological analysis. Therefore, generally a simple or four-quadrant abdominocentesis is attempted prior to DPL but if these techniques are nondiagnostic a DPL should be pursued.

iv. Abdominal fluid analysis:

1. Biochemical testing—The most reliable diagnostic test for bile peritonitis is the comparison of bilirubin concentration in the serum to that in the peritoneal effusion. If the bilirubin concentration in the effusion is two or more times greater than that in the serum, bile peritonitis should be suspected.

2. Cytology—In most cases an inflammatory exudate will be present. When evaluated cytologically, tan to bluish-green or black bile pigments may be visible either within macrophages or free. Bilirubin crystals may also be visualized.

3. Bacterial culture of the abdominal fluid should be attempted for both aerobic and anaerobic bacteria as septic biliary effusion markedly worsens prognosis and institution of antibiotic coverage based on culture and sensitivity testing at the earliest possible time is essential:

a. If septic bile peritonitis is suspected based on cytological and abdominal fluid biochemical findings, broad-spectrum antibiotics should be administered pending culture results.

v. Exploratory laparotomy:

1. If attempts at preoperative diagnosis of bile peritonitis resulting from trauma have failed but suspicion remains high, it is reasonable to perform an exploratory laparotomy.

2. Surgical treatment of EHBT trauma can be challenging and significant pre- and postoperative intensive care is often required for a successful outcome.

8. SURGICAL MANAGEMENT—TREATMENT OF UNDERLYING DEFECT

a. As soon as a diagnosis of bile peritonitis is made and patient stability has been achieved, surgical exploration is indicated to correct the underlying

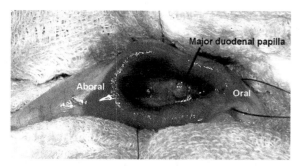

FIGURE 12.2   An antimesenteric duodenotomy has been created. This gives access to the major duodenal papilla.

defect and provide adequate lavage and drainage of the abdomen.

b. Thorough exploration of the abdominal cavity is indicated as concurrent injury to other organs sustained at the time of trauma may have occurred and must be evaluated.

c. Exploration of the EHBT should proceed cautiously as often many omental adhesions will be found in the area and care should be taken not to worsen any lacerations during initial evaluation.

d. If the site of leakage is difficult to localize, an antimesenteric duodenotomy can be performed followed by retrograde flushing of sterile saline into the CBD (Figure 12.2). Leakage of saline through the defect will usually be obvious.

e. The surgical treatment of traumatic EHBT lesions depends on the specific nature and location of the injury:

f. Gall bladder perforation:

   i. Although rarely the site of the lesion in traumatic cases perforation of the gall bladder can occur and should be treated by cholecystectomy:

      1. Removing the gall bladder has no known clinically relevant long-term side effects.

   ii. Dissection of the gall bladder from the hepatic fossa is performed. Some hemorrhage from hepatic parenchyma is expected and is best controlled with the use of a haemostatic agent such as oxidized regenerated cellulose (Surgicel©, Ethicon Inc., Somerville, NJ).

   iii. Once the gall bladder has been dissected free down to the cystic duct, double ligation of the cystic duct should be performed using 2–0 to 3–0 monofilament absorbable or nonabsorbable suture material. Application of hemoclips to the cystic duct to prevent bile leakage is also possible but may be less secure especially if clips are undersized.

   iv. Primary suturing of a gall bladder perforation with fine (4–0 to 5–0) monofilament absorbable suture material in a simple continuous pattern is also possible if the tissue is healthy and not too friable. However, dehiscence is possible making cholecystectomy the preferred option.

g. Cystic duct perforation/avulsion:

   i. In cases where the common bile duct is patent, simple cholecystectomy with double ligation distal to the lesion in the cystic duct may be possible.

   ii. If concurrent lesions in the common bile duct are present and biliary diversion is required, then primary closure of the cystic duct may be required prior to biliary diversion.

h. Hepatic duct injury:

   i. Isolated hepatic duct lacerations or avulsions have been reported and are best treated by simple ligation of the hepatic duct in question proximal and distal to the lesion.

   ii. Adequate collateral circulation of bile between hepatic divisions is present in dogs although atrophy of the hepatic lobe being drained by the injured hepatic duct in question can occur.

   iii. It is also possible to see a mild transient increase in concentrations of enzymes that reflect hepatocyte injury after hepatic duct ligation (e.g., alanine aminotransferase).

i. Common bile duct (CBD) perforation/avulsion:

   i. The two most common lesions are avulsion of the CBD from its duodenal attachment or perforating tears/lacerations of the CBD.

   ii. For avulsions either proximal ligation of the common bile duct with biliary diversion (cholecystoduodenostomy or cholecystojejunostomy) or re-implantation of the distal segment into the duodenum is possible but the latter is prone to dehiscence and stricture formation.

   iii. CBD tears can either be treated by primary closure of the tear or biliary diversion if the tear is located closer to the duodenal end and a sufficient number of hepatic ducts can have flow redirected toward a cholecystoenterostomy:

1. Primary closure:

   a. A simple continuous pattern of fine (4–0 to 5–0) monofilament absorbable suture material is used for simple tears.

   b. Tension-free suturing of healthy tissue must be ensured to avoid dehiscence. In one study, dehiscence after primary closure of common bile duct lesions occurred in 3 of 7 dogs (Watkins, 1983). Avulsions of the CBD can be treated with re-anastomosis but this will be very challenging in the normal nondistended CBD (normal diameter 2–4 mm in dogs and cats) that is most frequently encountered in cases of trauma.

2. Biliary diversion techniques:

   a. In all cases of CBD lacerations/avulsions, this author recommends biliary diversion in cases where the gall bladder, cystic duct, and proximal part of the CBD are intact as this will minimize the incidence of dehiscence and stricture formation.

   b. Cholecystoduodenostomy is the biliary diversion technique of choice in dogs and cats (Figure 12.3) (see Martin et al., 2003 for a more detailed description of this procedure):

   i. This procedure alters gastrointestinal physiology less than a cholecystojejunostomy where bile is permanently diverted away from the duodenum.

   c. Occasionally, tension-free mobilization of the duodenum to a location adjacent to the gall bladder is difficult and in these cases cholecystojejeunostomy is acceptable.

   d. With either technique postoperative complications such as ascending cholangitis, dehiscence, and stricture of the stoma are possible.

3. Biliary stenting:

   a. Whether to perform primary closure of CBD perforations over a biliary stent

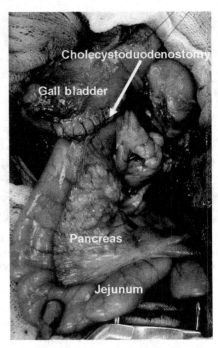

FIGURE 12.3 Intraoperative view of a completed cholecystoduodenostomy in a cat. A single layer simple continuous appositional suture pattern was used in this case.

remains controversial as no controlled randomized studies exist to compare results of treatment with or without stenting.

b. Stents made of red rubber catheters can be placed retrograde into the CBD to cross the lesion. The end of the stent exits through the major duodenal papilla into the duodenum. There they can be anchored to the duodenal mucosa with 1–2 sutures. (Figure 12.4).

c. Stent use may decompress the biliary system, thus decreasing likelihood of leakage and they may limit the formation of scar tissue.

d. The use of T-tube stents as well as straight stents that pass through the major duodenal papilla into the duodenum has been described in dogs.

e. Disadvantages may include an inhibitory effect on healing, ascending cholangitis from the duodenum and premature stent occlusion. The use of stents for management of obstructive

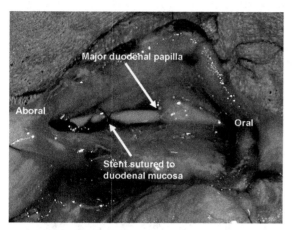

FIGURE 12.4 A biliary stent can be seen exiting the major duodenal papilla and anchored to the duodenal mucosa. An antimesenteric duodenotomy has been performed to give access to the papilla for stent placement.

biliary disease was generally well tolerated in dogs in one report; however a clear indication for and against stent use in traumatic cases is lacking (Mayhew et al., 2006). The use of biliary stents in cats may be associated with a higher incidence of early obstruction possibly due to the narrow gauge of stent that can be passed into the feline common bile duct (Mayhew and Weisse, 2008).

f. T-tube stents can be removed as soon as cholangiography has revealed patency and lack of leakage from the CBD. Straight stents residing in the duodenum will either pass out in the feces or can be removed endoscopically 1–3 months postoperatively.

9. SURGICAL MANAGEMENT—PERITONEAL LAVAGE AND ONGOING DRAINAGE

a. Correction of the underlying source of leakage is followed by liberal lavage of the peritoneal cavity with a warm balanced electrolyte solution until all gross debris has been removed.

b. Serious consideration should be given to providing ongoing drainage as due to the frequent delay in surgical treatment after diagnosis severe contamination of the peritoneal cavity is present in most cases.

c. Postoperative drainage can be accomplished in several ways:

i. Open abdominal drainage—arguably provides the greatest amount of drainage but is associated with high cost, the possibility of ascending nosocomial infection, and multiple anesthetic episodes. In one nonrandomized study, open peritoneal lavage was associated with an increased mortality rate in dogs with various causes of bile peritonitis (Ludwig et al., 1997).

ii. Closed suction Jackson–Pratt (Cardinal Health Inc., McGaw Park, IL.) or Blake (Ethicon Inc., Somerville, NJ) drains—provide excellent drainage with less risk of ascending infection and allow cytological and biochemical evaluation of peritoneal fluid collected from around the EHBT on a daily basis. This allows early detection of biliary leakage. Some residual phagocytosed bile may be seen on cytologic examination of peritoneal fluid over the first few days after EHBT repair.

iii. Passive drainage—The use of penrose drains to drain the peritoneal cavity is contraindicated as it has the significant disadvantage of providing less effective drainage and greater risk of ascending infection than aforementioned techniques.

10. COMPLICATIONS OF THERAPY AND PROGNOSIS

a. The morbidity and mortality in dogs and cats with EHBT trauma is high.

b. In one veterinary study of dogs with bile peritonitis, a 50% mortality rate was seen. In this study, sepsis was the most common cause of perioperative mortality (Ludwig et al., 1997).

c. Sepsis has been linked to EHBT in much experimental work due to the absence of bile salts in the intestine resulting in translocation of endotoxins into the portal and subsequently systemic circulation.

d. Other systemic complications observed include: hemorrhage, acute renal failure, decreased myocardial contractility, and hypotension.

e. When primary repair of bile duct lesions or cholecystoenterostomy has been performed, the most concerning postoperative complication is wound dehiscence.

f. When recurrence of bile peritonitis occurs due to dehiscence providing ongoing drainage alone has been reported to give a successful outcome in one report although most surgeons will consider re-exploration of the patient to be the safest option due to the possible development of sepsis, which gravely worsens the prognosis.

BIBLIOGRAPHY

Bacon NJ, White RAS. Extrahepatic biliary tract surgery in the cat: a case series and review. *J Small Anim Pract* 2003; 44: 231–235.

Fossum TW. *Small Animal Surgery*. St. Louis, Mosby, 2002; 475–486.

Hunt CA, Gofton N. Primary repair of a transected bile duct. *J Am Anim Hosp Assoc* 1984; 20: 57–64.

Ludwig LL, McLoughlin MA, Graves TK, *et al.* Surgical treatment of bile peritonitis in 24 dogs and 2 cats: a retrospective study (1987–1994). *Vet Surg* 1997; 25: 90–98.

Martin RA, Lanz OI, Tobias KM. Liver and biliary system. In: Slatter D, ed. *Textbook of Small Animal Surgery*. Saunders, Philadelphia, PA, 2003; 708–726.

Matthiesen DT. Complications associated with surgery of the extrahepatic biliary system. *Probl Vet Med* 1989; 1: 295–313.

Mayhew PD, Richardson RW, Mehler SJ, *et al.* Choledochal tube stenting for decompression of the extrahepatic portion of the biliary tract in dogs: 13 cases (2002–2005). *J Am Vet Med Assoc* 2006; 228: 1209–1214.

Mayhew PD, Weisse CW. Treatment of pancreatitis-associated extrahepatic biliary tract obstruction by choledochal stenting in seven cats. *J Small Anim Pract* 2008; 49: 133–138.

Mehler SJ, Mayhew PD, Drobatz KJ, *et al.* Variables associated with outcome in dogs undergoing extrahepatic biliary surgery: 60 cases (1988–2002). *Vet Surg* 2004; 33: 644–649.

Parchman MB, Flanders JA. Extrahepatic biliary tract rupture: evaluation of the relationship between the site of rupture and the cause of rupture in 15 dogs. *Cornell Vet* 1990; 80: 267–273.

Watkins PE, Pearson H, Denny HR. Traumatic rupture of the bile duct in the dog: a report of seven cases. *J Small Anim Pract* 1983; 24: 731–740.

TRAUMA-ASSOCIATED BODY WALL AND TORSO INJURY

Philipp D. Mayhew and William Culp

1. INTRODUCTION

a. Trauma can lead to injuries of the abdominal wall occurring alone or in concert with other abdominal injuries. These injuries can be caused by both blunt and penetrating trauma and will vary in severity (Figure 13.1):

   i. Body wall injuries may include minor injuries such as contusions or more severe injuries such as body wall rupture with subsequent herniation of the gastrointestinal tract structures as well as other organs, which in turn can lead to vascular compromise and necrosis.

b. The first challenge for the clinician is to recognize these injuries that are often overshadowed by more obvious trauma to the thorax, central nervous system, or extremities.

c. Correct prioritization of abdominal and other body system injuries is critical to successful management of the traumatized patient.

2. ABDOMINAL WALL HERNIATION

a. Abdominal wall herniation occurs most frequently due to either blunt trauma or animal bite wounds (Figure 13.2). Studies in the veterinary literature disagree as to which is the most common cause. Less common causes are gunshot or stab injury.

b. Blunt trauma likely causes a sudden dramatic rise in intra-abdominal pressure resulting in rupture of the weakest part of the abdominal wall musculature. Shear forces placed on the inelastic fibrous and tendinous attachments of muscles to bone can also result in wall defects and subsequent herniation.

c. In traumatically induced hernias, important pathological sequela include extreme pain and systemic inflammation induced by severe tissue trauma, the possibility of herniation of bowel or other abdominal organs and their subsequent strangulation. Full thickness body wall defects can result in evisceration.

d. Herniation of the abdominal wall following blunt trauma can occur at numerous sites: paracostal, lateral, inguinal, femoral, prepubic, and ventral:

   i. In one study, the most frequent sites in dogs were lateral paralumbar wall and prepubic ligament (Shaw et al., 2003).

   ii. The ventral body wall, femoral area, lateral paralumbar area, and cranial pubic ligament are the most common sites noted in cats.

e. There is debate whether some cases of hiatal hernias are the result of trauma. It is more likely that dogs with hiatal hernias have a preexisting weakness in the region of the lower esophageal sphincter that can become clinical after a traumatic event, although hiatal hernias are also seen in dogs that have not suffered trauma.

Manual of Trauma Management in the Dog and Cat, First Edition. Edited by Kenneth J. Drobatz, Matthew W. Beal and Rebecca S. Syring.
© 2011 John Wiley & Sons, Inc. Published 2011 by John Wiley & Sons, Inc.

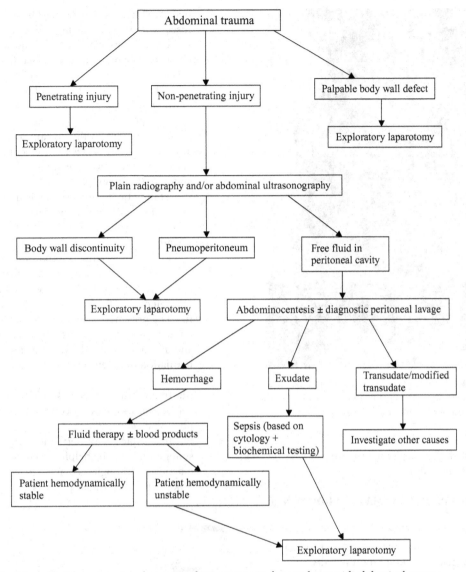

FIGURE 13.1   Flow chart demonstrating decision-making process in dogs and cats with abdominal trauma.

f. Inguinal hernias that appear after trauma may be associated with a preexisting weakness in the tissue bordering the entrance to the inguinal canal.

g. Diaphragmatic hernias are a common result of blunt trauma (see Chapter 6: Trauma-Associated Thoracic Injury).

h. It is difficult to predict whether or not organ strangulation and/or vascular compromise will occur in animals with body wall hernias. Some her-nias present with strangulation of hernia contents within days of trauma whereas other dogs have hernias that do not progress even over years.

i. Trauma-related hernias are more likely to stran-gulate due to inflammation, hematoma formation, and subsequent healing by fibrosis.

j. Hernias with small hernial rings are also more likely to scar down and cause strangulation sooner.

k. In one study of traumatic abdominal hernias in both dogs and cats, the small intestine was

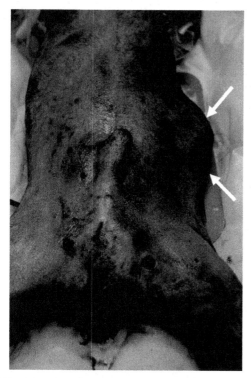

FIGURE 13.2 An obvious defect in the abdominal body wall can be seen and was palpable in this dog after sustaining bite wound injury (arrow).

herniated in 50% and omentum in 31–50% of cases (Shaw et al., 2003).

3. DIAGNOSIS OF TRAUMATIC ABDOMINAL WALL INJURY

a. Clinical signs:

i. In many cases, the clinical picture may be nonspecific and more representative of intercurrent traumatic injury. Lethargy, anorexia, and vomiting may be present. In one review of dogs with inguinal herniation, those dogs with strangulated nonviable intestine within their hernias were more likely to vomit than those without (Waters et al., 1993).

b. Physical examination:

i. In one study, only 65% of traumatic body wall hernias in dogs and cats were diagnosed at initial physical examination (Shaw et al., 2003).

ii. Careful palpation may reveal a palpable defect or an area of weakness in the body wall. Occasionally, an obvious outpouching of the

body wall may be visible, which can be confused with a soft tissue mass (Figure 13.2).

iii. Contents may be reducible allowing differentiation of a mass from a hernia. In some cases this will not be as obvious especially if the rent in the body wall is either small or if herniation of organs has not occurred.

iv. In ruptures of the prepubic tendon, the caudal abdominal wall may appear pendulous, although in many cases this defect is only noted at exploratory surgery or sometimes on lateral abdominal radiographs.

v. Traumatic inguinal hernia is uncommon and will usually present with a soft fluctuant mass in the groin area.

c. Imaging:

i. Plain radiography is important diagnostically to look for evidence of discontinuity in the body wall (Figure 13.3). Evidence of organ displacement into the hernia may also be visible.

ii. The presence of small intestinal loops containing gas pockets are usually easy to visualize and detect within body wall hernias; however, herniation of omentum may be more difficult to detect.

iii. In one study, only 42% of traumatic body wall hernias were detected with plain radiography (Shaw et al., 2003).

iv. If a suspicion for herniation exists, ultrasonography may be helpful in confirming a diagnosis, although its diagnostic accuracy is unknown in veterinary patients.

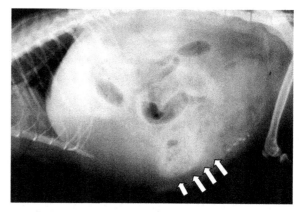

FIGURE 13.3 Loss of continuity of the ventral body wall can be seen in this cat with a traumatic abdominal wall hernia.

d. Surgical exploration:

i. Exploratory laparotomy is warranted in cases where the diagnosis cannot be firmly established based on the above criteria. Laparoscopic exploration of the abdomen could be used to diagnose abdominal wall defects giving the advantage of a minimally invasive approach.

4. TREATMENT—ABDOMINAL TRAUMA

a. Clear indications for performing surgical exploratory laparotomy on an emergent basis in dogs and cats having sustained abdominal trauma are as follows:

i. Evidence of septic peritonitis based on the visualization of intracellular bacteria or suggestive biochemical parameters in peritoneal effusions.

ii. Any form of penetrating injury from a projectile or severe bite wound.

iii. Evidence of intraperitoneal hemorrhage that is unremitting or resulting in an inability to hemodynamically stabilize the patient.

iv. Any evidence of a traumatic body wall hernia that contains herniated abdominal viscera.

b. In all cases, a thorough exploratory laparotomy should take place as intercurrent injury to other organs is always possible. In a study of traumatic body wall herniation, 33% of dogs and cats were found to have serious injuries to abdominal viscera including mesenteric avulsion, kidney avulsion, splenic laceration, bladder rupture, and various gastrointestinal tract perforations (Shaw et al., 2003).

5. TREATMENT OF TRAUMATIC BODY WALL HERNIAS

a. Body wall herniation in dogs and cats can vary from a very simple to a quite complex surgical technique.

b. Abdominal wall hernias:

i. In most dogs and cats, simple herniorrhaphy by apposition of tissue after debridement of necrotic/devitalized areas is satisfactory. Simple continuous appositional suturing with an absorbable monofilament suture material is advised.

ii. If large defects are encountered or defects where significant shear or crushing injury has

caused extensive necrosis or ischemic injury requiring debridement, closure without significant tension may be impossible. This can also occur in chronic cases where significant muscle contracture has resulted in enlargement of the original defect.

iii. If primary closure is impossible, reconstructive techniques need to be considered such as the use of muscle flaps, polypropylene mesh, or porcine intestinal submucosa (VET BiosisT™, Global Veterinary Products, Inc., New Buffalo, MI).

iv. The prospective surgeon should always realize going into such a case that the use of a reconstructive technique may be required.

c. Inguinal hernias:

i. The opening to the vaginal process must be sutured closed as much as possible but with enough space for the genitofemoral artery, vein and nerve, the external pudendal vessels, as well as the spermatic cord in males and round ligament in females to pass through.

ii. In more chronic cases, this type of hernia may also require a reconstructive surgery such as the cranial sartorius muscle flap to avoid recurrence.

d. Prepubic tendon rupture:

i. There is often little tissue left attached to the pubis, thus making this more of an avulsion injury from bone.

ii. If some ligamentous tissue remains attached to the pubis, interrupted tension relieving mattress suture placement between the edges of the torn ligament can be performed. However, more often the tissue is shredded and sutures that are placed are easily torn out when tension is applied. In these cases it is necessary to drill holes with a kirschner wire through the pubic bone along the desired insertion of the cranial pubic ligament and pass sutures of monofilament absorbable or nonabsorbable sutures through the holes that are then anchored in the avulsed ligament.

iii. If a significant distance is present between the pubis and the remainder of the cranial pubic ligament, a cuff of mesh can be used to bridge the defect. Polypropylene mesh (Prolene™ mesh, Ethicon, Somerville, NJ) or porcine small intestinal submucosa (VET BiosisT™, Global

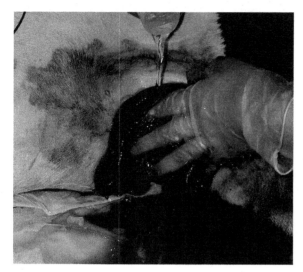

FIGURE 13.4 In this dog with an evisceration, thorough lavage of the herniated small intestinal loops is performed on an emergency basis prior to preparing the patient for laparotomy. (Photograph courtesy of Dr. Cynthia Otto.)

Veterinary Products, Inc., New Buffalo, MI) can be used for this purpose.

6. **EVISCERATION**

  a. This can result if a traumatic body wall defect penetrates muscle, subcutaneous tissues, and skin. It can also occur secondary to dehiscence of a celiotomy incision postsurgically.

  b. Despite the seemingly catastrophic nature of these injuries, many dogs and cats will survive if prompt treatment is pursued and organ damage is not too severe. In one recent study, 8 dogs and 4 cats that suffered major abdominal evisceration all survived to discharge from the hospital after the event (Gower et al., 2009).

  c. Immediate protection of herniated organs is mandatory to prevent further injury and avoid self-mutilation. Under sterile conditions herniated organs should be thoroughly lavaged, and returned to the abdominal cavity (Figure 13.4). They should be closely inspected for evidence of perforation, necrosis, or ischemic tissue injury.

  d. Resection and anastomosis of damaged bowel may be necessary.

  e. Collection of samples for bacterial culture and sensitivity testing should be performed prior to closure.

  f. Closure of the body wall defect in multiple layers should be performed initially from an intra-abdominal approach as described above. Closure from the outside should include more superficial muscles of the body wall followed by subcutaneous tissues and the skin:

   i. Depending on the degree of contamination, consideration should be given to the use of a drain.

   ii. If evisceration occurred very recently, thorough debridement and lavage may suffice. However, if the injury occurred more than a few hours prior to admission or if contamination is severe then active drainage, such as the use of a closed suction Jackson–Pratt drain should be considered.

   iii. The use of an open abdomen technique can also be considered in cases with severe contamination/active infection:

    1. In this technique, the linea alba is sutured loosely leaving a gap for ongoing drainage.

    2. The abdomen is then thickly wrapped with a nonadhesive, permeable dressing followed by roll cotton and the bandage is changed at least once daily.

    3. Re-exploration of the abdomen is usually performed at least once in the subsequent 2–3 days and a judgment has to be made regarding abdominal closure once the abdomen is considered to be sufficiently clean.

  g. Antibiotic therapy:

   i. Broad-spectrum antibiotic therapy should be initiated immediately upon identification of a penetrating abdominal wall injury. In the postoperative period, ongoing antibiotic therapy and general supportive care should be provided. Good empirical choices include the following: Ampcillin (22 mg/kg IV TID) and Cefoxitin (22 mg/kg IV TID) or a combination of Enrofloxacin (dogs; 10 mg/kg IV SID, cats; 5 mg/kg IV SID) and Ampicillin (22 mg/kg IV TID). These choices should be subsequently modified based on the results of bacterial culture and sensitivity testing.

   ii. Nonpenetrating abdominal wall injuries will only require antibiotic therapy in the perioperative period.

BIBLIOGRAPHY

Bjorling DE, Crowe DT, Kolata RJ, *et al*. Penetrating abdominal wounds in dogs and cats. *J Am Anim Hosp Assoc* 1982; 18: 742–748.

Gower SB, Weisse CW, Brown DC. Major abdominal evisceration injuries in dogs and cats: 12 cases (1998–2008). *J Am Vet Med Assoc* 2009; 234: 1566–1572.

Kolata RJ, Kraut NH, Johnston DE. Patterns of trauma in urban dogs and cats: a study of 1000 cases. *J Am Vet Med Assoc* 1974; 164: 499–502.

Kolata RJ, Johnston DE. Motor vehicle accidents in urban dogs: a study of 600 cases. *J Am Vet Med Assoc* 1975; 167: 938–941.

Shamir MH, Leisner S. Klement E, *et al*. Dog bite wounds in dogs and cats: a retrospective study of 196 cases. *J Vet Med* 2002; 49: 107–112.

Shaw SP, Rozanski EA, Rush JE. Traumatic body wall herniation in 36 dogs and cats. *J Am Anim Hosp Assoc* 2003; 39: 35–46.

Waters DJ, Roy RG, Stone EA. A retrospective study of inguinal hernia in 35 dogs. *Vet Surg* 1993; 22: 44–49.

TRAUMA-ASSOCIATED GASTROINTESTINAL INJURY

Philipp D. Mayhew and William Culp

1. INTRODUCTION

a. Trauma can lead to injuries of the gastrointestinal tract. These injuries can be caused by both blunt and penetrating trauma and will vary in severity:

  i. Primary gastrointestinal injuries can include the following:

  1. Minor bowel contusions/hematomas
  2. Mesenteric tears
  3. Vascular compromise/avulsion
  4. Penetrating wounds resulting in septic peritonitis

b. The first challenge for the clinician is to recognize these injuries. Recognition can be challenging because these injuries are often overshadowed by more obvious trauma to the thorax, central nervous system, or extremities.

c. Correct prioritization of abdominal and other body system injuries is critical to successful management of the traumatized patient.

2. PATHOPHYSIOLOGY

a. Trauma involving the abdominal cavity can result in multiple organ injury.

b. In urban dogs, gunshot injury is the most common cause of abdominal trauma accounting for a third of cases, followed by motor vehicle accidents and animal bite wounds. Sharp object injuries, falls

from a height (high-rise syndrome), and crush injuries are less common causes (Kolata et al., 1974).

c. Gastrointestinal perforation represents one of the most serious forms of injury but the possibility of other organ damage occurring concurrently must always be considered.

d. Gunshot injury:

  i. Injury to the bowel is not uncommon in animals with gunshot wounds that penetrate the abdominal cavity. In one study, approximately 17% of dogs with gunshot wounds sustained injury to the abdominal cavity (Fullington and Otto, 1997).

  ii. Young male dogs are at higher risk for injury secondary to gunshot wounds. This may be due to their propensity to roam and the perceived threat of aggressive behavior.

  iii. High-velocity weapons will result in the generation of significant waves of kinetic energy that are capable of causing injury well beyond the direct trajectory of the missile.

  iv. Multiple bowel perforation is often encountered making thorough exploration of the abdominal cavity in all cases of gunshot wound to the abdomen mandatory.

  v. Injuries to the cervical or thoracic esophagus may also result from gunshot injury but are rare. Injury to the thoracic esophagus in

Manual of Trauma Management in the Dog and Cat, First Edition. Edited by Kenneth J. Drobatz, Matthew W. Beal and Rebecca S. Syring.
© 2011 John Wiley & Sons, Inc. Published 2011 by John Wiley & Sons, Inc.

particular is rare due to its relatively protected position within the rib cage:

    1. These injuries may be difficult to detect initially but should be suspected in any dog with cervical pain and swelling of the neck and/or pneumomediastinum after gunshot trauma to those areas.

    2. Clinical signs associated with thoracic esophageal injuries are likely to initially be overshadowed by injuries to the lungs or vascular structures in the area.

e. Blunt trauma:

    i. Blunt trauma, most frequently caused by motor vehicle accidents or falling from heights, commonly causes injury to the brain, thorax, appendicular skeleton, spine, and solid organs within the abdomen. Bowel injuries are relatively rare following blunt trauma. Mesenteric tears and vascular compromise are more likely to occur following blunt trauma than intestinal perforation, although any of these injuries may occur (Figure 14.1).

    ii. Three different mechanisms that cause injury to the abdominal viscera may be involved:

        1. A sudden dramatic rise in intra-abdominal pressure ruptures hollow viscera or solid organs.

        2. Compression of abdominal viscera against the thoracic cage or thoracic spine.

        3. Sudden shearing forces leading to tears or avulsions of organs or vascular pedicles.

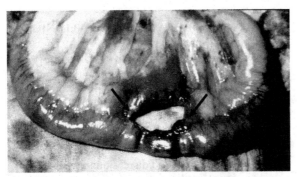

FIGURE 14.1 The result of a motor vehicle accident, this image demonstrates the potential for blunt trauma to lead to serious small intestinal injury (arrows). (Reprinted with permission: Tobias K, 2010, Slatter's Textbook of Small Animal Surgery, Saunders, 2010.)

    iii. The gastrointestinal tract is relatively free floating in the abdominal cavity and only has loose attachments to the body wall through the mesenteric root. Along with its considerable compressibility this may in part explain why blunt trauma is more likely to cause injury to solid organs or other less mobile structures than the gastrointestinal tract (see Chapter 11: Trauma-Associated Abdominal Parenchymal Organ Injury).

    iv. Abdominal injuries were noted in only 5.2% (31/600) dogs that were in motor vehicle accidents in one study (Kolata and Johnston, 1975). Of these abdominal injuries, the liver was the most frequently affected organ followed by injuries to the diaphragm, urinary tract, and spleen. Injury to the gastrointestinal tract was detected in only two dogs in this study.

    v. In dogs and cats suffering from falls from a height, gastrointestinal tract injuries are uncommon.

f. Animal bite wounds (see Chapter 20: Bite Wound Trauma):

    i. Bite wound injuries often have a greater component of shear and crushing injury than other types of wounds due to the way in which dogs will often bite their prey and then shake the other animal vigorously causing significant tearing and crushing.

    ii. The abdominal area is frequently injured during dog fights or dog on cat fights. In one study, 24% of dogs and 27% of cats that sustained bite wounds had injuries in the abdominal area (Shamir et al., 2002). Small dogs are more likely to have abdominal injury than larger dogs. Of dogs and cats that undergo wound exploration for bite wounds over the abdomen, 79% of wounds were noted to penetrate the abdomen, of which 65% had damage to internal organs. The most common gastrointestinal injuries are to the jejunum and mesentery but ileum, duodenum, cecum, and colon can also be injured (Shamir et al., 2002).

g. Sharp object injuries:

    i. These injuries can be high or low velocity in nature, examples of which include arrow injury, stab wounds, and penetrating stick foreign bodies from the oral cavity. These injuries tend to occur at a lower velocity than gunshot wounds and are, therefore, more likely to result in direct injury to the organs that they contact and carry less risk of injury distant from their trajectory. However, bowel perforations or vascular damage leading to ischemic necrosis of bowel can result.

h. Iatrogenic injury:

i. Iatrogenic injury to the esophagus can occur from manipulation of foreign bodies with endoscopy or when surgery is performed in the cervical area.

ii. Gastrointestinal perforation can also occur during endoscopic interventions, passing stomach tubes, enema administration, or diagnostic rectal examination.

3. PATHOPHYSIOLOGY—SEPTIC PERITONITIS

a. The inevitable result of bowel perforation is septic peritonitis.

b. Septic peritonitis initiates an acute inflammatory reaction that initially involves the activation of complement (especially C3a and C5a), thus inducing neutrophil chemotaxis and degranulation of basophils and mast cells.

c. Degranulation releases histamine and prostaglandins, which cause vasodilation and increased vascular permeability in turn leading to increased exudation of protein and fluid into the peritoneal cavity.

d. Tissue damage and bacterial infection leads to systemic and local release of cytokines TNF, IL-1, IL-6, IFN-γ amongst others.

e. Initially, peritoneal responses are self-protective: opsonization of contaminants by humoral and complement activity, chemotaxis of phagocytic macrophages and neutrophils aid clearance of bacteria, and fluid shifts into the peritoneal cavity lead to dilution of bacteria and debris.

f. In most cases, self-protective mechanisms are soon overwhelmed where the underlying source of contamination can no longer be controlled.

g. Hypovolemia and hypoproteinemia soon develop as fluid shifts from the intravascular space to the peritoneal cavity. Local defenses suffer as opsonins are diluted and phagocytic function is impaired.

h. Systemic hypotension impairs cardiac function due to decreased venous return of blood to the heart. Renal ischemia can lead to renal insufficiency and eventually acute renal failure. Tissue hypoxia causes anerobic metabolism to

occur in many tissues resulting in metabolic acidosis.

i. The role of bacteria in the development of peritonitis is crucial. It is known that perforation of the stomach and upper small intestine will lead to slower progression of clinical signs compared to colonic perforation, which causes severe peritonitis associated with high mortality.

j. The most likely reason for the severity of peritonitis when colonic leakage occurs is due to the overwhelming anerobic bacterial load (>99.9% anerobes) found in this location compared with the scant populations of acid-resistant bacteria and lack of anaerobes found in the stomach and upper small intestine.

k. In penetrating traumatic injuries to the abdominal cavity, bacterial populations can be the result of intestinal perforation but also due to inoculation from outside the body. While gunshot injuries were once considered most likely to be sterile, this has been shown not to be the case. In one canine study, 78% of cultured gunshot wounds were contaminated with bacteria (Fullington and Otto, 1997):

i. The most common bacterial isolates from gunshot wounds are enteric organisms, Staphylococci, and Clostridia.

ii. In penetrating bite wound injuries, the most common bacterial isolates are *Staphylococci, E. coli* and *Pasteurella* species.

l. It is likely that in animals with bowel perforation from penetrating injury, bacterial contamination can result from both intestinal sources as well as direct inoculation.

4. DIAGNOSIS OF TRAUMATIC BOWEL INJURY

a. Clinical signs:

i. Clinical signs of traumatic bowel injury alone are generally nonspecific in the immediate postinjury period. Relying purely on clinical signs for diagnosis will inevitably lead to significant delays in diagnosis and is discouraged.

ii. Signs such as vomiting, anorexia, lethargy, abdominal pain, and distension may all be seen in animals with injury to the gastrointestinal tract.

iii. Esophageal injury may lead to regurgitation, vomiting, lethargy, or evidence of respiratory distress caused by pleural

effusion/pyothorax in the case of thoracic
esophageal perforation.

b. Laboratory abnormalities:

   i. In the immediate posttrauma period, it is
likely that few abnormalities will be detected on
routine biochemical and hematological testing
unless major hemorrhage accompanies traumatic bowel injury. If perforation has occurred
and septic peritonitis or pyothorax develops,
hypoproteinemia, hypoglycemia, abnormal liver
enzyme concentrations, and leukocytosis with
or without a degenerative left shift may develop.

c. Imaging:

   i. Plain radiography:

     1. Evidence of free gas in the peri-
esophageal tissues in the neck or pneumomediastinum may indicate esophageal
perforation. Pleural effusion from pyothorax may also be present in more chronic
cases. It should be noted, however, that in
early cases, evidence of gas leakage may be
absent and esophageal injury should not be
ruled out if free gas is not seen.

     2. Loss of abdominal detail on plain radio-
graphs may indicate abdominal effusion,
a sample of which should be collected for
chemical and cytologic analysis. Localized
peritonitis can be present in the early stages
after injury and radiographic changes may
not be visible for 72 hours.

     3. In cases of pneumoperitoneum, the free
gas may have gained access to the peritoneal cavity from an open penetrating
injury. Suspicion for rupture of the gastrointestinal tract should be high when free
gas is detected radiographically in animals
following blunt trauma. Horizontal beam
radiographs with the patient in left lateral
recumbency is preferable to avoid confu-
sion of a possible gas cap with gas in the
stomach.

   ii. Radiographic contrast studies:

     1. If perforation of the esophagus, stomach
or small intestine is suspected but cannot
be confirmed using other means, contrast
radiographic contrast studies can be considered.

     2. Barium should not be used for this pur-
pose when gastrointestinal perforation is
possible as leakage of barium can cause
more severe peritonitis as well as granuloma and adhesion formation. An organic
nonionic iodinated contrast agent (e.g.,
Iohexol 350 mg/mL, Omnipaque™, GE
Healthcare Inc. Princeton, NJ) should be
used in these situations.

     3. For an esophagram, administer 20 mL
(dog) or 10 mL (cat) of iohexol mixed with
half to one cup of food.

     4. For evaluation of the stomach and
small intestine, administer 7–800 mgI/kg
of iohexol and dilute with water to reach
a whole volume of 10 mL/kg for dogs and
cats. Administer this by orogastric tube.
It is possible to miss small perforations
with contrast radiography as iodinated contrast agents are quickly reabsorbed by the
intestines.

   iii. Abdominal ultrasound:

     1. Abdominal ultrasound is a very useful
imaging modality to assess patients with
possible traumatic gastrointestinal injury
although its success is dependent on experience level.

     2. Ultrasonography allows prompt detec-
tion of free fluid in body cavities and allows
direct visualization of fluid pockets during
centesis, maximizing the chance of recovering a diagnostic sample (Figure 14.2).

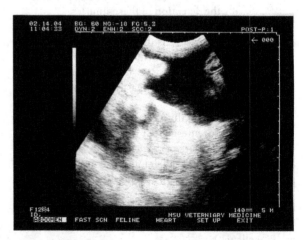

FIGURE 14.2 Ultrasound image demonstrating a free
pocket of fluid located adjacent to a bowel loop. This fluid
should be aspirated and evaluated cytologically and bio-
chemically and should undergo bacterial culture and sensitivity testing.

3. A new technique "focused assessment with sonography for trauma" (FAST) was recently described in veterinary patients. This widely used technique in humans allows a rapid ultrasonographic survey of the abdomen to be performed in the emergency room setting, soon after patients are admitted, to systematically assess for the presence of free fluid within the peritoneal cavity (see Chapter 3: Shock in the Trauma Patient).

4. Underlying bowel or mesenteric injuries may be detected with ultrasonography, although this will depend on severity of the injury and the degree of training of the ultrasonographer.

5. Ultrasound maybe used for evaluation of fluid or gas leakage from the cervical esophagus. If fluid pockets are seen ultrasound-guided aspiration of fluid for cytological and microbial culture and sensitivity testing is warranted.

iv. Computed Tomography (CT) and Magnetic Resonance Imaging (MRI):

1. No reports of advanced imaging for traumatic abdominal injury currently exist in the veterinary literature. However, CT is used extensively in humans for assessment of bowel and mesenteric injury and is associated with high sensitivity and specificity for the detection of these injuries.

d. Peritoneal fluid analysis:

i. Fluid analysis is the key to the prompt diagnosis of septic peritonitis, which in most cases of traumatic injury to the abdominal cavity will be the result of gastrointestinal tract rupture.

ii. Peritoneal fluid can be retrieved by simple abdominocentesis, four quadrant abdominocentesis, diagnostic peritoneal lavage, or via ultrasound-guided abdominocentesis.

iii. In cases of septic peritonitis, the character of the fluid is likely that of an exudate. Exudates have a high protein concentration (>3.0 g/dL) and high nucleated cell counts (>5000 cells/μL).

iv. A direct smear of the fluid and a smear of the sediment of abdominal fluid should be evaluated on an emergency basis for the following parameters:

1. Cellularity: Septic peritonitis will have a moderate to very cellular characteristic unless the contamination has just occurred:

a. Typically, if a direct smear is made of abdominal effusion white blood cell counts >5/high power field are suggestive of an inflammatory exudate that could be consistent with peritonitis. However, smear preparation and centrifugation will significantly affect the number of cells seen on direct smears.

b. Clumps of white blood cells are often indicative of elevation of white blood cell numbers.

c. It may take a minimum of three hours for substantial numbers of white blood cells to accumulate within the peritoneum.

d. Abdominal fluid cellularity may be minimal in animals that are immunosuppressed or that lack adequate numbers of white blood cell precursors and circulating white blood cells. When in doubt, a peripheral blood smear should be evaluated concurrently to verify that the patient has adequate numbers of white blood cells in circulation to mount a proper response to septic contamination of the abdominal cavity.

2. Types of cells present:

a. There are often both small numbers of red blood cells and larger numbers of white blood cells present in septic peritoneal effusions.

b. Neutrophils are the predominant white blood cell noted in septic peritonitis. These neutrophils will demonstrate variable degrees of degeneration (Figure 14.3). Macrophages will occur in higher numbers as the effusion becomes more chronic.

3. Presence of bacteria:

a. Identification of intracellular and extracellular bacteria within the neutrophils and/or macrophages of the peritoneal fluid samples is adequate to confirm the clinical diagnosis of septic peritonitis. (Figure 14.3).

b. In some cases, bacteria may not be readily identified but the suspicion for

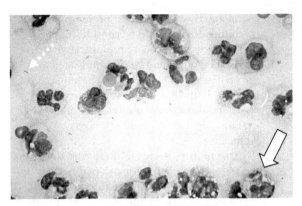

FIGURE 14.3 Cytological analysis of an effusion demonstrating degenerate neutrophils with extracellular (dashed arrow) and intracellular bacteria (solid arrow). This is an indication for immediate exploratory laparotomy. (Photomicrograph courtesy Dr. David Holt, University of Pennsylvania School of Veterinary Medicine, Philadelphia, PA)

intra-abdominal infection may remain high due to the results of other diagnostic tests. This may be due to early peritonitis or localized disease or the lack of skilled cytologists to evaluate the samples harvested. With a diagnosis of septic peritonitis requiring emergency surgical intervention this has prompted a search for other variables that can be measured more objectively.

4. Glucose concentration:

    a. Peripheral blood-to-peritoneal fluid glucose difference >20 mg/dL is 100% sensitive and specific for diagnosis of septic peritonitis in dogs and 86% sensitive and 100% specific in cats based on a study of 18 dogs and 12 cats (Bonczynski et al., 2003).

5. Lactate concentration:

    a. A peritoneal fluid lactate concentration >2.5 mg/dL has a 100% sensitivity and 91% specificity in dogs based on a study of 19 dogs. In cats, this parameter was not found to be helpful (Levin et al., 2004).

6. Nucleated cell count:

    a. A peritoneal fluid nucleated cell count above 13,000 cells/μL has an 86% sensitivity and 100% specificity in dogs and 100% sensitivity and specificity in

cats for diagnosis of septic peritonitis (Bonczynski et al., 2003).

7. Some caution should be used in interpreting the diagnostic characteristics of abdominal fluid glucose, lactate, and nucleated cell count. The information obtained using these parameters was determined in a study that compared animals with peritonitis to many animals with abdominal effusion that was not characterized by significant inflammation. It is possible that the changes in glucose, lactate, and nucleated cell counts demonstrated in this study may simply indicate the severity of inflammatory cell influx in the peritoneum, rather than being specific for intraperitoneal sepsis.

    e. Endoscopy:

    i. Endoscopic evaluation can be useful for evaluation of injury to the esophagus, stomach, and proximal duodenum. However, perforation can be missed using endoscopy alone and it does not allow assessment of vascular integrity.

    f. Surgical exploration:

    i. Exploratory laparotomy can be pursued as a diagnostic and therapeutic intervention in cases where traumatic bowel injury is suspected.

5. **TREATMENT—ABDOMINAL TRAUMA**

    a. Clear indications for performing surgical exploratory laparotomy on an emergent basis in dogs and cats having sustained abdominal trauma are as follows (see Figure 13.1 in Chapter 13: Trauma-Associated Body Wall and Torso Injury):

    i. Evidence of septic peritonitis based on the visualization of intracellular bacteria or suggestive biochemical parameters in peritoneal effusions.

    ii. Any form of penetrating injury from a projectile or severe bite wound.

    iii. Evidence of intraperitoneal hemorrhage that is unremitting or resulting in an inability to hemodynamically stabilize the patient.

    iv. Any evidence of a traumatic body wall hernia that contains herniated abdominal viscera.

    b. In all cases, a thorough exploratory laparotomy should take place as intercurrent injury to other organs is always possible. In a study of traumatic body wall herniation, 33% of dogs and cats were found to have serious injuries to abdominal viscera including mesenteric avulsion, kidney avulsion, splenic laceration, bladder rupture, and various gastrointestinal tract perforations (Shaw et al., 2003).

6. TREATMENT OF TRAUMATIC GASTROINTESTINAL PERFORATION

a. Esophagus:

   i. Small esophageal tears mostly occur after the endoscopic removal of esophageal foreign bodies or rarely after balloon dilation of esophageal strictures. Small esophageal tears may be successfully managed by temporarily diverting passage of food and water past the tear by placement of a gastrostomy tube:

      1. Animals should all be monitored very closely for evidence of leakage from the esophagus. Depending on location this may result in cellulitis and abscess formation within the cervical area or if the thoracic esophagus is the site of the leakage it may result in septic mediastinitis or pyothorax.

   ii. Larger tears, circumferential necrotic lesions, or traumatic avulsions usually result from chronic foreign body entrapment or transthoracic bite or projectile injuries. In these cases surgical exploration of the cervical and/or thoracic esophagus is warranted depending on the site of injury:

      1. A ventral midline approach is used for access to the cervical esophagus, a right sided 3rd–4th space intercostal thoracotomy is used for the cranial thoracic esophagus. For the caudal esophagus, a left-sided 7th–9th intercostal thoracotomy will provide good access.

      2. Necrotic tissue should be trimmed back to a healthy bleeding edge followed by closure using one or two layer interrupted or continuous appositional pattern using monofilament absorbable suture material.

      3. When resection and anastomosis are required, avoidance of excessive tension is mandatory. Resection of greater than 3–5 cm of esophagus increases risk of dehiscence and esophageal replacement techniques should be considered.

   iii. In all dogs and cats undergoing esophageal surgery, nutritional support via gastrostomy tube placement and medical management with sucralfate, H_2-antagonists or proton-pump inhibiting drugs should be considered.

   iv. In all cases the risk of postoperative stricture formation should be communicated to the owners and their development monitored for using both clinical signs (most frequently, regurgitation) and possibly elective endoscopic examination 4–6 weeks after injury.

b. Stomach:

   i. Due to its protected location partially inside the ribcage, traumatic stomach perforation is rare. Iatrogenic stomach perforation may occur with orogastric tube placement or with endoscopy, particularly when there is underlying gastric pathology such as gastric necrosis in dogs with gastric dilatation volvulus or infiltrative intestinal diseases.

   ii. Gastric perforation is most likely to occur with projectile injury. During exploration of the abdomen for such injuries, care should be taken to inspect the stomach very thoroughly as multiple perforations must not be missed.

   iii. Areas of necrotic stomach around the site of perforation are liberally trimmed and the stomach wall is closed using monofilament absorbable suture material. A simple continuous pattern in the mucosa is followed by an inverting cushing or continuous Lembert pattern in the seromuscular layer.

c. Small intestine:

   i. The small intestines are the most likely organ in the abdomen to be affected by penetrating trauma.

   ii. Like the stomach, the small intestine should be carefully evaluated for multiple areas of trauma especially from gunshot wounds, which can result in multiple perforations or even transections of small intestine.

   iii. Care must be taken not to miss small perforations on the mesenteric side where fat often obscures direct visualization of the intestinal wall.

   iv. General principles of management include debridement of necrotic tissue, restoration of intestinal continuity and function followed by liberal irrigation prior to closure of the abdomen.

   v. Simple mural hematomas can either be left untreated or oversewn with a simple

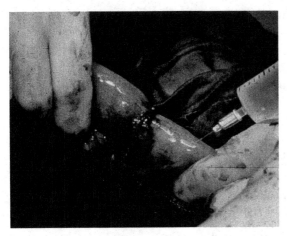

FIGURE 14.4 After an intestinal resection and anastomoses is complete, the site can leak-tested by injecting saline into the bowel lumen using a 22-gauge needle and syringe. (Photo courtesy of Dr. Lillian Aronson, University of Pennsylvania School of Veterinary Medicine, Philadelphia, PA)

interrupted or continuous inverting lembert suture pattern.

vi. Small penetrating injuries may be treated by trimming of the edges followed by closure using simple interrupted appositional sutures of monofilament absorbable suture. Sutures are placed approximately 2–3 mm apart.

vii. Closure can be tested by the injection of saline solution through a 22G needle into the intestinal segment concerned while the intestine oral and aboral to the injury is held closed with digital pressure or the use of doyen forceps (Figure 14.4). If saline leaks easily from the incision line, additional sutures are added at that location.

viii. When a transection of the intestine has occurred or there is a circumferential area of necrotic or ischemic tissue a resection and anastomosis must be performed (Figure 14.1):

1. Doyen forceps or the fingers of an assistant are used to prevent leakage of intestinal chyme during resection of the affected segment. Crushing carmalt clamps are placed across the limits of the intestine to be resected and including a small margin of healthy intestine at both ends.

2. Once the arteries and veins in the mesenteric arcades are ligated, the damaged intestine can be removed.

3. The anastomosis can be performed using a simple interrupted or continuous suture pattern of 3–0 to 4–0 monofilament absorbable suture. It is advisable to start placing sutures at the mesenteric side otherwise subsequent visualization of this area will be impaired.

4. Finally, rents in the mesentery must be closed using a continuous pattern of monofilament absorbable suture material starting at the base of the mesenteric root and terminating at the mesenteric wall of the anastomosis or vice versa:

a. Rents in the mesentery can be found in isolation after blunt or penetrating abdominal trauma and should always be closed to avoid herniation of bowel or other organs through them resulting in strangulation.

ix. If greater than 70% of the small intestine requires resection, "short bowel syndrome" can result leading to maldigestion and malabsorption. This can lead to chronic diarrhea and weight loss although in some dogs adaptation of the bowel will occur over time resulting in resolution of clinical signs. If this does not occur, surgical procedures are described to treat more severe cases.

d. Large intestine:

i. Colonic injury often results in severe peritonitis due to the high load of anerobic bacteria present in the hindgut.

ii. Perforation will result in rapid progression of septic peritonitis that may be more rapidly debilitating or more likely to be fatal compared to gastric or upper small intestinal perforation.

iii. Colonic resection and anastomosis is often necessary if there is perforation, as colonic injuries are usually associated with significant necrosis or vascular injury around the perforation.

iv. It may be possible to perform a local resection, similar to that previously described for the small intestine, when very small perforations are detected early. Care should be taken not to cause stricture formation from significant luminal narrowing associated with local resections.

v. In people, postoperative leakage occurs more frequently after colonic anastomosis than it does following small intestinal anastomosis. It is not known if this holds true in small animals. The reasons for this are not clear but may be associated with a more tenuous blood supply in the area of the distal colon and recto-colonic junction. In this area, care should be taken to preserve the cranial rectal branch of the caudal mesenteric artery.

vi. The blood supply to the ascending, transverse, and descending colon is segmental via vasa recta emanating from the right, middle, and left colic arteries, which anastomose distally with the cranial mesenteric artery.

vii. To preserve perfusion to a healing colonic anastomosis, it is recommended that each of the vasa recta supplying the section to be removed be ligated individually rather than ligating the colic arteries. Although slightly more time consuming, this is worthwhile.

viii. The anastomosis is performed by single layer simple interrupted or continuous suture pattern using a monofilament absorbable suture material.

ix. If resection of the ileo-cecocolic junction is required due to the location of traumatized bowel, it may be necessary to employ one of several techniques available for overcoming significant disparities in luminal size. The reader is referred elsewhere for a full summary of such techniques (Hedlund and Fossum, 2007).

e. Broad-spectrum antibiotic therapy should be initiated immediately upon identification or a high suspicion of gastrointestinal injury. In the postoperative period, ongoing antibiotic therapy and general supportive care should be provided. Good empirical choices might include the following: Ampcillin (22 mg/kg IV TID) and Cefoxitin (22 mg/kg IV TID) or a combination of Enrofloxacin (dogs; 10 mg/kg IV SID, cats; 5 mg/kg IV SID) and Ampicillin (22 mg/kg IV TID). These choices should be subsequently modified based on the results of bacterial culture and sensitivity testing.

BIBLIOGRAPHY

Bjorling DE, Crowe DT, Kolata RJ, et al. Penetrating abdominal wounds in dogs and cats. *J Am Anim Hosp Assoc* 1982; 18: 742–748.

Bonczynski JJ, Ludwig LL, Barton LJ, et al. Comparison of peritoneal fluid and peripheral blood pH, bicarbonate, glucose and lactate concentration as a diagnostic tool for septic peritonitis in dogs and cats. *Vet Surg* 2003; 32: 161–166.

Boysen SR, Rozanski EA, Tidwell AS, et al. Evaluation of a focused assessment with sonography for trauma protocol to detect free abdominal fluid in dogs involved in motor vehicle accidents. *J Am Vet Med Assoc* 2004; 225: 1198–1204.

Brown DC. Small intestines. In: Slatter D, ed. *Textbook of Small Animal Surgery*. 3rd edition. WB Saunders, Philadelphia, PA, 2003; pp. 644–664.

Connally HE. Cytology and fluid analysis of the acute abdomen. *Clin Tech Small Anim Pract* 2000; 15: 17–24.

Fullington RJ, Otto CM. Characteristics and management of gunshot wounds in dogs and cats: 84 cases (1986–1995). *J Am Vet Med Assoc* 1997; 210: 658–662.

Hedlund CS, Fossum TW. Surgery of the digestive tract. In: Fossum TW, ed. *Small Animal Surgery*. 3rd edition. WB Saunders, Philadelphia, PA, 2007; 339–530.

Holt DE, Brockman D. Large intestine. In: Slatter D, ed. *Textbook of Small Animal Surgery*. 3rd edition. WB Saunders, Philadelphia, PA, 2003; pp. 665–682.

Hosgood GL, Salisbury SK. Pathophysiology and pathogenesis of generalized peritonitis. *Probl Vet Med* 1989; 1: 159–167.

Kolata RJ, Johnston DE. Motor vehicle accidents in urban dogs: a study of 600 cases. *J Am Vet Med Assoc* 1975; 167: 938–941.

Kolata RJ, Kraut NH, Johnston DE. Patterns of trauma in urban dogs and cats: a study of 1000 cases. *J Am Vet Med Assoc* 1974; 164: 499–502.

Kyles AE. Esophagus. In: Slatter D, ed. *Textbook of Small Animal Surgery*. 3rd edition. WB Saunders, Philadelphia, PA, 2003; 573–592.

Levin GM, Bonczynski JJ, Ludwig LL, et al. Lactate as a diagnostic test for septic peritoneal effusions in dogs and cats. *J Am Vet Hosp Assoc* 2004; 40: 364–371.

Pavletic MM. Gunshot wound management. *Compend Contin Educ Pract Vet* 1996; 18: 1285–1299.

Shamir MH, Leisner S, Klement E, et al. Dog bite wounds in dogs and cats: a retrospective study of 196 cases. *J Vet Med* 2002; 49: 107–112.

Shaw SP, Rozanski EA, Rush JE. Traumatic body wall herniation in 36 dogs and cats. *J Am Anim Hosp Assoc* 2003; 39: 35–46.

Waters DJ, Roy RG, Stone EA. A retrospective study of inguinal hernia in 35 dogs. *Vet Surg* 1993; 22: 44–49.

TRAUMA-ASSOCIATED OCULAR INJURY

Deborah C. Mandell

1. INTRODUCTION

a. Many different types of trauma can cause a variety of ocular injuries. There is blunt ocular trauma and penetrating ocular trauma.

b. The most important aspects in treating ocular injuries are to:
  - **i.** Prevent loss of vision
  - **ii.** Prevent loss of the eye
  - **iii.** Alleviate pain
  - **iv.** Prevent long-term complications

c. Most ocular injuries occur concurrently with head trauma and these injuries should always be addressed and stabilized prior to treating the eye (see Chapter 7: Traumatic Brain Injury).

d. Other major body system abnormalities should be rapidly assessed and treatment instituted.

e. If significant head trauma is present, then a rapid assessment of the anterior part of the globe should be performed and a more complete ophthalmic examination performed once the animal is stable. The rapid examination includes evaluating the following:
  - **i.** The globe—intact or proptosed
  - **ii.** Periorbital structures—severity of swelling, hemorrhage/bruising, lacerations, abrasions
  - **iii.** Conjunctiva—hemorrhage, lacerations
  - **iv.** Sclera and cornea—intact, ulcer, laceration, rupture
  - **v.** Anterior chamber—anterior uveitis, hyphema

  - **vi.** Pupil size, responsiveness, symmetry (see Chapter 7: Traumatic Brain Injury)

f. A sterile, water-based lubricant or topical antibiotic ointment can be placed on the globe every 1–2 hours until a more thorough examination can occur.

g. Once the animal is deemed stable, a complete ophthalmic examination, including repeating the initial examination and performing a fundic examination should follow. Evaluating for the direct and indirect pupillary light reflex (PLR), menace response, and if a dazzle response is present is extremely important. Diagnostic tests such as fluorescein staining and intraocular pressure measurement can also be performed at this time.

h. Instillation of a topical anesthetic (0.5% proparacaine) may facilitate the examination.

i. If surgery is to be performed on the eye, smaller instruments or ophthalmic specific instruments and suture material should be used and will make the surgery much easier. Some instruments to include in an ophthalmic surgical pack (Figure 15.1):
  - **i.** Lid retractor
  - **ii.** Stevens tenotomy scissors
  - **iii.** Colibri forceps
  - **iv.** Castroviejo needle holders for fine suture material
  - **v.** Adson tissue forceps (small)
  - **vi.** Mayo scissors

Manual of Trauma Management in the Dog and Cat, First Edition. Edited by Kenneth J. Drobatz, Matthew W. Beal and Rebecca S. Syring.
© 2011 John Wiley & Sons, Inc. Published 2011 by John Wiley & Sons, Inc.

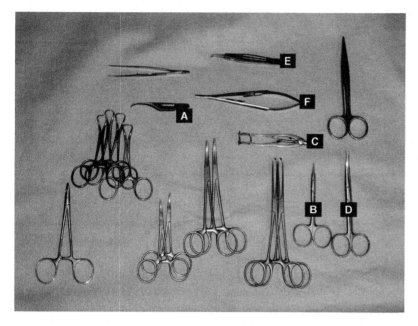

FIGURE 15.1   An ophthalmic surgery pack. This pack contains Colibri forceps—A; tenotomy scissors—B; eyelid retractor—C; strabismus scissors—D; iris tissue forceps—E; Castroveijo needle holders—F; along with other instruments not specific for ophthalmic surgery.

vii.   Strabismus scissors
viii.   Curved Metzenbaum scissors
ix.   Curved mosquito and Kelly hemostats
x.   Small needle holders
xi.   Surgical loupes

j.   In any injury that results in perforation of the cornea, or may lead to perforation of the cornea, the use of topical ointments should be avoided. The petroleum or oil base is extremely irritating to the uvea and can lead to intraocular inflammation. In this situation, topical solutions rather than ointments should be used.

k.   If trauma, induced ocular injury has limited the ability to visualize the posterior segments of the eye, ultrasound should be used to evaluate the lens, vitreous, retina, and sclera. A 7.5–12 MHz transducer with B mode ultrasound should be used. Coupling gel is placed after topical anesthetic is instilled in the eye. Computed tomography (CT) may also be used to diagnose orbital fractures, foreign objects, etc.

l.   An ophthalmologist should always be consulted if one is available, if the owners are interested, if there is a disease process that is not responding to treatment or if more than one disease process is occurring in the same eye. If intraocular or corneal surgery is needed (i.e., due to corneal laceration, perforation, iris prolapse,

penetrating foreign body), a veterinary ophthalmologist will have more experience, an operating microscope available, and will be able to use finer suture material for a more positive outcome.

2.   PROPTOSIS (Figure 15.2)
a.   Proptosis is forward displacement of the globe with the eyelids trapped behind the globe.

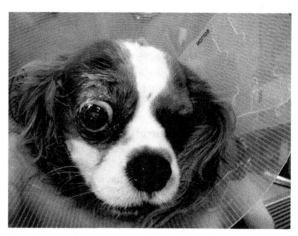

FIGURE 15.2   A 1 year old Cavalier King Charles spaniel with a mild proptosis. It is reasonable to attempt replacement with temporary tarsorrhaphy in these animals.

b. The two options for treatment are enucleation or replacement with temporary tarsorrhaphy. This decision is based on the following:

    i. Integrity of the globe

    ii. Integrity of the extraocular muscles

    iii. Integrity of cornea

    iv. Owner's decision and compliance

c. Replacement with temporary tarsorrhaphy is for cosmetic purposes only—to save the eye, not to save vision. The majority of dogs and cats do not regain vision if the proptosis is severe.

d. Brachycephalic dogs with lagophthalmic eyes (shallow orbits, prominent globes) are at the most risk for proptosis. Even minor trauma can lead to proptosis in these breeds. Since it does not take a lot of force to proptose these eyes, the injury to the eye may not be as severe and the prognosis for vision can be better.

e. For dolichocephalic dog breeds and cats, it takes a much greater force to proptose the eye. Therefore, significant head trauma is usually concurrently present. The patient with head trauma should always be stabilized prior to addressing the eye.

f. If the globe is ruptured, more than two extraocular muscles are damaged or avulsed from the sclera (see Figure 15.3), the cornea is damaged (i.e., road dirt embedded in the cornea), or the owners would not be able to medicate the eye, then enucleation is warranted. The degree of proptosis

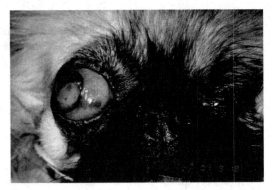

FIGURE 15.4 A 4-year old Lhasa Apso one month post replacement with temporary tarsorrhaphy after a proptosis. Notice the dorsolateral strabismus, lagophthalmos, and exposure keratitis. A permanent partial tarsorrhaphy to decrease the palpebral fissure or enucleation are options at this point.

may provide some idea regarding the amount of extraocular muscle damage.

g. The owners should be warned that enucleation may still be needed if replacement with temporary tarsorrhaphy fails or complications ensue.

h. Complications and sequelae of globe replacement include the following (Figure 15.4):

    i. Re-proptosis.

    ii. Exposure keratitis secondary to corneal denervation.

    iii. Dorsolateral strabismus due to rupture of the medial rectus muscle (it is the shortest). This can gradually improve over time.

    iv. The need for second surgery and possible enucleation.

    v. Abscess or infection of the globe.

    vi. Corneal ulceration or abrasion.

    vii. Phthisis bulbi if more than three extraocular muscles are damaged. This occurs because the vascular supply to the anterior part of the globe will be compromised (the blood vessels come in with the extraocular muscles).

i. If the globe is intact, the cornea is intact and minimally diseased, the majority of the extraocular muscles are intact and the owners understand and agree to the potential sequelae, then replacement with temporary tarsorrhaphy can be performed.

j. The globe can be flushed with 0.9% saline or sterile eyewash to clean any debris.

k. Replacement with temporary tarsorrhaphy:

    i. Copious amounts of sterile water-based lubricant are placed on the eye.

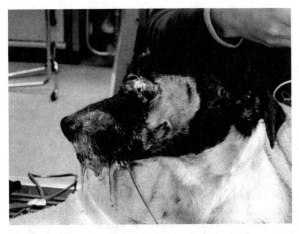

FIGURE 15.3 A 6-year old Jack Russell terrier with a severe proptosis with more than three extraocular muscles severed. The severity of the proptosis necessitated enucleation of the eye.

ii. The animal is placed under general anesthesia. Anesthetics that can increase intracranial pressure should be avoided (e.g., ketamine) (see Chapter 5: Analgesia in the Trauma Patient).

iii. The periorbital area is clipped and gently cleaned with povidine–iodine solution (NOT scrub) diluted 1:10–1:50. This is nonirritating to the periorbital skin and nontoxic to the cornea and conjunctival epithelium. Chlorhexidine is more irritating and is toxic to the cornea.

iv. A lateral canthotomy can be performed to increase exposure.

v. Horizontal mattress sutures using 3–0 or 4–0 nylon or silk with tension relieving stents are preplaced as shown in Figure 15.5. These are then used to replace the globe.

vi. Alternatively, a stay suture using 2–0 nylon 0.5–1 cm away from the upper and lower eyelid margins can be used to replace the globe and the horizontal mattress sutures can be placed after replacement.

vii. The sutures (either mattress or stay sutures) are lifted out and up while using a scalpel handle to gently push the globe back into the orbit.

viii. Once the globe is replaced, the sutures are crossed and held to prevent re-proptosis.

ix. The horizontal mattress sutures are placed as follows:

1. The suture is placed through a stent. The stents can be made out of pieces of sterile rubber bands, IV tubing, or red rubber catheters.

2. Starting 6–8 mm away from the eyelid margin, the suture is placed through the upper eyelid, comes out at the Meibomian glands and enters the lower eyelid margin at the Meibomian glands, exits 6–8 mm away from the margin, goes through another stent and then the needle direction is reversed (Figure 15.5).

3. An area is left open at the medial canthus for placement of medications.

4. Once all of the mattress sutures are placed, the sutures are tied to bring the eyelids together.

5. By placing the sutures this manner, the eyelids are everted, which protects the cornea (Figure 15.6).

x. The lateral canthotomy can be closed with 4–0 monofilament absorbable suture in a simple interrupted pattern.

xi. Aftercare consists of the following:

1. Topical antibiotic ointment or solution (neopolygramacidin, tobramycin or gentamicin ophthalmic solution 0.3%) every 6 hours. In cats, the neomycin can cause severe chemosis and anaphylaxis has been

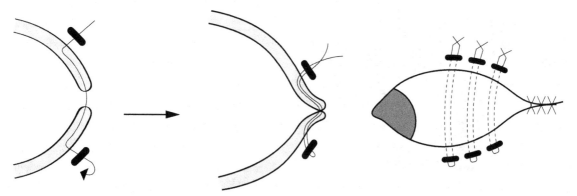

FIGURE 15.5 Replacement with temporary tarsorrhapy. Horizontal mattress sutures using 3–0 or 4–0 nylon or silk with tension relieving stents are placed as follows: The suture is placed through a stent. Starting 6–8 mm away from the eyelid margin, the suture is placed through the upper eyelid, comes out at the Meibomian glands and enters the lower eyelid margin at the Meibomian glands, exits 6–8 mm away from the margin, goes through another stent and then the needle direction is reversed. An area is left open at the medial canthus for placement of medications. Once all of the mattress sutures are placed, the sutures are tied to bring the eyelids together. (Reprinted with permission: Drobatz K and Costello M, 2010, Feline Emergency and Critical Care Medicine, Wiley-Blackwell, Ames, IA.)

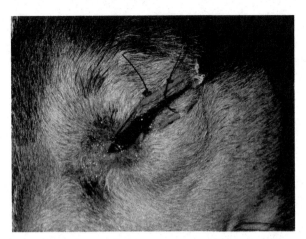

FIGURE 15.6 Post replacement with temporary tarsorrhaphy with stents.

reported in one cat (Plunkett, 2000), thus tobramycin or gentamicin is preferred. Solutions are usually easier for owners to apply.

2. Topical 1% atropine solution twice a day.

3. Systemic antibiotics (amoxicillin–clavulanic acid 15–20 mg/kg orally twice a day).

4. An Elizabethan collar must be worn at all times.

5. A short weaning course of anti-inflammatory doses (0.5 mg/kg prednisone twice a day for 3 days, then once a day for three days, then every other day for three treatments) of corticosteroids to control the swelling and decrease damage to the optic nerve.

6. Cold compresses can be applied for 15 minutes 4 times a day for 24 hours, then replaced with warm compresses to help reduce swelling.

7. Tramadol (1–4 mg/kg PO BID-QID) can be sent home for analgesia.

8. The owners must keep the area clean and dry and prevent build up of discharge.

xii. The sutures are removed in 10–14 days. If the proptosis was severe, the sutures can be removed one at a time a few days apart to monitor for complications.

xiii. Once all of the sutures are removed, the cornea should be fluorescein stained.

xiv. If there is extensive exposure keratitis or a larger palpebral fissure, then a permanent partial lateral or medial tarsorrhaphy can be performed.

xv. The prognosis for vision is guarded to grave, especially in cats and dolichocephalic dog breeds. If it occurred in a brachycephalic breed or was a mild proptosis, vision may return.

xvi. The prognosis for an acceptable cosmetic outcome (saving of the eye) is good.

3. ENUCLEATION (Figures 15.7a–g)

a. The animal is placed under general anesthesia when deemed stable. Anesthetic agents that can increase intracranial pressure should be avoided (e.g., ketamine) (see Chapter 5: Analgesia in the Trauma Patient).

b. A lateral canthotomy can be performed to maximize exposure if necessary.

c. A lid retractor can be placed to help increase exposure if the periorbital swelling is not severe (severe swelling will make the lid retractor impossible to use).

d. The subconjunctival approach is the most common and easiest approach for an enucleation, especially if performing an enucleation due to proptosis. In this approach, the globe is removed and then the eyelid margins are removed.

e. Starting 5 mm from the limbus, the conjunctiva and Tenon's capsule are dissected from the sclera, that is, the dissection should be between the sclera and conjunctiva/Tenon's capsule, starting 5 mm from the limbus.

f. Any extraocular muscles that are still attached are dissected off of the sclera using tenotomy or curved Metzenbaum scissors.

g. The sclera is followed back to the optic nerve and vessels.

h. Any necrotic or damaged tissue or muscle should be removed with the globe.

i. Extreme care must be taken, especially in cats, not to pull on the globe as it is being removed. The optic chiasm is much shorter in cats. Excessive traction on the globe as it is being removed can lead to blindness in the contralateral eye.

j. The optic nerve and vessels are clamped with Kelly or mosquito hemostats with the curve facing up, 5 mm behind the globe.

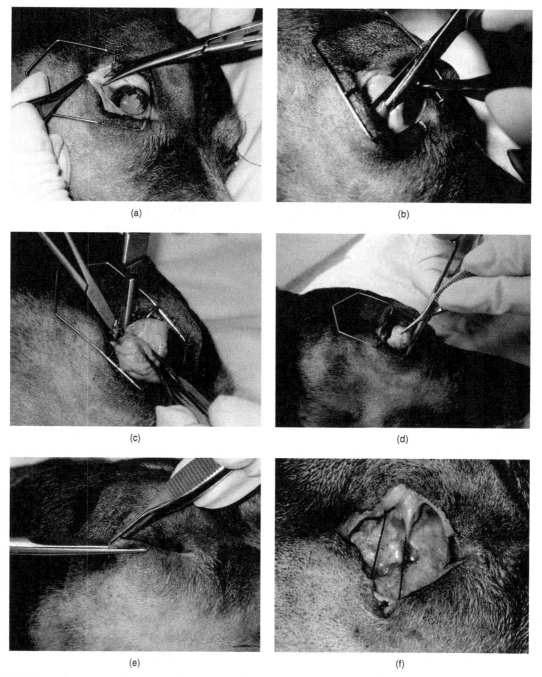

FIGURE 15.7 Subconjunctival enucleation. (a) An incision is made in the bulbar conjunctiva, which is extended circumferentially around the globe. (b) Dissect the extraocular muscles at their attachment to the globe. (c) Place hemostats behind the back of the globe to clamp the optic nerve and vessels. Make sure not to pull up/out on the globe excessively. Cut the globe off of the hemostats, on the side closest to the surgeon. (d) Take the third eyelid and gland out. (e) Remove the upper and lower eyelids, about 5–8 mm from the margin. (f) A large horizontal mattress suture with 0-2-0 PDS can be placed from upper and lower periosteum. This creates a shelf to help prevent sinking of the skin. (g) Post enucleation.

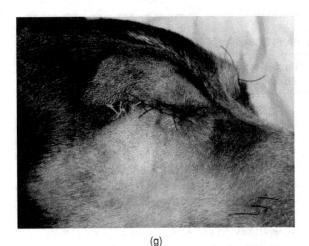

(g)

FIGURE 15.7   (*Continued*)

k. One or two ligatures using 3–0 PDS can be placed under the hemostats although this is not necessary and many ophthalmologists do not perform this step.

l. Using a #10 or #15 scalpel, the globe is dissected off of the hemostats on the side closest to the surgeon.

m. The back of the globe must be inspected to ensure that all of the sclera and choroid have been removed. A black piece of tissue will be seen on the hemostats and/or a hole will be seen on the back of the globe if not completely removed. This tissue must be removed before closing or there can be persistent drainage.

n. The hemostats are removed. The area can be packed with gel foam or direct pressure with gauze sponges can be applied if post enucleation hemorrhage is persistent.

o. The third eyelid and gland must be removed in its entirety to prevent persistent production and drainage of tears.

p. 3–4 mm of the upper and lower eyelid margins should be removed using Mayo scissors or a scalpel.

q. A large horizontal mattress suture using 2–0 PDS is placed from the periosteum in the upper orbit to the periosteum in the lower orbit. This cannot be closed but creates a shelf to help prevent sinking of the skin.

r. The subcutaneous tissue is closed with 3–0 to 4–0 PDS in a simple interrupted or continuous pattern.

s. The skin and lateral canthotomy are then closed with 3–0 to 4–0 nylon, monofilament absorbable, or silk in a simple interrupted pattern.

t. Systemic antibiotics (amoxicillin–clavulanic acid orally 15–20 mg/kg twice daily) are given for 14 days.

u. Pain management (see Table 15.1) can include systemic analgesics (buprenorphine 0.01 mg/kg IV/SQ every 4–6 hours while in the hospital and then systemic nonsteroidal anti-inflammatory medication and/or tramadol (1–4 mg/kg PO BID-QID) to go home as needed (see Chapter 5: Analgesia in the Trauma Patient).

v. Cold compresses can be applied for 15 minutes four times a day for the first 24 hours and then replaced with warm compresses to reduce swelling.

w. The sutures are removed in 10–14 days.

x. Complications include abscess formation or infection, subcutaneous emphysema (air may enter the orbit through the nasolacrimal duct during respiration), and orbital depression or sinking.

4. PERIORBITAL/SUBCONJUNCTIVAL SWELLING AND HEMORRHAGE (Figure 15.8)

a. Periorbital swelling and hemorrhage can be present with or without concurrent ocular damage.

b. However, severe swelling can prevent the animal from being able to close the eyelids and protect the cornea.

c. Therefore, even if the globe is intact and healthy, the swelling can lead to corneal abrasions or ulcers secondary to exposure if not recognized.

d. The eye should be fluorescein stained at presentation to determine the presence and extent of corneal injury. If a corneal abrasion or ulcer is present, then topical antibiotic ointment (triple antibiotic ointment in dogs and erythromycin ointment (0.3%) in cats) should be started three to four times a day.

e. Two treatment options have been advocated:

    i. Temporary tarsorrhaphy to protect the cornea (see above, Proptosis)

    ii. Application of a sterile lubricant with or without topical antibiotics to protect the cornea while the swelling is resolving.

    iii. The decision is based on the stability of the patient and if the eyelids can actually be moved and closed. Some swelling is so severe that the eyelids cannot be pulled over the globe.

TABLE 15.1
TOPICAL AND SYSTEMIC MEDICATIONS USED IN OCULAR INJURY AND DISEASE

DRUG	Mechanism of Action	Potential Side Effects/Complications	Dose, Route, and Frequency
Topical antibiotics Erythromycin 0.3%	Binds to 50S ribosomal unit of susceptible bacteria	Hypersensitivity	$1/4$ inch topically every 8 hours
Neopolygramicidin suspension		Neomycin associated with anaphylaxis in one cat; can also cause chemosis in local irritation.	1 drop topically every 6–8 hours
Neopolybacitracin ointment		Neomycin associated with anaphylaxis in one cat; can also cause chemosis in local irritation.	$1/4$ inch topically every 6–8 hours
Oxytetracycline with polymixin B	Binds to 30S and 50S ribosomal units	Local irritation	$1/4$ inch topically every 8 hours
Gentamicin suspension/ointment 0.3%	Irreversibly binds to 30S ribosomal unit	Ototoxicity and nephrotoxicity rare	1 drop or $1/4$ inch topically every 4–8 hours
Tobramycin suspension 0.3%	Irreversibly binds to 30S ribosomal unit	Ototoxicity and nephrotoxicity rare	1 drop topically every 4–8 hours
Ciprofloxacin suspension 0.5%	Inhibits bacterial DNAgyrase preventing DNA supercoiling synthesis	Hypersensitivity	1 drop topically every 1–6 hours
Cefazolin (reconstitute to 50 mg/mL with 0.9% NaCl; remove 3.75 mls from artificial tear solution and replace with 3.75 mls cefazolin; stable for 10 days)	Inhibits mucopeptide synthesis in cell wall	Hypersensitivity	1 drop topically every 1–6 hours
Systemic antibiotics Amoxicillin–clavulonic acid (Clavamox®)	Inhibits mucopeptide synthesis in cell wall	Vomiting/anorexia/diarrhea	15–20 mg/kg orally every 12 hours
Enrofloxacin	Inhibits bacterial DNA-gyrase	Can lead to idiosyncratic reaction leading to retinal degeneration in cats—not recommended in cats	10–15 mg/kg orally once a day in DOGS only
Doxycycline	Inhibits 30S ribosomal unit	Vomiting/anorexia/diarrhea	10 mg/kg orally every 24 hours
Topical corticosteroids Prednisone acetate 1%	Inhibits arachadonic acid	Inhibits corneal healing	1 drop topically every 6–8 hours
Neopolydexamethasone 0.5%	Inhibits arachadonic acid with an antibiotic	Inhibits corneal healing Neomycin can lead to severe reaction in cats	1 drop topically every 6–8 hours

(Continued)

TABLE 15.1
(CONTINUED)

DRUG	Mechanism of Action	Potential Side Effects/Complications	Dose, Route, and Frequency
Systemic corticosteroids Prednisone	Inhibits arachadonic acid	Immunosuppression Polyuria/polydipsia/ polyphagia	Anti-inflammatory: 0.5 mg/kg orally twice a day initially
Topical nonsteroidal anti-inflammatory drugs Flurbiprofen 0.3%	Inhibits cyclooxygenase, phopholipase A2, and prostaglandin synthesis	Inhibits corneal healing Hypersensitivity	1 drop topically every 6–8 hours
Systemic nonsteroidal anti-inflammatory drugs Meloxicam 1.5 mg/mL	Inhibits cyclooxygenase, phopholipase A2, and prostaglandin synthesis	Vomiting/anorexia/diarrhea Azotemia Not recommended for use in cats	0.1 mg/kg orally once daily (dogs only)
Carboprofen (Rimadyl®)	Inhibits cyclooxygenase, phopholipase A2, and prostaglandin synthesis	Vomiting/anorexia/diarrhea Azotemia	2.2 mg/kg orally twice a day NOT in cats
Deracoxib (Deramaxx®)	Inhibits cyclooxygenase, phopholipase A2, and prostaglandin synthesis	Vomiting/anorexia/diarrhea Azotemia	1–2 mg/kg orally once a day NOT in cats
Drugs that increase aqueous drainage Mannitol	Osmotic diuretic leading to decrease in amount of aqueous and vitreous humor	Dehydration, hypernatremia, initial hypervolemia	1–2 g/kg intravenously over 20–30 minutes, can be repeated in 4–6 hours
Latanoprost (Xylatan®)	Prostaglandin analog; increased drainage through alternate uveoscleral route	Miosis, anterior uveitis	1 drop topically every 12 hours
	Leads to miosis, which opens drainage angle	Hypersensitivity	
Drugs that decrease aqueous production Dorzolamide (Trusopt®)	Carbonic anhydrase inhibitor	Local irritation	1 drop topically every 8–12 hours
Methazolamide	Carbonic anhydrase inhibitor	Anorexia, vomiting, diarrhea	2 mg/kg orally every 12 hours
Timolol	β-blocker	Bronchoconstriction rare	1 drop topically every 8–12 hours

TABLE 15.1
(CONTINUED)

DRUG	Mechanism of Action	Potential Side Effects/Complications	Dose, Route, and Frequency
Drugs to induce mydriasis			
Atropine 1%	Cycloplegia; parasympatholytic, paralyzes sphincter muscle	Closes drainage angle; can increase IOP	1 drop topically every 6–12 hours to maintain pupil dilation
Tropicamide 1%	Cycloplegia; parasympatholytic, paralyzes sphincter muscle	Potential to increase IOP less than with atropine (short duration of action)	1 drop topically every 6–8 hours
Epinephrine (dipivefrin)	Sympathomimetic; stimulates dilator muscle	Can increase aqueous drainage/decrease production	1 drop topically every 8–12 hours
Phenylephrine	Sympathomimetic; stimulates dilator muscle	Can increase aqueous drainage/decrease production	1 drop topically every 8–12 hours
Topical anesthetics			
Proparacaine 0.5%	Sodium channel blocker, anesthetizes cornea	Inhibits corneal healing if applied frequently, decreases blink reflex	1 drop topically, can repeat 3 times in 5 minutes
Tetracaine 0.5%	Sodium channel blocker, anesthetizes cornea	Inhibits corneal healing if applied frequently, decreases blink reflex	1 drop topically, can repeat 3 times in 5 minutes
Drugs for pain relief			
Tramadol		May cause sedation	1–4 mg/kg orally every 6–12 hours
Nalbuphine 1.2%	Topical opioid		1 drop topically every 8–12 hours
Buprenorpine	Partial opioid agonist/antagonist	May cause sedation	0.01–0.02 mg/kg intravenously/ subcutaneously/ intramuscularly every 6–8 hours
Anticollagenases			
Autologous serum	Contains α macroglobulins as antiprotease	Must keep refrigerated	1 drop topically every 1–2 hours
Acetylcysteine	Metal chelating agent that binds to zinc, which is a cofactor for collagenases		1 drop topically every 1–2 hours Make into a 5–10% solution diluting with artificial tears

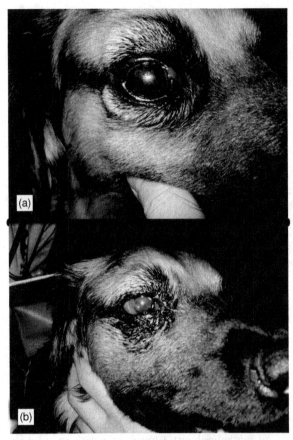

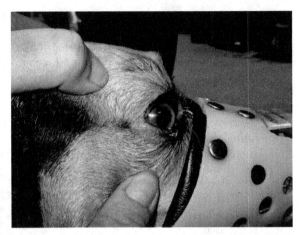

FIGURE 15.9 A 5-year old mixed breed that was accidentally hit in the head with a bat. There is anterior uveitis with a swollen "fluffy" iris and aqueous flare. The IOP was 6 mm Hg.

FIGURE 15.8 (a) A 4-year old mixed breed hit by car with severe periorbital swelling and hemorrhage and complete hyphema. Topical antibiotic ointment alternating with topical artificial tears was instituted. (b) The same dog three days later. The swelling has dramatically subsided and the dog was now able to close his eyelids to protect his cornea.

iv. If topical medications are used without a temporary tarsorrhapy, then the eye should be rechecked and fluorescein stained in 2–3 days.

5. **TRAUMATIC ANTERIOR UVEITIS**

   a. Traumatic anterior uveitis (Figure 15.9) occurs secondary to disruption of the blood-aqueous barrier.

   b. Clinical signs include a miotic pupil, swollen, red or "fluffy" iris, aqueous flare, hyphema, blepharospasm, and conjunctival hyperemia.

   c. An intraocular pressure (IOP) measurement should be performed. IOP will be low (<10 mm Hg, normal 15–25 mm Hg) in anterior uveitis secondary to decreased production of aqueous humor.

   d. The cornea should be fluorescein stained to rule out a concurrent corneal ulcer.

   e. If fluorescein stain is negative:

   i. Topical corticosteroids (Prednisone acetate, 1%) should be administered three to four times a day.

   ii. Topical atropine (1%) should also be administered twice a day or as needed to keep the pupil dilated. This controls pain by preventing ciliary body spasm and prevents synechia.

   iii. The eye should be reevaluated in one week and the topical steroids can be weaned over the course of two weeks, if there are no signs of anterior uveitis.

   f. If there is a concurrent corneal ulcer then topical corticosteroids are contraindicated:

   i. Topical nonsteroidal anti-inflammatory medications (flurbiprofen 0.3% three to four times a day) can be used instead of topical corticosteroids:

   1. Topical nonsteroidal anti-inflammatory medications (NSAIDs) can also delay healing and if there is a deep corneal ulcer they should be used cautiously. The eye should be reevaluated in 2 days. If the corneal ulcer is not healing or progressing, then discontinue the use of the topical nonsteroidal medication.

ii. Topical atropine (1%) twice a day should be started.

iii. Topical antibiotics should be started at four times a day. In dogs, triple antibiotic ointment or solution, tobramycin (0.3%) solution or gentamicin ointment or solution can be used. In cats, erythromycin ointment is preferred (unless the cornea is perforated or in danger of perforating) due to the potential of the neomycin in triple antibiotic formulations leading to chemosis, irritation, and possible anaphylaxis. Topical tobramycin or gentomycin can also be used.

iv. Systemic NSAIDs (see Table 15.1) should be started, especially if topical NSAIDs are not being used.

g. If the IOP measurement is normal or elevated with concurrent signs of anterior uveitis then the patient also has secondary glaucoma (see below):

    i. Topical atropine, which closes the drainage angle and can increase intraocular pressure, is contraindicated.

    ii. An epinephrine-like or sympathomimetic topical medication (e.g., dipivefrin 0.1%), which dilates the pupil yet does not close the drainage angle can be used two times a day. This may increase drainage of aqueous humor and decrease production of aqueous humor as well.

    iii. Treatment is also needed to treat the secondary glaucoma (see below):

        1. Topical carbonic anhydrase inhibitors (CAI) (e.g., dorzolamide) should be used three times a day.

        2. Topical beta-blockers (e.g., timolol) should also be used three times a day if available. Cosopt® (Merck, Sharpe, and Dohme Corp.) contains both dorzolamide and timolol. This preparation is also available in a generic form.

        3. Oral CAI such as methazolamide (2 mg/kg PO BID) may be needed as well if the topical medications are not controlling the intraocular pressure.

        4. The intraocular pressure should be rechecked in 24 hours and then, if improved, in one week to assess treatment.

h. A traumatic anterior uveitis that is complicated with a concurrent corneal ulcer or secondary glaucoma should be reevaluated frequently (every 3–5 days depending on severity).

i. Anterior uveitis secondary to lens injury can be extremely intense and difficult to treat:

    i. It is due to disruption of the anterior lens capsule and leakage of antigenic lens protein into the anterior chamber.

    ii. Clinical signs of a lens injury include fibrin on the lens, a fibrin strand leading from the lens or an opacity on the lens along with signs consistent with anterior uveitis. It will be easier to see lens injury with slit lamp magnification.

    iii. Topical corticosteroids should be used if there is no concurrent corneal ulcer.

    iv. Topical nonsteroidal anti-inflammatory medication (flurbiprofen 0.3%, three to four times a day) can be started if there is a concurrent corneal ulcer. However, this can delay corneal healing and the eye should be rechecked in 1–2 days to ensure that the ulcer is not progressing.

    v. Systemic corticosteroids at anti-inflammatory doses (prednisone 0.5 mg/kg twice a day) are needed to help control the inflammation.

    vi. Topical atropine should be used at two to four times a day, to maintain a dilated pupil.

    vii. If the anterior uveitis is difficult to control or the eye is developing secondary glaucoma, then the lens may need to be extracted by an ophthalmologist. Consultation with an ophthalmologist is advised.

6. HYPHEMA

a. Hyphema refers to blood in the anterior chamber secondary to disruption of the blood aqueous barrier and leakage of red blood cells. The blood can come from the iris, ciliary body, choroid, and/or retina.

b. If possible, a fundic examination should be performed to look for concurrent retinal hemorrhage or detachment.

c. An IOP measurement should be taken. Secondary glaucoma is a common sequela to hyphema.

d. Atropine (1%, twice a day) can be initiated to prevent synechiae if the IOP is low and can be followed and monitored frequently. If the IOP is normal or elevated, then atropine should not be used (see j below).

e. If the hyphema fills the entire anterior chamber, then presence of an indirect pupillary light response (PLR) in the unaffected eye should be evaluated. If there is a negative indirect PLR, then prognosis for vision is guarded and intraocular damage secondary to the trauma is suspected (e.g., retinal detachment).

f. Ultrasound of the eye should be used to evaluate all intraocular structures if not visible.

g. If there is mild to moderate hyphema, it will most likely resolve over time (7–21 days).

h. If a large blood clot forms, especially if it is leading to secondary glaucoma, an ophthalmologist can be consulted about infusing tissue plasminogen activator (TPA) into the anterior chamber (intracameral) to promote thrombolysis. This is usually advocated within 2–3 days of clot formation. This is not without risks such as corneal endothelial damage, therefore, an ophthalmologist should be consulted to determine if appropriate.

i. The use of topical corticosteroids has not been conclusively shown to be of benefit, although some ophthalmologists advocate the use of topical corticosteroids for a secondary anterior uveitis (iridocyclitis) (secondary to mediators released from blood cells).

j. If there is an elevated IOP and constricted pupil, then a sympathomimetic drug (e.g., dipivefrin 0.1%) can be used two times a day to dilate the pupil. Topical medications to control the IOP should also be started (dorzolamide TID, timolol TID). The eye should be rechecked in 24–48 hours.

7. GLAUCOMA

a. Glaucoma can occur secondary to a traumatic anterior uveitis, lens-induced injury and secondary anterior uveitis, anterior lens luxation or hyphema. An intraocular pressure reading >25 mm Hg is indicative of glaucoma. A normal to elevated intraocular pressure reading with anterior uveitis is consistent with secondary glaucoma.

b. Clinical signs such as buphthalmia may not be present.

c. An IOP measurement should be taken on any eye that has sustained injury (except a corneal perforation or rupture of the globe).

d. The options for decreasing intraocular pressure are to increase drainage (mannitol, latanoprost) and decrease aqueous humor production (CAI inhibitors, beta-blockers)

e. Glaucoma secondary to anterior lens luxation:

   i. If there is an anterior lens luxation (see below) and the IOP is >35 mm Hg, then emergency treatment should be instituted.

   ii. Mannitol (1–2 g/kg) intravenously over 20–30 minutes is given to increase aqueous and vitreous drainage:

      1. Use cautiously in dehydrated or hypovolemic patients or in patients with heart or kidney disease.

      2. A repeated IOP reading should be taken 1 hour post mannitol administration.

      3. Dose can be repeated in 4 hours if needed.

      4. Animals that are receiving repeated doses of mannitol must have their electrolytes, packed cell volume, and total solids monitored every 6–8 hours to prevent deleterious side effects (dehydration, hypernatremia, etc).

   iii. Prostaglandin analogs (e.g., latanoprost) are contraindicated if there is an anterior lens luxation (due to trapping of the lens in the anterior chamber secondary to the miosis).

   iv. Topical carbonic anhydrase inhibitors (CAI) (e.g., dorzolamide) three times a day should be started. Timolol, a topical beta blocker, should be added three times a day if available. Cosopt® (Merck, Sharpe, and Dohme Corp.) contains both dorzolamide and timolol. This preparation is also available in a generic form.

   v. Oral CAI such as methazolamide (2 mg/kg PO BED) may be needed to control the IOP.

   vi. Lens extraction should be performed as soon as possible for the best chance of return of vision.

   vii. Owners must be warned that secondary glaucoma may still occur in the future secondary to intraocular surgery. The eye will have to be closely monitored.

f. Glaucoma secondary to an anterior uveitis or hyphema:

   i. Mannitol is usually not used in glaucoma secondary to anterior uveitis, it is usually not acute glaucoma and not used in glaucoma secondary to hyphema due to the potential of increasing the hemorrhage.

   ii. Topical carbonic anhydrase inhibitors (CAI) (e.g., dorzolamide) three times a day should be started Cosopt® (Merck, Sharpe, and Dohme Corp.) contains both dorzolamide and timolol. This preparation is also available in a generic form.

iii. Topical atropine is contraindicated if the IOP is elevated (atropine-induced mydriasis closes the drainage angle and increases the IOP).

iv. An epinephrine-like or sympathomimetic topical medication (e.g., dipivefrin 0.1%) can be used to induce mydriasis in anterior uveitis and secondary glaucoma. It will dilate the pupil and not cause closure of the drainage angle. It may increase aqueous drainage and decrease aqueous production. It is used two times a day.

v. If secondary to anterior uveitis, then treatment for the uveitis must be started with topical corticosteroids (e.g., prednisone acetate 1%) four times a day (once a concurrent corneal ulcer is ruled out).

vi. The eye and IOP should be rechecked in 24–48 hours to determine success of treatment.

g. Glaucoma secondary to lens injury and lens-induced uveitis:

i. Treatment for glaucoma and the intense lens-induced uveitis must be started as soon as possible.

ii. Topical corticosteroids (e.g., prednisone acetate 1%) four times a day must be started once a concurrent corneal ulcer is ruled out.

iii. Atropine is contraindicated. A sympathomimetic topical medication (e.g., dipivefrin 0.1%) three times a day can be used to induce mydriasis. The sympathomimetic medication can also lower the IOP.

iv. Topical CAI's (e.g., dorzolamide) and timolol should be used three times a day.

v. Systemic corticosteroids at an anti-inflammatory dose (prednisone 0.5 mg/kg twice a day) are usually needed.

vi. In most cases, if the lens induced uveitis led to glaucoma, the lens should be extracted as soon as possible to try to save the eye. Consultation with an ophthalmologist is advised.

8. LENS LUXATION (Figure 15.10)

a. A lens luxation can occur secondary to blunt head trauma.

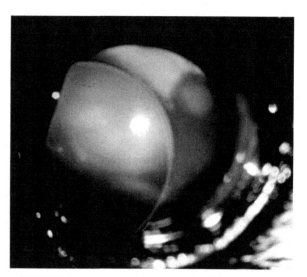

FIGURE 15.10   An anterior lens luxation. (Reprinted with permission: Drobatz K and Costello M, 2010, Feline Emergency and Critical Care Medicine, Wiley-Blackwell, Ames, IA.)

b. An anterior lens luxation is a surgical emergency due to the development of secondary glaucoma:

i. Clinical signs of an anterior lens luxation include movement of the iris (iridodonesis), corneal edema (where the lens is touching the cornea), anterior uveitis, increase or decrease (asymmetry) in the depth of the anterior chamber, and possibly visualization of the edge of the lens, especially dorsally.

ii. An IOP measurement should be taken. If greater than 35 mm Hg, then mannitol (1–2 g/kg IV over 20 minutes) should be started (see Glaucoma above).

iii. Topical antiglaucoma medications (dorzolamide, timolol) should be started three times a day. Latanoprost is contraindicated. (see Glaucoma above).

iv. The lens should be extracted as soon as possible.

v. The owners should be warned that secondary glaucoma is a potential sequela to any intraocular surgery.

c. A posterior lens luxation is not an emergency. However, consultation with an ophthalmologist should be considered due to the potential of retinal detachment from changes in the vitreous or direct contact of the lens capsule or the lens moving into the anterior chamber in the future.

9. LACERATIONS

a. Lacerations can occur in the eyelids, in the conjunctiva or in the cornea and sclera.

b. Eyelid lacerations:

i. Keep the cornea lubricated if any tissue rubs or touches the cornea.

ii. Under general anesthesia, gently clean the wound with diluted povidine–iodine solution (1:10–1:50), debriding as little tissue as possible.

iii. If a laceration involves the eyelid margins, the margins must appose each other completely to prevent corneal irritation and ocular discomfort. The Meibomian glands are good landmarks to line up with each other to ensure proper alignment:

1. Using 4–0 absorbable monofilament suture or silk (or the smallest suture material available) in a cruciate or a figure-of-eight pattern, start 3–4 mm away from one margin placing the suture half thickness, cross over the wound and go into the eyelid about 2–3 mm away from the Meibomian glands, come out of the Meibomian glands on that side, go into the Meibomian glands on the *other* side of the wound, come out 2–3 mm from the Meibomian glands, cross

over and come out 3–4 mm away from the eyelid margin (Figure 15.11).

2. Close the remainder of the laceration with a simple interrupted pattern, with the sutures spanning half of the thickness of the conjunctiva (do not go full thickness through the eyelid).

iv. If the laceration was full thickness, close it in two layers (conjunctiva then skin), taking care to appose the eyelid margins as described above.

v. Take care to preserve the lacrimal puncta if the laceration is at the ventral medial canthus to prevent epiphora and conjunctivitis. If involving the puncta, consultation with an ophthalmologist is advised.

vi. Systemic broad-spectrum antibiotics such as amoxicillin–clavulonic acid (15 mg/kg BID orally) should be started. Topical antibiotics are not needed due to the abundant blood supply to the eyelids.

vii. An Elizabethan collar should be worn for 7–10 days.

c. Third eyelid lacerations:

i. If only the conjunctiva (or top layer) was damaged, then surgery is not needed to repair the laceration due to an adequate blood supply and rapid healing.

ii. If the membrane of the third eyelid gland was lacerated, then a simple continuous pattern

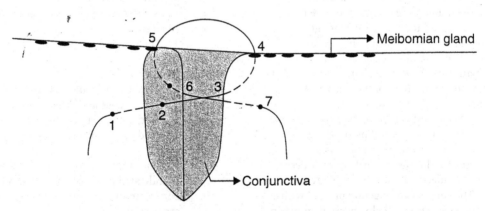

FIGURE 15.11 Suture placement for an eyelid laceration: (1) Enter the eyelid about 3–4 mm away from the margin. (2) Exit through the middle of the eyelid width. (3) Enter the other eyelid (other part of the laceration) about 2–3 mm from the margin. (4) Exit through the Meibomian glands. (5) Enter first eyelid through the Meibomian glands. (6) Exit through the middle of the eyelid width. (7) Enter and exit the other eyelid about 3–4 mm away from the margin. (Reprinted with permission: Drobatz K and Costello M, 2010, Feline Emergency and Critical Care Medicine, Wiley-Blackwell, Ames, IA.)

can be used with 4–0 absorbable monofilament suture or silk to close the laceration.

iii. If a piece of the third eyelid was damaged or torn during the injury, then surgery is needed to repair it. The damaged tissue should be removed. Then the bulbar conjunctiva and the palpebral conjunctiva (both surround the third eyelid gland on either side) are closed to each other (over the gland), closing the defect. Take care to preserve the leading margin of the third eyelid.

d. Conjunctival lacerations:

i. Most conjunctival lacerations do not require surgery to close them and can be allowed to heal by second intention due to rapid healing. Some may only require to debride the area.

ii. However, if there is large defect, then the conjunctiva can be closed with 6–0 monofilament absorbable suture in a simple interrupted pattern, being sure to bury the knots or have the knots on the bulbar conjunctival side to prevent corneal or conjunctival irritation.

iii. If there is any necrotic tissue, this needs to be debrided.

iv. Topical antibiotics (triple antibiotic solution in dogs, erythromycin ointment in cats or tobramycin solution in dogs or cats) should be used three times a day for 5–7 days.

e. Corneal lacerations are treated according to the depth of the laceration (Figure 15.12a–c):

i. A thorough examination must be performed under the eyelids and under the third eyelid to make sure a foreign body is not present causing the laceration. Instillation of a topical anesthetic (proparacaine 0.5%) will facilitate visualization and movement of the third eyelid gland.

ii. A Seidel test can be performed to check for a full thickness laceration or leakage of aqueous humor. Fluorescein dye is applied to the cornea and if there is leakage of aqueous humor, rivulets will form from the dye.

iii. The cornea can be gently pressed with a cotton-tipped swab to help check the integrity of the cornea.

iv. Partial thickness corneal lacerations may heal with medical therapy. Treatment includes topical antibiotics and topical atropine if needed (see Corneal Ulcer below).

v. Full thickness corneal lacerations (Figure 15.12b) may need surgery to debride and close the edges:

1. The cornea can be sutured with 6–0 to 9–0 absorbable suture material (Vicryl, PDS) in a simple interrupted pattern.

2. The suture should go 1/2 to 2/3 the depth of the cornea and NOT go full thickness through the cornea.

3. The anterior chamber can be reinflated if necessary with sterile saline or balanced salt solution using a 25 gauge (or smaller) needle entered at the limbus (Figure 15.12c).

4. A conjunctival flap should follow corneal repair (see below).

5. Topical broad-spectrum antibiotics (ciprofloxacin 0.5%) every 3–4 hours and topical atropine (1%) every 8–12 hours are started.

6. Systemic antibiotics (amoxicillin–clavulanic acid 15–20 mg/kg orally twice a day) and systemic anti-inflammatory medication (prednisone 0.5 mg/kg PO BID for 3 days then SID for 3 days, then EOD for three treatments if the lens capsule was damaged or a NSAID if the lens capsule is intact—see Table 15.1) should be used as well.

vi. Cat scratches are common causes of corneal lacerations:

1. The cat claw is notorious for penetrating the cornea and touching the anterior lens capsule.

2. If the lens capsule has been damaged, then an intense and difficult to treat lens induced anterior uveitis (see above) may follow due to leakage of foreign lens protein.

3. Since topical corticosteroids are contraindicated in a corneal laceration, oral corticosteroids at anti-inflammatory doses are indicated.

4. The owners must be warned that the lens may need to be removed if complications ensue.

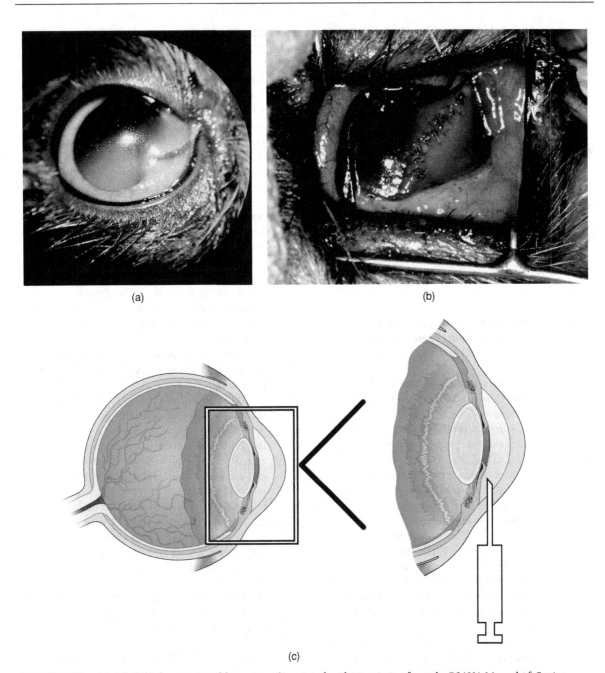

(a)

(b)

(c)

FIGURE 15.12   (a) A full thickness corneal laceration. (Reprinted with permission from the BSAVA Manual of Canine and Feline Emergency and Critical Care, King and Boag, 2007.) (b) Post suturing of a full thickness corneal laceration. (c) Placement of syringe filled with sterile saline or balanced salt solution (BSS) for reinflation of the anterior chamber.

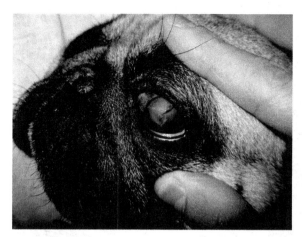

FIGURE 15.13   A 2-year-old Pug with an iris prolapse in the center of the cornea secondary to another Pug dog fight.

vii.   The iris can prolapse through the cornea in a corneal laceration (Figure 15.13). A visible piece of the iris will be seen through the cornea (iris prolapse):

    1.   Topical broad-spectrum antibiotics (ciprofloxacin 0.5%) every 2–4 hours are started.

    2.   Topical atropine (1%) two to four times a day is specially important to try to pull the iris back into the anterior chamber or minimize the amount of iris prolapsing through the defect.

    3.   Systemic antibiotics (amoxicillin–clavulanic acid 15–20 mg/kg orally twice a day) and systemic anti-inflammatory medication should be used as well (NSAIDs if the anterior lens capsule was not disrupted or corticosteroids if the anterior lens capsule was disrupted—see above).

    4.   Surgery as soon as possible to replace and possibly debride the iris may be needed for the best outcome for vision and the eye. This would be followed by suturing the cornea and then placing a pedicle conjunctival flap/graft or other stabilizing procedure.

viii.   Scleral lacerations are frequently full thickness (see Scleral rupture) and require enucleation.

10. FOREIGN BODIES

    a.   The most common foreign bodies to become lodged in the eye include little pieces of wood, sticks, grass awns, and glass. They can become embedded in the conjunctiva, cornea, or sclera.

    b.   Clinical signs include an acute onset of blepharospasm, epiphora, rubbing at the eye, lethargy and corneal edema if involving the cornea.

    c.   A foreign body under the upper, lower, or third eyelid typically causes a vertical or straight corneal ulcer or laceration. These areas need to be extensively searched for the foreign object (see Corneal laceration).

    d.   The foreign body may be seen grossly or a slit lamp or magnification may be necessary to visualize the foreign body.

    e.   Topical anesthetic (proparacaine 0.5%) should be instilled to facilitate the examination.

    f.   Conjunctival foreign bodies may be removed with tissue or Colibri forceps if the foreign object is large enough:

        i.   If the animal is calm, then topical anesthetic may be all that is required. If not, sedation is indicated.

        ii.   If the area of the conjunctiva is damaged secondary to the foreign body, it should be debrided.

        iii.   A blade or needle may be needed if the foreign object is small and an ophthalmologist can use magnification and more specific instruments if needed.

        iv.   The area is flushed with copious amounts (about 4 oz) of sterile saline or eyewash.

        v.   Topical antibiotic ointment (triple antibiotic ointment in dogs or erythromycin ointment 0.3% in cats) should be used three to four times a day.

        vi.   The eye should be reevaluated in one week.

    g.   Corneal foreign bodies can span into the stroma or penetrate full thickness:

        i.   After placement of topical anesthetic (proparacaine 0.5%), the eye can be gently flushed with copious amounts (about 4 oz) of sterile eyewash or sterile saline to dislodge the object.

        ii.   If the object is not dislodged, a 25 g needle can be used to try to lift the foreign body out of the superficial corneal tissue. An incision may be needed over the foreign body and Colibri or tissue forceps may be needed to grasp the object. Extreme care must be taken to not push the object deeper into the stroma or into the anterior chamber.

iii. Foreign bodies that span into the anterior chamber may require surgery on the cornea after the object is removed. Debriding and suturing of the cornea along with a conjunctival graft may be needed:

1. If an ophthalmologist is not available, the cornea can be sutured using 6–0 to 9–0 absorbable suture (vicryl, PDS) in a simple interrupted pattern. The sutures should go $\frac{1}{2}$ to $\frac{2}{3}$ the depth of the cornea.

2. The anterior chamber can be reinflated if necessary with sterile saline or balanced salt solution using a 1 cc syringe with a 25 g needle placed at the limbus (Figure 15.13c).

3. A conjunctival flap should then follow if there is concern about corneal integrity or it is felt that added support is necessary (see below).

4. Topical ciprofloxacin every 4 hours and systemic antibiotics (amoxicillin–clavulonic acid 15–20 mg/kg PO BID) are started as discussed for a perforated corneal ulcer.

5. Topical atropine (1%) is used twice a day.

6. Systemic nonsteroidal anti-inflammatory medication should be used for 5–7 days as well (see Table 15.1).

11. CORNEAL ULCERS

a. Corneal ulcers are one of the most common traumatic injuries. The trauma can be blunt (e.g., hit by car), secondary to an animal fight, or secondary to a foreign object (embedded or not).

b. Clinical signs include blepharospasm, ocular discharge, conjunctival hyperemia, corneal edema, and possibly a miotic pupil.

c. A corneal ulcer is diagnosed based on results of a fluorescein stain:

i. A Seidel test can be performed to check for a full thickness laceration or leakage of aqueous humor. Fluorescein dye is applied to the cornea and if there is leakage of aqueous humor, rivulets will form from the dye.

ii. The cornea can be gently pressed with a cotton tipped swab to help check the integrity of the cornea.

d. Treatment depends on the depth of the corneal ulcer.

e. A *superficial* corneal abrasion involves the corneal epithelium and a superficial ulcer starts to involve the stroma:

i. Treatment includes topical antibiotics (triple antibiotic ointment or solution in dogs, erythromycin ointment 0.3% in cats) three times a day. If there is a miotic pupil secondary to iridocyclospasm, then topical atropine (1%) once or twice a day is indicated.

ii. Most noncomplicated superficial ulcers should heal and re-epithelialize within 5 days. Another fluorescein stain should be performed at this time.

f. *Diffuse superficial abrasions or ulcers* can occur secondary to shampoos or other caustic material getting underneath the eyelids:

i. These can span the entire corneal epithelium.

ii. The eye should be flushed with copious amounts (about 4 oz) of sterile saline or eyewash.

iii. Topical antibiotics (triple antibiotic ointment or solution in dogs, erythromycin ointment 0.3% in cats) as in a superficial ulcer 4–6 times a day are started.

iv. Addition of topical autologous serum (1 drop every 2–4 hours) to help aid in reepithelization (it is epitheliotrophic) should be considered:

1. Collect 5–10 mL of the patient's blood in a red top tube and centrifuge it.

2. The serum is then pipetted into another red top tube, all aseptically. This serum must be refrigerated.

v. These may take longer than one week to heal, depending on the extent of the abrasion or ulcer. The eye should be rechecked and fluorescein stained in weekly intervals.

g. A *deep* corneal ulcer spans into the corneal stroma. Many times, they can be visualized grossly before fluorescein stain (Figure 15.14):

i. Treatment involves topical broad-spectrum antibiotics (gentamicin or tobramycin 0.3%) four times a day and topical atropine 1% twice a day for the iridocyclospasm if a miotic pupil is present.

ii. An Elizabethan collar must be worn at all times.

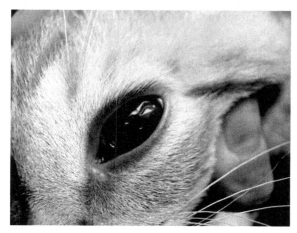

FIGURE 15.14   A deep corneal ulcer secondary to a cat fight in a 6-month-old kitten. This was treated with ciprofloxacin drops every 4 hours and atropine drops every 12 hours and healed without complications. (Reprinted with permission: Drobatz K and Costello M, 2010, Feline Emergency and Critical Care Medicine, Wiley-Blackwell, Ames, IA.)

    iii.   If more than 80% of the stroma is involved, then a conjunctival graft (see below) or other surgery for support is indicated.
    iv.   The eye should be rechecked in one week and then weekly to monitor progression.
    v.   Deep corneal ulcers can take up to three weeks to heal.
    vi.   Deep corneal ulcers can become infected and become *melting ulcers* (Figure 15.15)

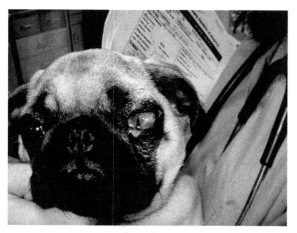

FIGURE 15.15   A melting perforated corneal ulcer in a 4-month-old Pug. Notice the white slimy film over the ulcer that is characteristic of a melting ulcer.

rapidly due to bacteria that invade the cornea. Most commonly, these are Gram negative collagenase producing bacteria such as *Proteus* spp. and *Pseudomonas* spp.:
    1.   Clinical signs include a white thick film that covers or surrounds the corneal ulcer.
    2.   Cytology and aerobic culture and sensitivity should be performed.
    3.   Topical antibiotic therapy must include coverage for Gram negative bacteria and must be applied every 1–2 hours. Topical ciprofloxacin is a very good broad-spectrum antibiotic for melting ulcers. Also topical cefazolin can be made (see Table 15.1) to increase the spectrum of coverage. If ciprofloxacin is not available, then cefazolin drops and gentamicin drops can be used.
    4.   Topical anticollagenase therapy must be started and applied every 1–2 hours:
        a.   This can be achieved with autologous serum, or acetylcysteine.
        b.   Mix the acetylcysteine in an artificial tears solution bottle, diluted to a 5–10% solution.
        c.   To make the autologous serum, collect 5–10 mL of the patients blood in a red top tube and centrifuge it. The serum is then pipetted into another red top tube, all aseptically. This serum must be refrigerated.
    5.   Systemic antibiotics must be started. Doxycycline has excellent antiprotease properties and has been shown to concentrate in the tear film, making it an excellent choice for a systemic antibiotic for melting or infected ulcers. Amoxicillin–clavulonic acid can be used as well.
  h.   A *descemetocele* is a deep corneal ulcer that spans to Descemet's membrane and is only one cell layer away from rupturing (Figure 15.16):
    i.   Fluorescein stain will show a clear or black area in the center (Descemet's membrane) of the ulcer that does not take up stain.
    ii.   It is considered a surgical emergency. A conjunctival graft or other surgery (corneal graft from donor, corneoscleral transposition) for support should be performed as soon as possible, if possible.

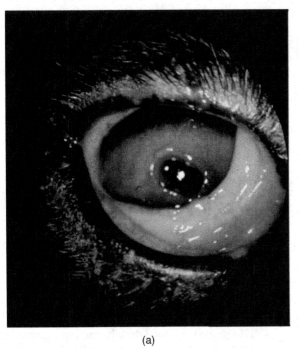
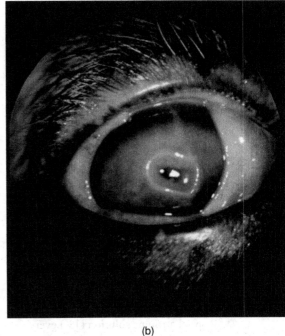

(a)   (b)

FIGURE 15.16 Image A represents a classic descemetocele. Image B is the same descemetocele after Fluorescein stain. Notice the clear area in the center.

iii. Medical management is started until surgery can be performed. Topical solutions should be used instead of ointments due to the potential of the cornea perforating. The oil base of ointments can cause severe intraocular inflammation:

1. Topical broad-spectrum antibiotic solution (ciprofloxacin 0.5%) every 2–3 hours.

2. Topical atropine (1%) solution two to four times a day for iridocyclospasm and to prevent synechiae.

3. Systemic antibiotics such as amoxicillin–clavulonic acid (15 mg/kg BID) orally or ampicillin (22 mg/kg TID) intravenously should be started.

4. Systemic nonsteroidal anti-inflammatory medication should be started (Table 15.1).

5. An Elizabethan collar must be worn at all times.

6. Strict cage rest.

7. If the animal is very painful or too difficult to medicate, then systemic pain medications +/− sedation is warranted (buprenorphine 0.01 mg/kg IV/SQ or

butorphanol 0.2–0.4 mg/kg IV/SQ every 4–6 hours).

8. Due to the potential of corneal rupture, care must be taken for gentle restraint; neck leads and jugular venipuncture must be avoided.

i. A *perforated corneal ulcer* is also a surgical emergency (Figure 15.17):

i. Clinical signs include a misshapen cornea, decreased depth to the anterior chamber, a fibrin clot sealing the defect, fibrin in the anterior chamber, and an obvious perforation in the cornea. An *iris prolapse* (Figure 15.13) may also be present (see above, Corneal laceration).

ii. A conjunctival graft or other protective surgery should be performed as soon as possible, if possible.

iii. Medical management includes the following:

1. Topical broad-spectrum antibiotics (ciprofloxacin 0.5%) every 2–3 hours. Also, topical cefazolin can be made (see Table 15.1) to increase the spectrum of coverage.

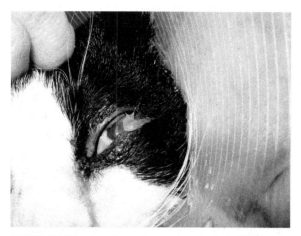

FIGURE 15.17   A perforated cornea in a 5-year-old cat. (Reprinted with permission: Drobatz K and Costello M, 2010, Feline Emergency and Critical Care Medicine, Wiley-Blackwell, Ames, IA.)

2. Topical atropine solution (1%) every 4–6 hours. This is particularly important if the iris is prolapsed through the defect.

3. Systemic broad-spectrum antibiotics such as amoxicillin–clavulonic acid (15–20 mg/kg BID) orally or ampicillin (22 mg/kg TID) intravenously.

4. Oral anti-inflammatory medication:

    a. If the anterior lens capsule is intact, then nonsteroidal anti-inflammatory drugs (see Table 15.1) are indicated.

    b. If the anterior lens capsule has been damaged, then anti-inflammatory doses of corticosteroids are indicated (prednisone 0.5 mg/kg PO BID for 3 days then SID for 3 days then every other day for 3 treatments). Clinical signs that may be seen to indicate that the lens was damaged include fibrin extending from the lens or an opacity on the lens capsule. If the anterior lens capsule was damaged, the foreign lens protein can leak out and lead to a massive, difficult to treat, lens-induced uveitis. The owners should be warned that the lens may need to be removed if the anterior uveitis cannot be controlled with medical therapy or secondary complications such as glaucoma occur.

    5. An Elizabethan collar must be worn at all times.

    6. Strict cage rest must be enforced as well as no neck leads, no jugular venipuncture, and gentle restraint.

  iv. The cornea can seal with aggressive medical management and prognosis for the eye may be good, depending on the severity of the perforation. The prognosis for vision also depends on the severity of the perforation, how much cornea is affected, and if the anterior lens capsule was involved.

12. RETINAL DETACHMENT AND/OR HEMORRHAGE

  a. Retinal detachment or hemorrhage (Figures 15.18 and 15.19) can occur secondary to blunt or penetrating trauma.

  b. A retinal detachment (Figure 15.18) occurs when the neuroretina separates from the underlying retinal pigmented epithelium:

    i. In trauma, a retinal detachment can occur if there is a break or tear in the retina leading to vitreous fluid accumulation under the neuroretina, leading to a severe detachment (rhegmatogenous detachment).

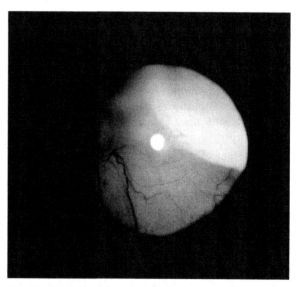

FIGURE 15.18   Retinal detachment. Notice the balloon of retinal tissue. (Reprinted with permission: Drobatz K and Costello M, 2010, Feline Emergency and Critical Care Medicine, Wiley-Blackwell, Ames, IA.)

ii. Penetrating ocular trauma can also lead to retinal detachment where there is a pulling force in the vitreous detaching the retina (tractional detachment).

c. Clinical signs can include any other sign of ocular trauma, especially hyphema. There may also be absence of a menace response and absence of a direct and indirect PLR.

d. Retinal detachments may be seen with a focal light source directed through a dilated pupil if severe and/or complete. The retinal vessels will appear to balloon out toward the lens.

e. A fundic examination will show the retinal hemorrhage(s) grossly as red or brown areas in the tapetal fundus (Figure 15.19). In a retinal detachment, a cloudy area may be seen in the retina. A crisp view of the optic nerve and/or vessels will not be seen.

f. Ultrasound of the eye can help diagnose retinal detachments if the fundus is not visible. A 7.5–12 MHz transducer with B mode ultrasound should be used. Coupling gel is placed after topical anesthetic is instilled in the eye (Figure 15.20).

g. Partial retinal detachments may heal over time.

h. Prognosis for vision depends on if the animal is visual at presentation and if there is an indirect PLR in the unaffected eye. In the absence of an indirect PLR, the prognosis for vision is guarded to poor.

i. There is no specific oral or topical treatment. Crate rest should be enforced.

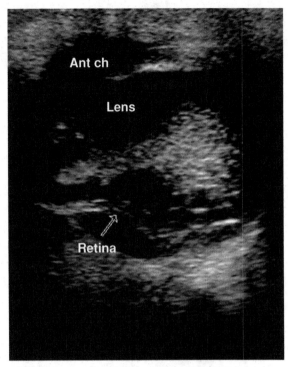

FIGURE 15.20 Ultrasound of an eye showing retinal detachment and hemorrhage in the posterior chamber.

j. There are veterinary ophthalmologists who perform retinopexy. This uses a diode or argon laser or cryotherapy to reattach the retina. This needs to be performed within 4 weeks of the detachment to have the best chance of regaining vision. The surgery is not without potential complications and an ophthalmologist should be consulted to determine if the patient is a candidate for this procedure.

13. SCLERAL RUPTURE

a. The globe can rupture at any part of the sclera secondary to blunt trauma, including the part that is not visible. The most common site is near the optic nerve.

b. Clinical signs include blindness with a negative menace and negative direct and indirect PLR, hyphema, subconjunctival hemorrhage, and eyelid and conjunctival swelling.

c. The eye may look smaller or collapsed.

d. An IOP reading can be low.

e. Ultrasound of the eye is used to help diagnose a scleral rupture and should be performed in any eye

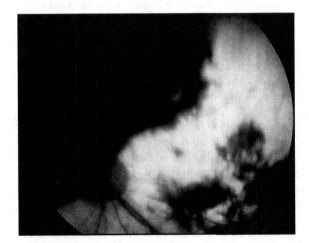

FIGURE 15.19 Retinal hemorrhage.

where the intraocular structures are not visible. An area of ill-defined scleral margins can be seen along with echoic material in the anterior and posterior chamber and vitreous.

f. Treatment usually consists of enucleation, although there are no studies to determine long-term prognosis in a scleral rupture that is not enucleated. Most likely, the eye will become phthisical.

g. Since cats are prone to develop post traumatic sarcomas secondary to an ocular trauma (see below), enucleation may be the best option for cats.

14. POST TRAUMATIC SARCOMA

a. Can occur in cats secondary to any ocular trauma, trauma to the lens, post intraocular surgery, and chronic uveitis.

b. The cause is unknown but the tumor is a highly malignant type of neoplasia:

    i. It invades the optic nerve and retina.

    ii. It metastasizes to regional lymph nodes and distant sites.

c. Clinical signs include hyphema, an intraocular mass, anterior uveitis, and glaucoma.

d. Ultrasound can be used to diagnose an intraocular mass.

e. Chest radiographs should be performed to rule out pulmonary metastatic disease.

f. Exenteration is recommended:

    i. Exenteration refers to surgery to remove the entire contents of the orbit.

    ii. All tissue should then be submitted for biopsy.

g. The long term prognosis is guarded to poor due to the likelihood of metastatic disease, especially if there is evidence of extrascleral extension on histopathology of the globe.

15. CONJUNCTIVAL GRAFT/FLAP PLACEMENT
(Figures 15.21 and 15.22)

a. A conjunctival flap or graft is performed when extra support is needed for the cornea. The flap will supply fibroblasts to promote corneal healing and provide a blood supply to deliver anticollagenases and systemically administered antibiotics to the lesion.

b. A conjunctival graft or flap is indicated for deep corneal ulcers where the ulcer spans more

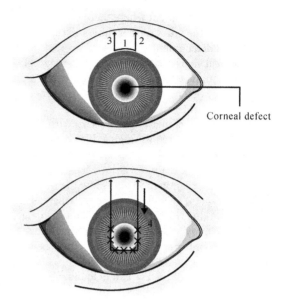

Corneal defect

FIGURE 15.21 Conjunctival pedicle flap/graft: (1) An incision in made in the conjunctiva about 2 mm away from the limbus, parallel to the limbus (horizontal). It should be wide enough to cover the defect. (2) The incision is extended caudally. The conjunctiva is then dissected and freed off of the bulbar fascia. (3) Another incision is made and extended caudally, on the other side of the horizontal incision. (4) The pedicle flap is stretched over the defect and sutured to the cornea. The sutures should span $\frac{1}{2}$ to $\frac{2}{3}$ the depth of the cornea.

than 50% of the stroma, descemetoceles, and any corneal perforations (i.e., laceration, foreign body, etc).

c. Many ophthalmologists do not recommend the use of third eyelid flaps or temporary tarsorrhapies for deep corneal ulcers, descemetoceles, or perforated corneas because they do not provide a blood supply and they impair monitoring of the lesion.

d. Ideally, an ophthalmologist should be consulted, as there are other alternative surgeries that an ophthalmologist can perform to protect the cornea instead (e.g., corneoscleral transposition).

e. A very common type of conjunctival graft is the pedicle flap.

f. The two most important aspects of conjunctival flap surgery are that the flap is thin and free of tension. The animal will be more uncomfortable and painful if the flap is too thick and the flap will

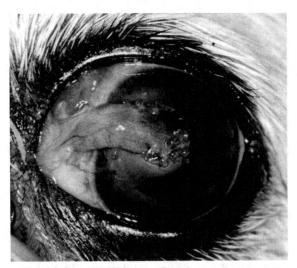

FIGURE 15.22 Post conjunctival pedicle flap placement.

viii. Stretch the flap (still connected caudally) over the defect. If there is any tension, make the flap longer, again, taking care to keep the flap thin as it is being made.

ix. Once the flap can be stretched over the defect without any tension, the flap is sutured to the cornea on three sides of the defect.

x. Simple interrupted sutures of 6–0 to 9–0 absorbable suture (vicryl, PDS) going 1/2 to 2/3 the depth of the stroma are placed. Do not go full thickness or penetrate the cornea.

g. Topical antibiotics and topical atropine as discussed for a deep corneal ulcer are then started.

h. The pedicle portion can be trimmed in about a month (close to the limbus) to uncover normal cornea. This is easier than trying to remove the sutures.

BIBLIOGRAPHY

Blocker T, van der Woerdt A. The feline glaucomas: 82 cases (1995–1999). *Vet Ophthalmol* 2001; 4 (2): 81–85.

Brooks DE. Glaucoma in the dog and cat. *Vet Clin North Am Small Anim Pract* 1990; 20 (3): 775–797.

Budelsky CL, Dubielzig RR. Follow-up study on cats previously diagnosed with post traumatic sarcoma and possible effects on lifespan. Abstracts: 33rd Annual Meeting of the American College of Veterinary Ophthalmologists. Denver, CO, USA. October 9–13, 2002. *Vet Ophthalmology* 2002; 5 (4): 283–301.

Cho, J. Surgery of the Globe and Orbit. *Top Comp Anim Med* 2008; 23 (1): 23–37.

Colitz CM. Feline uveitis: diagnosis and treatment. *Clin Tech Small Anim Pract* 2005; 20: 117–120.

Collius BK, Moore CP. Diseases and surgery of the canine anterior uvea. In: Gelatt KN, ed. *Veterinary Ophthalmology*. 3rd edition. Lippincott Williams & Wilkins, Baltimore (MD), 1999; 755–795.

Dietrich U. Feline glaucomas. *Clin Tech Small Anim Pract* 2005; 20: 108–116.

Dziezyc J, Hager DA. Ocular ultrasonography in veterinary medicine. *Semin Vet Med Surg (Small Anim)* 1988; 3: 1–9.

Gilger BC, Hamilton HL, Wilkie DA, van derWoerdt A. Traumatic ocular proptosis in dogs and cats – 84 cases (1980–1993). *J Am Vet Med Assoc* 1995; 206: 1186–1190.

Glaze MB, Gelatt KN. Feline ophthalmology. In: Gelatt KN, ed. *Veterinary Ophthalmology*. 3rd edition. Lippincott Williams & Wilkins, Baltimore, MD, 1999; 997–1052.

Gionfriddo JR. The causes, diagnosis, and treatment of uveitis. *Vet Med* 1995; 90: 278–284.

Gionfriddo JR. Recognizing and managing acute and chronic cases of glaucoma. *Vet Med* 1995; 90: 265–275.

be more likely to breakdown if it is placed under tension:

i. Under general anesthesia, the periorbital area is gently clipped and scrubbed with diluted povidine–iodine solution (1:10–1:50).

ii. At the dorsal or lateral conjunctiva, forceps are used (Colibri forceps should be used) to pick up the conjunctiva directly above or closest to the site of the corneal defect.

iii. An incision in made in the conjunctiva parallel to the limbus, about 2 mm from the limbus.

iv. The incision should extend the length of the corneal defect, so that it will cover the width of the defect.

v. An incision is made perpendicular to the first incision, going caudally up the conjunctiva.

vi. The conjunctiva is dissected away from the bulbar fascia of the sclera (Tenon's capsule) using blunt dissection, taking extreme care to keep it thin as it is being dissected free (this gets more difficult as it extends back).

vii. Another incision is made on the other side of the parallel incision to free the flap. The one side can be stretched to see if the length is sufficient to cover the defect. Alternatively, the pedicle can be dissected following the curve of the limbus (instead of going up the conjunctiva, curve the incisions to make the flap).

Giuliano EA. Feline ocular emergencies. *Clin Tech Small Anim Pract* 2005; 20: 135–141.

Hendrix DVH. Disease and surgery of the canine conjunctiva. In: Gelatt KN, ed. *Veterinary Ophthalmology*. 3rd edition. Lippincott Williams & Wilkins, Baltimore, MD, 1999; 619–634.

Komaromy AM, Brooks DE, Kallberg ME, *et al*. Hyphema. Part I. Pathophysiologic considerations. *Compend Contin Educ Pract Vet* 1999; 21: 1064–1069, 1091.

Komaromy AM, Brooks DE, Kallberg ME, *et al*. Hyphema. Part II. Diagnosis and treatment. *Compend Contin Educ Pract Vet* 2000; 22: 74–79.

Mandell DC, Holt E. Ophthalmic Emergencies. *Vet Clin North Am Small Anim Pract* 2005; 35: 455–480.

Mandell DC. Ophthalmological emergencies. In: King L, Boag A, eds. *BSAVA Manual of Canine and Feline Emergency and Critical Care*. 2nd edition. British Small Animal Veterinary Association, 2007; 147–158.

Massa KL, Gilger BC, Miller TL, *et al*. Causes of uveitis in dogs: 102 cases (1989–2000). *Vet Ophthalmol* 2002; 5 (2): 93–98.

Moore PA. Feline corneal disease. *Clin Tech Small Anim Pract* 2005; 20: 83–93.

Narfstrom K, Ekesten B. Diseases of the canine ocular fundus. In: Gelatt KN ed. *Veterinary Ophthalmology*. 3rd edition. Lippincott Williams & Wilkins, Baltimore, MD, 1999; 869–933.

Nelms SR, Nasisse MP, Davidson MG, Kirshner SE. Hyphema associated with retinal disease in dogs: 17 cases (1986–1991). *JAVMA* 1993; 202: 1289–1292.

Paul TA, Ward DA. Clinical features, etiologies and outcomes of hyphema in dogs: a retrospective study (1999–2002). Abstracts: 34th Annual Meeting of the American College of Veterinary Ophthalmologists, Coeur D'Alene, ID, USA. October 22–25, 2003. *Vet Ophthalmol* 2003; 6 (4): 351–366.

Plunkett SJ. Anaphylaxis to ophthalmic medication in a cat. *J Vet Emerg Crit Care* 2000; 10 (3): 169–171.

Rainbow ME, Dziezyc J. Effects of twice daily application of 2% dorzolamide in intraocular pressure in normal cats. *Vet Ophthalmol* 2003; 6 (2): 147–150.

Rampazzo A, Eule C, Speier S, *et al*. Scleral rupture in dogs, cats and horses. *Vet Ophthalmol* 2006; 9 (3): 149–155.

Sapienza JS. Feline lens disorders. *Clin Tech Small Anim Pract* 2005; 20: 102–107.

Severin GA. *Veterinary Ophthalmology Notes*. 2nd edition. Colorado State University, Fort Collins, CO, 1976.

Strubbe DT, Gelatt KN. Ophthalmic examination and diagnostic procedures. In: Gelatt KN, ed. *Veterinary Ophthalmology*. 3rd edition. Lippincott Williams & Wilkins, Baltimore, MD, 1999; 427–466.

Vainisi SJ, Wolfer JC. Canine retinal surgery. *Vet Ophthalmol* 2004; 7 (5): 291–306.

Van Der Woerdt A. Lens induced uveitis. *Vet Ophthalmol* 2000; 3 (4): 227–234.

Whitley RD, Gilger BC. Diseases of the canine cornea and sclera. In: Gelatt KN, ed. *Veterinary Ophthalmology*. 3rd edition. Lippincott Williams & Wilkins, Baltimore, MD, 1999; 635–673.

Whitley RD, Hamilton HL, Weigand CM. Glaucoma and disorders of the uvea, lens and retina in cats. *Vet Med* 1993; 88: 1164–1173.

Whitley RD, Whitley EM, McLaughlin SA. Diagnosing and treating disorders of the feline conjunctiva and cornea. *Vet Med* 1993; 8: 1138–1149.

Willis AM, Diehl KA, Robbin TE. Advances in topical glaucoma therapy. *Vet Ophthalmol*. 2002; 5 (1): 9–17.

TRAUMA-ASSOCIATED MUSCULOSKELETAL INJURY TO THE HEAD

Alexander M. Reiter and John R. Lewis

1. INTRODUCTION

a. In head trauma patients, stabilizing the cardiovascular and respiratory systems and preventing or limiting secondary brain injury are of utmost priority (see Chapter 7: Traumatic Brain Injury).

b. Unless immediate surgical intervention is necessary to prevent further deterioration, definitive repair of injuries under general anesthesia can be delayed until the patient has been stabilized.

c. Following initial stabilization, a history is obtained from the owner, including the time elapsed since the trauma, progression of clinical signs, medications administered, and pertinent medical history.

d. Extraoral examination may reveal obvious wounds and asymmetry of the head and neck, hemorrhage, discharge from mouth, nose, eyes and ears, displaced or fractured teeth and bones, and swellings.

e. Intubation through a pharyngostomy or tracheostomy site allows intraoperative evaluation of the occlusion, particularly when multiple comminuted jaw fractures are present. Temporary tracheostomy is also useful during postoperative recovery of an animal with airway obstruction.

f. Pre-, intra-, and postoperative monitoring should emphasize blood pressure, oxygenation and ventilation, and serial neurologic evaluation (see Chapter 4: Monitoring of the Trauma Patient).

g. Initially, the mouth is flushed with dilute chlorhexidine digluconate (0.1–0.2%), and the injured sites are carefully debrided to remove blood clots, foreign material, and necrotic tissue.

h. Injured vessels are ligated to prevent further blood loss, and soft tissue lacerations are sutured (or closed after orthopedic repair) (see Chapter 17: Trauma-Associated Soft Tissue Injury to the Head and Neck).

i. Antibiotic therapy may be considered in selected cases to treat or prevent infection (ampicillin 22 mg/kg IV q 2 hours or cefazolin 20 mg/kg IV q 2 hours intraoperatively; amoxicillin/clavulanic acid 14 mg/kg PO BID, clindamycin 11 mg/kg PO BID, or cephalexin 25 mg/kg PO BID postoperatively).

j. Trauma-associated musculoskeletal injury mainly affects the bones and joints of the head rather than the musculature attached to bones. Mechanical trauma is often the primary reason for injury, though thermal and chemical injuries are possible. Injuries of maxillofacial and mandibular structures usually include tooth fractures, tooth displacement injuries, fractures of the jaw, joint injuries, and palate defects.

k. Nasoesophageal, esophagostomy, and gastrostomy tubes are rarely needed to bypass the oral cavity of patients undergoing major oral and maxillofacial surgery. Some cats may benefit from

Manual of Trauma Management in the Dog and Cat, First Edition. Edited by Kenneth J. Drobatz, Matthew W. Beal and Rebecca S. Syring.
© 2011 John Wiley & Sons, Inc. Published 2011 by John Wiley & Sons, Inc.

TABLE 16.1
DIAGNOSTIC, TEMPORARY FIRST-AID AND SURGICAL PROCEDURES THAT EMERGENCY CLINICIANS SHOULD BE ABLE TO PERFORM IN PATIENTS WITH MUSCULOSKELETAL INJURIES OF THE HEAD

- Management of airway obstruction, including temporary tracheostomy
- Placement of nasoesophageal and esophagostomy tubes
- Inspection and palpation of extra- and intraoral structures of the head
- Radiography of the head
- Recognition and differentiation of wear, fractures, and displacement injuries of teeth
- Fabrication and placement of tape muzzles
- Circumferential wiring for mandibular symphysis separation and parasymphyseal fractures
- Differentiation of TMJ luxation from open-mouth jaw locking
- Reduction of rostrodorsal TMJ luxation with a wood dowel
- Reduction of open-mouth jaw locking by manual opening the mouth, unlocking the coronoid process from the zygomatic arch, and closing the mouth

placement of an esophagostomy tube to ensure proper nutrition and medication during the immediate postoperative period.

l. Surgery for many musculoskeletal injuries of the head is performed by a veterinary dentist or oral surgeon. The emergency clinician usually performs temporary first-aid treatment; however, minor trauma may already be addressed by means of definitive surgery in the emergency room setting (Table 16.1).

2. DIAGNOSTIC TOOLS

a. Inspection—Extraoral tissues and oral cavity are inspected for lacerations, asymmetry, swellings, fractured and displaced teeth, hemorrhage, and discharge from orifices of the head.

b. Palpation—The head is palpated both extra- and intraorally for asymmetry, discontinuity, crepitus, and emphysema; evaluate range of mandibular opening.

c. Diagnostic imaging—Familiarity with normal head anatomy, including anatomy of teeth, jaws, temporomandibular joints, and attached soft tissue structures, is imperative in order to diagnose pathology and establish a treatment plan:

i. Radiography:

1. Dental radiographs—Obtain radiographs to assess tooth injuries and further define jaw fracture sites; most jaw fractures can be satisfactorily assessed with size 2 and 4 dental film and intraoral imaging techniques; size 4 dental film can also be utilized to evaluate injuries to the zygomatic arch, mandibular ramus, temporomandibular joint (TMJ), and tympanic bulla in cats and small dogs.

2. Standard medical radiographs—For caudal mandibular and maxillary fractures in medium-sized and large dogs; contrast radiography to be considered for trauma to the salivary gland-duct complex.

ii. Computed tomography—For patients with moderate to severe head trauma on presentation, failure of improvement, or deterioration of clinical signs; often indicated for caudal mandibular and maxillary fractures and TMJ injury.

iii. Magnetic resonance imaging—Preferred imaging technique for assessment of soft tissue trauma such as intracranial structures.

3. DENTOALVEOLAR TRAUMA

a. Anatomy and physiology of the tooth and periodontal tissues (Figure 16.1):

i. Gingiva protects the connective tissue attachment apparatus of the tooth. Periodontal ligament attaches the tooth to the bone and acts as shock absorber. Alveolar bone surrounds the alveolar socket.

ii. The dental hard tissues are enamel (covering the crown), cementum (covering the root), and dentin (representing the bulk of hard substance between the enamel and cementum and the pulp).

iii. The pulp is situated in the pulp cavity, which consists of the pulp chamber in the crown and the root canal in the root(s). Odontoblasts line the inside of the pulp cavity, producing predentin that later becomes mineralized dentin.

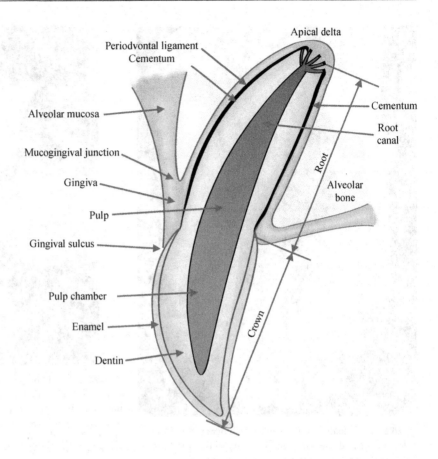

FIGURE 16.1 Anatomy of the tooth and periodontal tissues.

iv. The innermost dentin is the "youngest", and the outermost dentin is the "oldest" produced dentin. Dentin apposition along the inside of the pulp cavity continues throughout life of permanent teeth, unless irreversible pulpitis or pulp necrosis occurs. Therefore, healthy teeth of young adult animals have a fairly wide pulp cavity, while that of old animals is narrow.

v. Comparing the radiographic appearance of the root canal width between ipsi- and contralateral teeth is a very effective means to determine pulp vitality of teeth with suspected endodontic pathology. A nonvital tooth (necrotic pulp) stops producing dentin. Thus, its pulp cavity will appear larger compared to that of vital teeth of similar size (Figure 16.2).

vi. Periapical pathology results when pulpal infection and inflammation extend through the apical foramina into the periapical region of the tooth.

b. Tooth wear:

i. Usually a slow process that can expose dentin but allows the pulp to respond with formation of dentinal sclerosis and reparative (tertiary) dentin; rapid tooth wear removes enamel and dentin faster than odontoblasts in the pulp cavity can form dentin; pulp exposure is diagnosed visually and confirmed by palpation with a pointed dental instrument that "falls" into an opening of the tooth; an open pulp cavity may reveal pink soft tissue (recent exposure) or dark necrotic tissue (old exposure) at the worn tooth surface (Figure 16.3).

ii. Causes:

1. Attrition—Caused by contact of a tooth with another tooth (e.g., a maloccluding tooth contacts another tooth when the mouth is closed).

2. Abrasion—Caused by contact of a tooth with objects of non-oral origin (e.g., chronic chewing on abrasive materials); police dogs are prone to fracture of canine

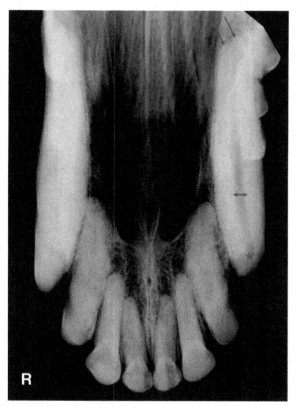

FIGURE 16.2   Radiograph obtained with dental film from a dog. Compared with the right maxillary canine tooth, the left maxillary canine tooth shows periapical radiolucency and apical root resorption (small arrows), a relatively large pulp cavity (double-ended arrow), and a structural crown defect (asterisk), indicating that the left maxillary canine tooth is nonvital. (Copyright 2010 Alexander M. Reiter, University of Pennsylvania.)

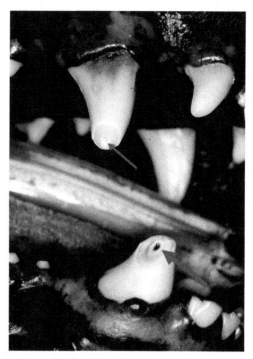

FIGURE 16.3   Photograph of canine teeth from a dog. The right maxillary canine tooth shows abrasive wear of its tip; however, the process was slow enough to allow formation of dentinal sclerosis and reparative (tertiary) dentin (small arrow). The pulp cavity of the right mandibular canine tooth became exposed (black spot) and succumbed to prolonged chronic inflammation (large arrow). (Copyright 2010 Alexander M. Reiter, University of Pennsylvania.)

teeth if their distal tooth surfaces are weakened by wear from chewing on cage bars ("cage biter teeth").

3. Erosion—Caused by contact of a tooth with a chemical substance (e.g., demineralization of the tooth's surface due to acids from silage feeding in cattle, chronic regurgitation/vomiting, etc.).

iii. Treatment:

1. Remove the cause of tooth wear (extraction of maloccluding teeth, removal of abrasive materials, modification of abnormal chewing behavior, etc.).

2. Clean, polish, and condition the defect, and cover exposed dentin with unfilled resin (materials may be purchased from Henry Schein® at www.henryschein.com or Shipp's Dental and Specialty Products at www.drshipp.com).

3. Endodontic treatment is indicated for teeth with pulp exposure, irreversible pulpitis, pulp necrosis, and periapical disease (see p 263).

4. Protect structurally weak teeth whose crowns are at risk of fracture (e.g., place metal crowns on cage biter teeth in active police dogs).

c. Tooth fractures (Figure 16.4):

i. They are classified based on location (crown, crown and root, or root) and tissues involved (uncomplicated = no pulp exposure; complicated = with pulp exposure):

1. Crown infraction—Incomplete fracture of enamel without loss of tooth structure;

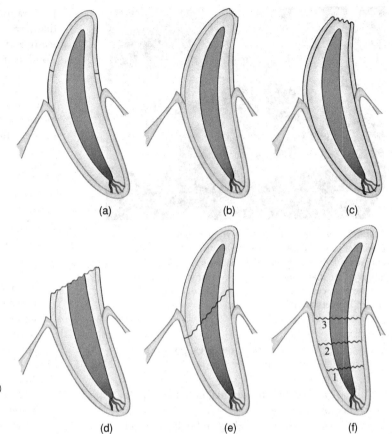

FIGURE 16.4   Tooth fractures. (a) Crown infraction. (b) Uncomplicated crown fracture—enamel only. (c) Uncomplicated crown fracture—enamel and dentin. (d) Complicated crown fracture—with pulp exposure. (e) Crown-root fracture. (f) Root fractures; note that apical root (1) and mid-root (2) fractures have a good to fair prognosis, while coronal root (3) fractures have a poor prognosis.

represents a weak point through which bacteria can challenge the pulp.

2. Uncomplicated crown fracture—Fracture of enamel only or enamel and dentin without pulp exposure; denuded dentin creates a pathway for stimuli to pass through dentinal tubules to the pulp.

3. Complicated crown fracture—Fracture of enamel and dentin with pulp exposure; if acute, bleeding occurs from the torn pulp; if left untreated this always results in pulp necrosis:

   a. Common in canine teeth of dogs and cats due to motor-vehicle trauma, falls from great heights, kicks, and hits.

   b. Common in carnassial teeth of dogs due to chewing on hard objects (e.g., nylon bones, cow hooves, ice cubes); maxillary fourth premolars typically show "slab" fractures where a vestibular portion

has separated from the rest of the tooth (Figure 16.5).

   c. Common in all teeth of cats due to odontoclastic resorption weakening the tooth structure.

4. Crown-root fracture—Fracture of enamel, dentin, and cementum, often with pulp exposure; if a crown-root fracture cannot be made into a crown fracture by periodontal surgery or orthodontic extrusion, the tooth should be extracted.

5. Root fracture—Fracture of cementum and dentin, usually with pulp exposure; the coronal segment is displaced and pulp necrosis may result, but generally the apical segment is not displaced and has an intact blood supply:

   a. Apical root and midroot fractures: good to fair prognosis (splinting and root canal therapy of the coronal segment).

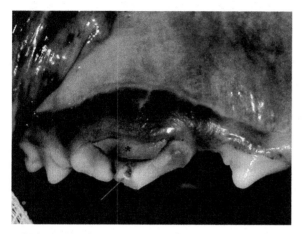

FIGURE 16.5 Photograph of the right maxillary fourth premolar tooth of a dog, exhibiting a "slab" fracture that extends subgingivally. The slab (asterisk) is still attached to gingiva. The main cusp of the crown is fractured off, exposing the pulp cavity (arrow). (Copyright 2010 Alexander M. Reiter, University of Pennsylvania.)

      b. Coronal root fractures: poor prognosis (extract tooth).
  d. Thermal injury:
    i. Causing pulp hyperemia, pulpitis, or pulp necrosis.
    ii. Caused by poor scaling and polishing techniques, restorative cavity and crown margin preparations, careless use of thermocautery, diathermy, electrosurgery and laser units near teeth, and electric cord injuries.
  e. Tooth displacement injuries:
    i. Concussion and subluxation—Normal or slightly increased mobility and sensitivity to percussion, but no displacement; monitor radiographically to determine pulp vitality.
    ii. Luxation—Clinically or radiographically evident displacement of the tooth within its alveolus:
        1. Lateral and extrusive luxation—most common; often associated with fracture of the alveolus (Figures 16.6a and 16.6b).
        2. Intrusive luxation—rare; associated with trauma that forced a tooth into the nasal cavity, resulting in chronic rhinitis and nasal discharge; sometimes noticed in retired Greyhound racing dogs; tooth extraction necessitates surgical exposure of the nasal cavity through an intraoral approach.
    iii. Avulsion (exarticulation)—Complete extrusive luxation refers to a tooth that is no longer situated in its alveolar socket(s):
        1. After automobile accidents, falls from heights, fighting with other animals, or when a tooth gets caught in a fence.

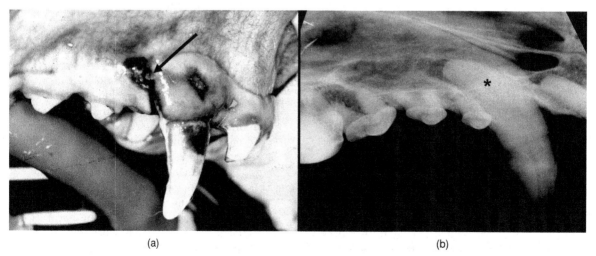

(a)   (b)

FIGURE 16.6 Right maxillary canine tooth in a dog with lateral and extrusive luxation. (a) Photograph; note the lacerated gingival tissues (arrow). (b) Radiograph obtained with dental film; note the extrusive displacement of the tooth from its alveolar socket (asterisk). (Copyright 2010 Alexander M. Reiter, University of Pennsylvania.)

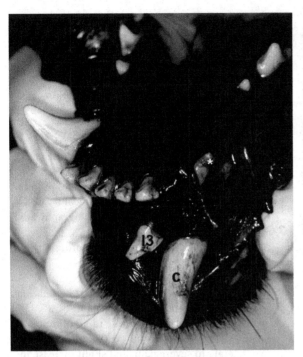

FIGURE 16.7   Photograph of the left rostral mandible of a dog with avulsed third incisor tooth (I3) and canine tooth (C), which are out of their alveolar sockets but remain attached to gingiva. The root apex of the third incisor (asterisk) is visible clinically. (Copyright 2010 Alexander M. Reiter, University of Pennsylvania.)

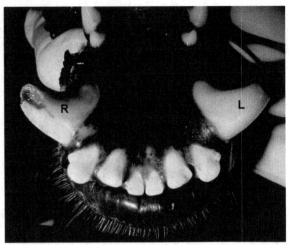

FIGURE 16.8   Photograph of mandibular canine teeth in a dog. The crown of the right canine (R) is acutely fractured (bleeding pulp). The fracture of the crown of the left canine (L) is old (black debris at fracture site). (Copyright 2010 Alexander M. Reiter, University of Pennsylvania.)

    2. The most commonly avulsed teeth in dogs are incisors and canines (Figure 16.7).
f. Clinical signs of endodontic disease:
    i. Crown discoloration—Progressive tooth discoloration (pink, red, purple, gray, or brown) and/or periapical radiolucency can reasonably be interpreted as indicative of pulp necrosis; transillumination may be helpful (vital teeth rather translucent, nonvital teeth more opaque).
    ii. Crown defects—A fine-tipped dental explorer will find irregularities in the crown surface or catch in an open pulp chamber; recent pulp exposure reveals bleeding pulp, while an old exposure shows black debris and necrotic pulp (Figure 16.8).
    iii. Tooth mobility—Directly proportional to the integrity of root attachment; crown-root and root fractures often result in mobility of a crown segment.

    iv. Swelling and sinus tract:
    1. Incipient intraoral swelling is detected by digital palpation of alveolar mucosa overlying the apices of tooth roots and comparison with the tooth on the contralateral side.
    2. Facial swellings and extraoral sinus tracts originating from diseased maxillary fourth premolar teeth in cats and dogs are located ventral to the medial canthus of the eye.
    3. Intraoral sinus tracts usually drain at the mucogingival junction.
    4. Swellings and sinus tracts due to endodontic disease have a history of responsiveness to antibiotics and recurrence when antibiotic therapy is discontinued.
    5. Sinus tracts can be traced with a gutta-percha cone, and a radiograph is obtained to locate their source.
    v. Reduced biting pressure—Noted during eating, play, or training; reluctance to eat hard or fibrous food; preference to chew food on the unaffected side; increased plaque and calculus build-up on the affected side (Figure 16.9).
    vi. Regional lymphadenopathy and fever—With acute apical abscess.

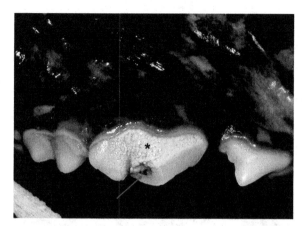

FIGURE 16.9 Photograph of the right maxillary fourth premolar tooth with a complicated crown fracture (arrow) in a dog. Note the increased plaque and calculus build-up on this tooth (asterisk). This may be due to a combination of roughness of the fracture site surface (which then becomes more plaque-retentive) and preference to chew food on the unaffected side (which eliminates abrasive cleansing of teeth on the affected side). (Copyright 2010 Alexander M. Reiter, University of Pennsylvania.)

vii. Pain response—Percussion at the occlusal surface of several healthy teeth and the suspect tooth with a finger or the handle of a dental mirror; pain response may indicate pulpitis or extension of infection/inflammation into the periapical region.

g. Pathophysiology and radiographic signs:

i. Pulpitis—Inflammation of the pulp:

1. Reversible pulpitis—Thermal stimuli (usually cold) cause a pain response that subsides as soon as the stimulus is removed; removal of the irritant resolves the pulpitis.

2. Irreversible pulpitis—This may be acute, subacute, or chronic, partial or total, infected or sterile; acutely inflamed pulp is symptomatic (prolonged episodes of pain); chronically inflamed pulp is usually asymptomatic; reddish cauliflower-like growth of pulp tissue through an open pulp chamber is occasionally seen in young animals.

ii. Pulp necrosis:

1. Resulting from an irreversible pulpitis or a traumatic event that causes long-term interruption of the blood supply to the pulp.

2. Partial or total (total necrosis before it affects the apical periodontal ligament is asymptomatic).

3. Spread of infection/inflammation through apical foramina leads to periapical disease.

iii. Acute apical periodontitis:

1. Painful inflammation around the apex before the bone begins to resorb.

2. Resulting from an extension of pulpitis and pulp necrosis into periapical tissues.

3. May be unremarkable radiographically.

iv. Acute apical abscess:

1. Painful, purulent exudate around the apex.

2. May be unremarkable radiographically (or have slightly widened periodontal space around apex).

3. Clinical signs include rapid onset of slight to severe swelling (cellulitis), moderate to severe pain, and slight increase in tooth mobility; fever and general malaise are present in advanced cases.

v. Chronic apical periodontitis (granuloma):

1. Generally asymptomatic; demineralization of bone causing diffuse or circumscribed radiographically evident lesions.

2. Sinus tracts may yield frank suppuration; as pressure from pus is relieved by drainage or antibiotic therapy, the sinus tract may close temporarily; if pressure from pus builds up again, the sinus tract returns.

3. Proliferation of epithelial rests of Malassez in the periodontal ligament may create a periapical cyst.

vi. Phoenix abscess:

1. Acute exacerbation of chronic apical periodontitis.

2. Symptoms identical to those with acute apical abscess.

vii. Periapical osteosclerosis:

1. Excessive mineralization of periapical bone of a vital tooth caused by low-grade pulpal irritation.

2. Asymptomatic and benign; does not require endodontic therapy.

viii. Condensing osteitis (focal sclerosing osteomyelytis):

1. Excessive mineralization of periapical bone of a nonvital tooth caused by long-standing and low-toxic exudation from an infected pulp.

2. Requires endodontic therapy.

ix. Osteomyelitis:

1. Can arise directly from an endodontic infection.

2. Live bacteria pass the apex and multiply in the bone, resulting in localized or wide-spread infection of the bone.

3. If left untreated, the acute form may progress to a chronic form and bone necrosis.

x. Pulp mineralization:

1. Greatest endodontic significance of pulp mineralization is that it may hinder root canal access and shaping.

2. Diffuse mineralization (often a pathologic process related to various forms of injury).

3. Pulp stones (denticles) that form around epithelial cells remnants.

h. Treatment:

i. Fractured teeth, endodontic disease, and periapical disease:

1. Vital pulp therapy—Partial pulpectomy, pulp capping/dressing, and restoration; primarily utilized for very recent fractures (1–2 days old) of permanent teeth in young adult cats or dogs (less than 18–24 months of age), or after intentional surgical crown reduction; antibiotic administration (ampicillin 22 mg/kg IV q 2 hours intraoperatively; amoxicillin/clavulanic acid 14 mg/kg PO BID for 5 days postoperatively) is warranted, if pulp vitality is to be retained.

2. Apexification procedure—Complete pulpectomy, root canal fill with calcium hydroxide paste, and temporary restoration; to stimulate formation of a closed apex with hard tissue in incompletely developed permanent teeth with necrotic pulp or in fully developed permanent teeth that have "open" apices due to apical root resorption; antibiotic therapy is usually not warranted.

3. Standard root canal therapy—Utilized if the pulp is exposed for longer periods of time (e.g., when vital pulp therapy is no longer an option), has become necrotic, or when periapical disease has developed; pre-, intra-, and postoperative dental radiography is of utmost importance; the goal of treatment is the removal of pulp tissue and diseased dentin and providing a hermetic seal at the root apex (cleaning, shaping, disinfecting, and obturating the pulp cavity); antibiotic therapy is usually not warranted.

4. Partial tooth resection—Considered to be a useful treatment for periodontally and/or endodontically involved carnassial teeth affected individually or in the line of a jaw fracture (retained crown-root segments aid as anchorage for jaw fracture repair devices).

5. Surgical root canal therapy—Performed when standard root canal therapy does not resolve periapical disease; the procedure involves apicoectomy and retrograde root canal filling.

ii. Luxated and avulsed teeth:

1. Immediate antibiotic therapy (ampicillin 22 mg/kg IV q 2 hours intraoperatively; amoxicillin/clavulanic acid 14 mg/kg PO BID, clindamycin 11 mg/kg PO BID, or doxycycline 10 mg/kg PO SID for 4–6 weeks postoperatively).

2. Success of replantation is influenced by the speed with which the tooth is replanted:

a. An avulsed tooth should ideally be replanted within 15–20 minutes.

b. If extraoral dry time was 20–60 minutes, some periodontal ligament cells may still be vital.

c. If extraoral dry time was greater than 60 minutes, all periodontal ligament cells have died, and replantation has a poor prognosis that could lead to the loss of the tooth.

3. If replantation cannot be accomplished within 15–20 minutes, the tooth should be placed in a transport medium until arrival of the patient and tooth at the veterinary dentist. Periodontal ligament cells on the tooth surface may remain vital in:

a. Fresh milk for up to 6 hours.

b. Hank's Balanced Salt Solution (Save-A-Tooth, 3M-Health Care, St. Paul, MN) for up to 24 hours.

4. Prior to replantation, the tooth should be soaked for 5 minutes in a doxycycline solution (1 mg doxycycline in 10 mL lactated Ringer's solution); do not touch the root surface with instruments.

5. The alveolar socket should be rinsed with doxycycline solution; do not curette the socket with instruments.

6. Then the tooth is repositioned/replanted, lacerated soft tissues are sutured, and a splint is applied; in humans, the splint is semi-rigid to allow for physiologic movement (a wire or nylon suture attached with composite to the replanted tooth and two adjacent teeth); in companion animals, the splint may be more rigid to avoid accidental tooth displacement during the postoperative period.

7. In 1–2 weeks, the splint is removed, and endodontic therapy is performed with calcium hydroxide paste fill.

8. In another 2 weeks, standard root canal therapy is performed.

9. Complications:

   a. Dentoalveolar ankylosis (bony fusion between the tooth and alveolar bone) and root replacement resorption (gradual replacement of the tooth with bone).

   b. If endodontic treatment fails, inflammatory root resorption leading to rapid destruction of the tooth is an inevitable consequence.

4. JAW FRACTURES

a. The mandibles, maxillae, and incisive bones contain teeth, with tooth roots sometimes reaching into the ventral mandibular cortex in small-breed dogs.

b. The ventral third of the mandible includes the mandibular canal; in the upper jaw, the infraorbital canal penetrates the maxilla in the area of the fourth premolar and molar teeth; both canals contain a neurovascular bundle, supplying teeth, bones, and surrounding soft tissues.

c. Mandibular fractures occur more frequently than maxillary fractures.

d. Traumatic versus pathologic:

   i. Traumatic jaw fractures are secondary to automobile trauma, falls, kicks, hits, gunshots, and fights with other animals.

   ii. Pathologic jaw fractures are secondary to severe periodontal disease, oral neoplasia, and metabolic abnormalities (e.g., hyperparathyroidism).

   iii. In many cases, both traumatic and pathologic criteria play a role; for example, mandibular fractures often occur after trauma in areas with loss of alveolar bone around teeth due to periodontal disease (Figures 16.10a and 16.10b).

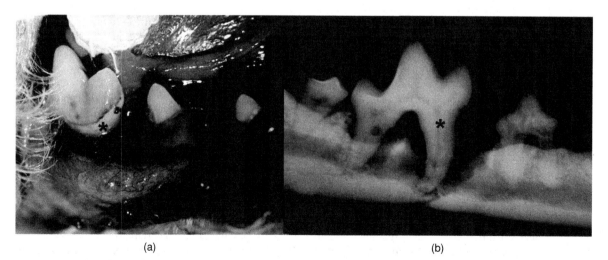

(a)   (b)

FIGURE 16.10 Pathologic right mandibular fracture at the level of the mesial root (asterisks) of the first molar tooth in a dog. (a) Photograph. (b) Radiograph obtained with dental film; note that the fracture site shows severe alveolar bone loss due to preexisting periodontitis. (Copyright 2010 Alexander M. Reiter, University of Pennsylvania.)

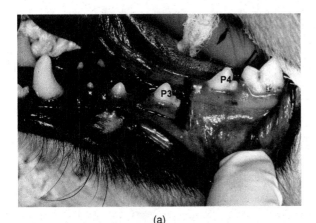

(a)

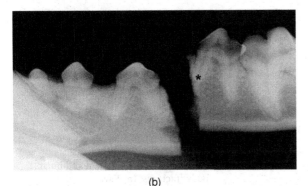

(b)

FIGURE 16.11 Left mandibular fracture between the third and fourth premolar teeth (P3 and P4) in a dog. (a) Photograph. (b) Radiograph obtained with dental film; note that the fracture line runs in a slightly caudoventral direction (unfavorable fracture), also exposing the apex of the mesial root of the fourth premolar (asterisk). (Copyright 2010 Alexander M. Reiter, University of Pennsylvania.)

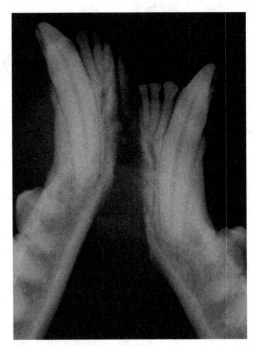

FIGURE 16.12 Radiograph obtained with dental film of a cat with separation of the mandibular symphysis after falling from a window. High-rise trauma patients typically present with head, thorax, and limb injuries. Head injuries include mandibular symphyseal separation and perisymphyseal fracture, fractured teeth (maxillary canines and fourth premolars), traumatic cleft palate, temporomandibular joint luxation, and fracture of the condylar process of the mandibular ramus. (Copyright 2010 Alexander M. Reiter, University of Pennsylvania.)

e. Mandibular fractures:
   i. Unilateral mandibular fractures may result in a shift of the lower jaw toward the side of injury or cause other malocclusion; bilateral mandibular fractures may result in a dropped-lower-jaw appearance.
   ii. Common sites for mandibular fracture in dogs include the region of the premolars and molars (particularly at distal roots of mandibular first molars) and the area immediately distal to the canines (Figures 16.11a and 16.11b); in cats, the mandibular symphysis (symphyseal separation and perisymphyseal fracture) (Figure 16.12) and the condylar process of the mandibular ramus are frequently involved; a bilateral rostral mandibular fracture is sometimes seen with trauma in animals that fall and land on their chin.
   iii. An oblique mandibular body fracture, with the fracture line running in a rostroventral direction, is relatively stable, as the masticatory muscle forces will hold the fracture segments in apposition to a large extent (favorable fracture); a mandibular body fracture with the fracture line running in a caudoventral direction is unstable, as the muscular forces will lead to considerable displacement of the fracture segments (unfavorable fracture) (Figure 16.13).
   iv. Bilateral pathologic mandibular fractures often are considered orthopedic disasters; they sometimes occur iatrogenically upon manual opening of the mouth or during tooth

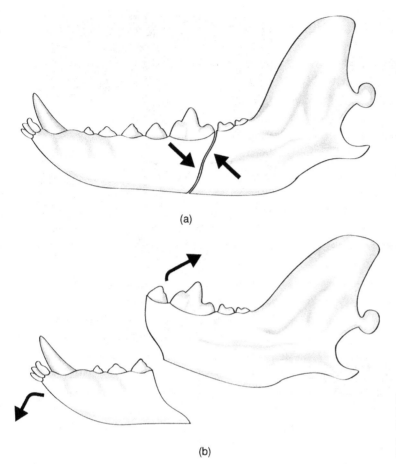

(a)

(b)

FIGURE 16.13 Oblique mandibular body fractures. (a) Favorable, if the fracture line runs in a rostroventral direction. (b) Unfavorable, if the fracture line runs in a caudoventral direction.

extraction, particularly in small dogs with severe periodontal disease.

v. Fractures of the mandibular ramus are relatively stable because the surrounding muscle mass usually prevents gross displacement of the fracture segments.

vi. Condylar process fractures may occur after automobile trauma or falling from a height; they often heal as pain-free and functional nonunion without surgical intervention, but comminuted fractures could result in TMJ ankylosis in immature and young adult cats and dogs; if joint ankylosis prevents mouth opening and interferes with food ingestion, uni- or bilateral condylectomy is performed; the prognosis after corrective condylectomy is guarded to poor if the animal is very young, as the cut bony surfaces are inclined to reankylose.

f. Maxillary fractures:

i. Fractures of the upper jaw are often multiple, may remain in alignment, or may be depressed.

ii. Airway obstruction may be life-threatening in brachycephalic dogs and those that have pre-existing respiratory problems; such animals should be placed in an oxygen cage, the nostrils should be cleaned of dried bloody discharge and kept unobstructed, and ability to ventilate should be monitored (see Chapter 4: Monitoring of the Trauma Patient). Intubation, and/or tracheostomy, to secure a patent airway may be necessary to facilitate patient stabilization.

iii. Epistaxis, facial swelling (edema), pain, and asymmetry are the usual physical findings, with or without crepitus and subcutaneous emphysema.

iv. Fractures of the incisive, nasal, frontal, maxillary, and palatal bones and the bones that

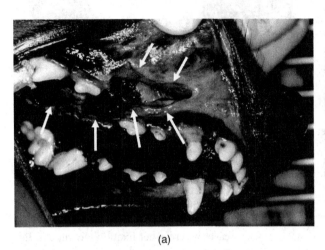

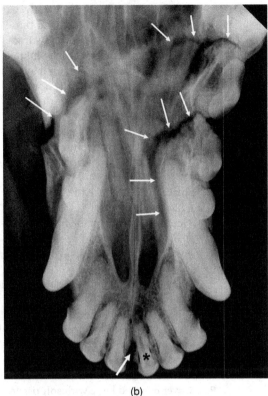

(a) (b)

FIGURE 16.14 Maxillary fractures in a dog after automobile trauma. Note the torn soft tissues and the presence of multiple, comminuted, and unstable fractures of the incisive, maxillary, nasal, and palatine bones, exposing the nasal cavity (arrows). (a) Photograph. (b) Radiograph obtained with dental film; note that the left maxillary third incisor tooth (asterisk) was nonvital prior to the automobile trauma (large pulp cavity compared to other incisors). (Copyright 2010 Alexander M. Reiter, University of Pennsylvania.)

form the zygomatic arch (zygomatic and temporal bones) often do not require surgical repair other than suturing of torn soft tissues; severely comminuted, depressed, and grossly unstable upper jaw fractures require surgical intervention (Figures 16.14a and 16.14b).

v. A common injury of the upper jaw is a unilateral separating fracture of the body and alveolar process of the maxilla, so that the rostrolateral portion of the upper jaw is highly mobile and the nasal cavity is exposed.

vi. Some cats with head trauma present with traumatic cleft palate or a unilateral separation of the temporal bone from the parietal bone.

vii. Combined fractures of the zygomatic arch and the mandibular ramus can result in excess callus formation and ankylotic fusion in young animals, resulting in decreased range of mandibular opening.

g. Teeth in jaw fracture lines:

i. Jaw fracture stabilization and postoperative occlusion are unfavorably influenced by extraction of structurally intact and periodontally healthy teeth associated with fracture lines. These teeth contribute to proper alignment of fracture segments and provide surface areas for anchorage of fracture repair devices.

ii. Teeth with fracture lines extending along the periodontal space toward the root apex have the poorest long-term prognosis; however, rather than extracting such teeth when they are otherwise structurally intact, they may be left in place and carefully monitored for any evidence of periodontal or endodontic pathology.

iii. Severely mobile teeth, teeth with advanced periodontitis or periapical disease, and those that interfere with reduction of the jaw fracture should be extracted, as they may inhibit bone healing; partial tooth resection may be an alternative to complete tooth extraction.

h. Surgical treatment is aimed at repairing hard and soft tissue injuries, establishing normal masticatory function and providing acceptable cosmesis:

  i. Basic principles of jaw fracture repair:

    1. Utilize noninvasive techniques, if possible.

    2. Anatomically reduce the fracture and restore occlusion.

    3. Neutralize forces on the fracture line and stable fixation.

    4. Avoid soft tissue entrapment by the fixation technique.

    5. Avoid further trauma to teeth and other soft and hard tissues.

    6. Properly assess tissue vitality.

    7. Remove diseased teeth and devitalized tissue at the fracture site.

    8. Avoid excessive elevation of soft tissue from bone surfaces.

    9. Cover exposed bone with soft tissue.

    10. Rapidly restore function.

  ii. Techniques:

    1. Maxillomandibular fixation (MMF)—Achieved with adhesive tape muzzling (see description below) or maxillomandibular bridging (bilateral resin bridge that bonds maxillary and mandibular canines or carnassial teeth together); MMF provides proper occlusal alignment and stabilization of caudal mandibular fractures, pathologic mandibular body fractures, or chronic TMJ luxation:

      a. Fitting the patient with an in-clinic fabricated adhesive tape muzzle is an easy, inexpensive, and noninvasive technique that can also be used as temporary first-aid treatment of jaw fractures, when stabilizing medical management is necessary before surgical intervention.

      b. Muzzling provides dental interlock and stabilization of minimally displaced stable fractures (e.g., fractures of the mandibular ramus), fractures occurring in young animals (in which bone healing

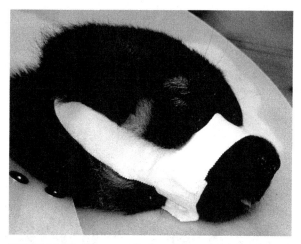

FIGURE 16.15 Photograph of a puppy with bilateral mandibular fractures. Treatment included suturing of torn soft tissues and wearing of a tape muzzle for two weeks. (Copyright 2010 Alexander M. Reiter, University of Pennsylvania.)

happens rapidly), pathologic mandibular fractures (so that a functional, if not rigid, fibrous union is achieved), chronic TMJ luxation, and additional support in cases where other fixation techniques did not achieve optimal stabilization (Figure 16.15):

    i. First, a layer with the adhesive side of the tape outward is formed into a loop, encircling the upper and lower jaws. A second layer is then added, with the adhesive side facing inward, directly on top of the first layer. The muzzle is applied snug enough for the dental interlock to be maintained, but loose enough to permit the tongue to protrude and allow prehension of water and semi-liquid food; the gap between maxillary and mandibular incisors should be 5–10 mm in cats and small dogs and up to 15 mm in mid-sized to large dogs (Figure 16.16).

    ii. A loop ventral to the ears and around the neck is added (also adhesive side out for the first layer, then adhesive side in for the second layer).

    iii. Muzzling in cats and short-nosed dogs is possible by providing an

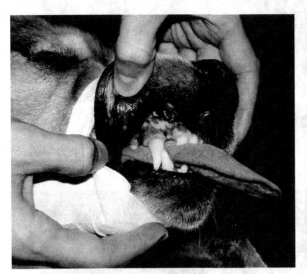

FIGURE 16.16 Photograph of a dog with right caudal mandibular fracture treated with osseous wiring and muzzling. A tape muzzle can provide additional support in cases where other fixation techniques do not achieve optimal stabilization. The muzzle should be applied snug enough for the dental interlock to be maintained, but loose enough to permit the tongue to protrude and allow prehension of water and semi-liquid food. (Copyright 2010 Alexander M. Reiter, University of Pennsylvania.)

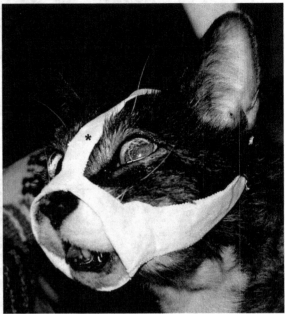

FIGURE 16.17 Photograph of a cat with right mandibular fracture after gunshot trauma. Muzzling in cats and short-nosed dogs is possible by providing an additional middle layer (asterisk) running over the forehead, which will effectively keep the tape "helmet" in position. (Copyright 2010 Alexander M. Reiter, University of Pennsylvania.)

additional middle layer running over the forehead, which will effectively keep the muzzle in position (Figure 16.17); alternatively, the muzzle can be sutured to skin to prevent slippage.

c. It is best to fabricate and discharge the patient with a couple of tape muzzles, thus allowing change of a "dirty" muzzle as needed.

d. Complications with muzzling include dermatitis, heat prostration, dyspnea in brachycephalic patients, and aspiration pneumonia.

2. Circumferential wiring—Involves placing a wire around a bone or bones; the most common indication for circumferential wiring in small animals is mandibular symphyseal separation or perisymphyseal fracture (Figures 16.18a–j):

a. Make a stab incision at the ventral midline in the chin area.

b. Insert a gauge 18 or 20 needle between bone and soft tissues of the mandible distal to the canine teeth (keep the needle as close to the bone as possible), through which a 20 or 22 gauge orthopedic wire is passed.

c. Remove the needle and reinsert it on the other side and pass the oral wire end through the needle.

d. Remove the needle, and while the mandibles are stabilized in proper alignment, twist the ends in a pull-and-twist fashion until the lower jaw is stable.

e. Trim the wire and bend the twisted wire end caudally, so that the skin covers it.

f. Remove the wire in 4 weeks by cutting the exposed wire loop in the mouth, bending up the cut wire ends, locating the twisted knot under the chin (the skin may need to be incised again), and pulling the wire out; leaving the wire in place for longer or overtightening bears

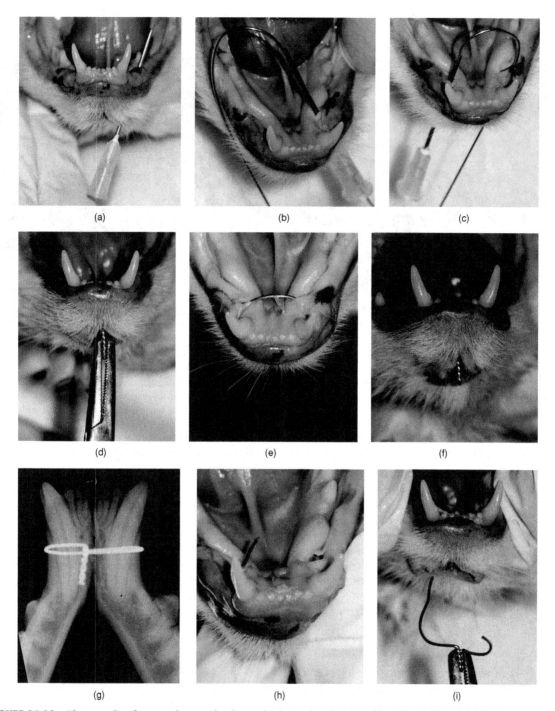

FIGURE 16.18 Photographs of a cat cadaver and radiograph obtained with dental film of cat in Figure 16.12, demonstrating repair of mandibular symphyseal separation by means of circumferential wiring. (a) A stab incision is made at the ventral midline in the chin area, and a gauge 18 needle is inserted and advanced between bone and soft tissues of the mandible distal to the canine teeth. (b) A 22 gauge orthopedic wire is passed through the needle. (c) The needle is removed and reinsert on the other side, and the oral wire end is passed through the needle. (d–f) The needle is removed, and the wire ends are twisted in a pull-and-twist fashion until the lower jaw is stable. (g–h) The twisted wire end is bent caudally, so that the skin covers it. A radiograph should always be obtained after repair is completed. (i–j) The wire is removed in about 4 weeks by cutting the exposed wire loop in the mouth, bending up the cut wire ends, locating the twisted knot under the chin, and pulling the wire out. (Copyright 2010 Alexander M. Reiter, University of Pennsylvania.)

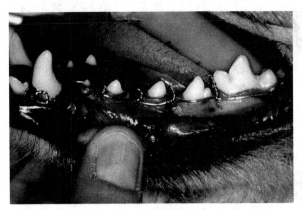

FIGURE 16.19 Photograph of interdental wiring (Stout multiple loop technique) utilized for reduction of the left mandibular body fracture in the dog shown in Figure 16.11. (Copyright 2010 Alexander M. Reiter, University of Pennsylvania.)

the risk of tissue necrosis and exposure of canine tooth roots.

3. Interdental wiring:

   a. Effective alignment of fracture segments is achieved with various techniques of interdental wiring (e.g., Stout multiple loop or Risdon technique), which make use of the dental crowns as anchoring points and provide additional retention surface for splint materials (Figure 16.19).

   b. At least two teeth in each fracture segment should be included into the wiring procedure. The size of the orthopedic wire used in cats may range from gauge 24–28, and in dogs from gauge 22–26.

   c. Interdental wiring should always be performed together with intraoral splint application.

4. Intraoral splint:

   a. Splinting with chemically cured resin (e.g., Protemp™ 3 Garant™, 3M ESPE Dental Products, St. Paul, MN) is an easy, noninvasive, versatile, and inexpensive technique for the repair of jaw fractures when teeth are present for anchorage of the splint.

   b. Interdental wiring should be performed prior to splint application to stabilize and align the fracture segments.

   c. The teeth should be cleaned, acid-etched, and air-dried prior to application of the resin, which is primarily added to the lingual surface of the mandibular teeth and the buccal surface of the maxillary teeth.

   d. Once the resin has set, the splint is trimmed to allow for closure of the mouth and then polished (Figure 16.20).

5. Osseous wiring—Osseous wiring can be used alone or in combination with interdental wiring and intraoral splint application and may present a viable technique of fracture stabilization in edentulous areas of the jaws; disadvantages include need for significant soft tissue elevation and potential iatrogenic trauma to tooth roots and neurovascular structures in mandibular and infraorbital canals.

6. Percutaneous (external) skeletal fixation—Useful in fractures associated with extensive soft tissue injuries, severe comminution, missing bone fragments, and edentulous bone segments; similar disadvantages as for osseous wiring.

7. Bone plating—Provides rigid stabilization of jaw fractures and rapid return to normal function; similar disadvantages as for osseous wiring in addition to high cost of equipment.

8. Partial mandibulectomy and maxillectomy—Performed when extensive trauma, infection, or necrosis precludes reduction or adequate jaw fracture fixation; salvage procedures for bilateral pathologic mandibular body fractures involve extraction of all diseased teeth and rostral mandibulectomy with rostral advancement of the lip commissure (commissuroplasty), resulting in a smaller oral aperture, providing support for the tongue, and permitting adequate alimentation with a soft diet.

5. JOINT INJURIES

a. The head contains three joints, left and right temporomandibular joints (TMJs) and mandibular symphysis.

b. The TMJ is formed by the condylar process of the mandible and the mandibular fossa of the

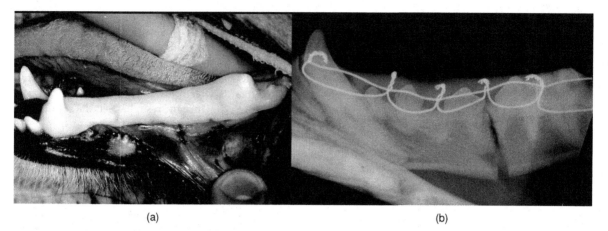

(a)   (b)

FIGURE 16.20   Completed intraoral splint for repair of the left mandibular body fracture in the dog shown in Figures 16.13 and 16.21. (a) Photograph. (b) Radiograph obtained with dental film. (Copyright 2010 Alexander M. Reiter, University of Pennsylvania.)

temporal bone. Bony support for the mandibular condyle within the mandibular fossa is provided caudoventrally by the retroarticular process of the temporal bone and rostrodorsally by a small unnamed process of the temporal bone (Figure 16.21).

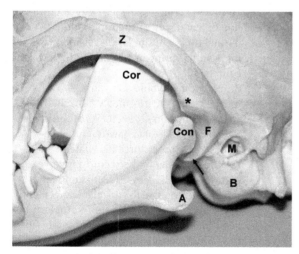

FIGURE 16.21   Photograph (lateral view) of a dog skull, showing the condylar (Con), angular (A), and coronoid (Cor) processes of the mandibular ramus; mandibular fossa (F), retroarticular process (arrow) and small unnamed process (asterisk) of the temporal bone; zygomatic arch (Z); tympanic bulla (B) and external acoustic meatus (M). (Copyright 2010 Alexander M. Reiter, University of Pennsylvania.)

c. Lower jaw movements are mostly in unison, but the synchondrosis at the mandibular symphysis allows independent movements of the mandibular rami, permitting TMJ luxation to occur without fracture.

d. Mandibular symphyseal separation.

e. An animal that presents with a history of TMJ injury may either not be able to open or to close the mouth. Thus, most TMJ disorders and their differentials can be placed in one or the other category:

  i. Unable to close the mouth:

  1. TMJ luxation +/− associated fracture of bones forming the joint.

  2. Open-mouth jaw locking (TMJ subluxation/luxation with coronoid process displacement).

  3. Fracture of the zygomatic arch/coronoid process +/− excessive callus formation.

  4. Trigeminal neuropathy (mandibular neurapraxia).

  5. Neurogenic atrophy of muscles of mastication.

  6. Neoplasia.

  ii. Unable to open the mouth:

  1. TMJ ankylosis.

  2. TMJ osteoarthritis.

  3. Craniomandibular osteopathy (CMO).

  4. Fracture of zygomatic arch/coronoid process +/− excessive callus formation.

  5. Masticatory myositis.

6. Tetanus.
7. Ocular disease.
8. Space-occupying retroorbital lesion.
9. Foreign bodies.
10. Ear disease.
11. Neoplasia.

f. Other clinical signs include pain on prehension and mastication of food; pain on palpation of the TMJ, ear canal, zygomatic arch, and ocular structures; swelling of the TMJ area and surrounding tissues; decreased range of TMJ motion; enophthalmos/exophthalmos; masticatory muscle atrophy; and malocclusion.

g. Radiographic evaluation of the TMJ is traditionally performed with standard medical radiographic film and extraoral imaging techniques (in cats and small dogs, the size 4 dental radiographic films may also be utilized). Dorsoventral (or ventrodorsal) and right and left lateral oblique are standard views; sometimes, it may be helpful to add an open-mouth view to the series:

    i. Dorsoventral (or ventrodorsal): ventral (or dorsal) recumbency; the mouth is closed with the palate parallel to the radiographic film; the x-ray beam is centered between the joints.

    ii. Lateral oblique views: lateral recumbency; the mouth can be open or closed; the joint imaged must be the TMJ closest to the film/table (Figure 16.22); either nose-up or axial rotation of the head, or a combination of both:

        1. Nose-up rotation: Initially, the sagittal plane of the head is positioned parallel to the radiographic film, then the nose is elevated approximately 15–30°. The joint to be examined should appear rostral to the opposite joint and—with the exception of the thin ramus of the opposite mandible—be free from superimposition with other skeletal structures or the endotracheal tube.

        2. Axial rotation: Initially, the sagittal plane of the head is positioned parallel to the radiographic film, then the head is rotated laterally approximately 15–30°. The joint to be examined should appear ventral to the opposite joint and be free from superimposition with other skeletal structures or the endotracheal tube.

        3. Combination of nose-up and axial rotation: Initially, the sagittal plane of the head

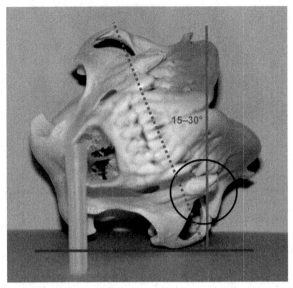

FIGURE 16.22 The technique of obtaining a lateral oblique view of the temporomandibular joint (TMJ) is demonstrated on a dog skull. The joint imaged must be the TMJ (black circle) closest to the film/table (blue line). In the axial rotation technique, the skull is rotated laterally approximately 15–30° (angle between the red line, which is the direction of the x-ray beam, and the dashed red line, which indicates the dorsal plane). (Copyright 2010 Alexander M. Reiter, University of Pennsylvania.)

is positioned parallel to the radiographic film, then the head is rotated laterally and the nose is elevated.

    iii. Open-mouth frontal view: The animal is in dorsal recumbency with its nose pointed upward. The mouth is open with the hard palate and the mandible angled approximately 30–35° to the central x-ray beam, which is directed perpendicular to the radiographic film and passes through the middle of an imaginary line drawn between the two joints.

    iv. When radiographs do not provide enough detail of the TMJ, computed tomography (CT) and magnetic resonance imaging (MRI) may be necessary.

h. TMJ luxation:

    i. With rostrodorsal luxation, the mandibular condyle moves rostrally and dorsally, causing the lower jaw to shift laterorostrally to the contralateral side and inability of the animal to close its mouth fully due to tooth-by-tooth contact (Figure 16.23); the laterorostral shift may

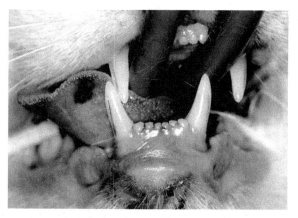

FIGURE 16.23 Photograph of a cat with rostrodorsal luxation of the left mandibular condyle, causing the lower jaw to shift laterorostrally to the right side and inability of the animal to close its mouth fully due to tooth-by-tooth contact. This distinguishes it from open-mouth jaw locking where the mouth is held wide open without contact between mandibular and maxillary teeth. (Copyright 2010 Alexander M. Reiter, University of Pennsylvania.)

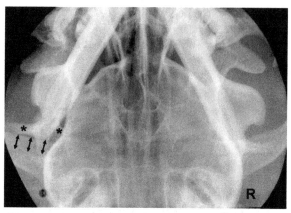

FIGURE 16.24 Radiograph obtained with dental film (dorsoventral view) of the head of the patient in Figure 16.25. Note the rostral displacement of the left mandibular condyle (asterisks point toward lateral and medial poles of the condyle) and increased width of the left temporomandibular joint space (double-ended arrows). (Copyright 2010 Alexander M. Reiter, University of Pennsylvania.)

go unnoticed in cats and dogs with large upper lips, obscuring visualization of the oral orifice, or if the mandibular body also is fractured.

ii. Cats have a higher incidence of luxation due to decreased mandibular symphyseal movement and shorter jaw length, compared to dogs.

iii. The well, developed retroarticular process resists caudal displacement of the mandibular condyle; fracture of this process may be obligatory for caudal luxation to occur.

iv. A dorsoventral radiographic view best demonstrates luxation, revealing increased width of the joint space and rostral displacement of the mandibular condyle (Figure 16.24).

v. Acute treatment—Reduction of luxation is obtained by placing a wood dowel (pencil in smaller animals) between the upper and lower carnassial teeth on the affected side only (dowel acts as a fulcrum) and closing the lower jaw against the dowel while simultaneously easing the jaw caudally (Figure 16.25); the reduction is often unstable, and a tape muzzle for 2 weeks may be indicated to prevent the animal from opening the mouth wide and reduce the likelihood of recurring displacement.

vi. Definitive surgery—Chronic luxation is treated by unilateral condylectomy.

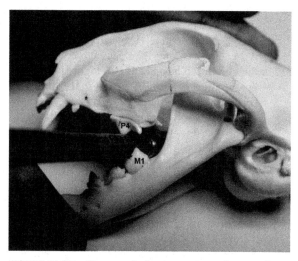

FIGURE 16.25 Photograph demonstrating reduction of rostrodorsal luxation of the left mandibular condyle (asterisk) on a feline skull. A hexagonal wooden pencil is placed between the maxillary fourth premolar (P4) and mandibular first molar (M1) on the affected side only, and the lower jaw is closed against the dowel while simultaneously easing the jaw caudally. The same treatment is contraindicated in animals with open-mouth jaw locking. F = mandibular fossa of the temporal bone. (Copyright 2010 Alexander M. Reiter, University of Pennsylvania.)

i. Open-mouth jaw locking:
  i.   Predominantly reported in Bassett hounds and Persian cats, TMJ dysplasia is a rare congenital or trauma-associated condition, affecting bony and/or soft tissues of one or both joints.
  ii.   Predisposition:
    1. Shallow mandibular fossa.
    2. Underdeveloped retroarticular process and/or articular eminence.
    3. Abnormally angled and flattened mandibular condyles.
    4. Slack lateral ligament.
    5. Excessively mobile mandibular symphysis.
    6. Brachycephalic head conformation.
  iii. Radiographic features of dysplasia:
    1. Flattening of the mandibular condyle and fossa.
    2. Hypoplastic or misshapen retroarticular process.
    3. Widened irregular joint space with periarticular osteophytosis.
    4. Increased obliquity of the articular surface of the mandibular condyle.
  iv.   Open-mouth jaw locking can occur without TMJ dysplasia as sequelae to traumatic events that caused flattening of or excessive callus formation at the zygomatic arch, malunion fracture of the mandibular body, and increased mandibular symphyseal laxity.
  v.   Dysplasia may result in periods of open-mouth jaw locking, with yawning often precipitating an event:
    1. The coronoid process of the mandible will flare laterally, locking onto or lateral to the zygomatic arch.
    2. The animal presents with its mouth wide open; in contrast to classic TMJ luxation there is no tooth-by-tooth contact (Figures 16.26a and 16.26b).
    3. An ipsilateral protuberance on the lateroventral aspect of the zygomatic arch may be palpable and sometimes even visible.
    4. Locking occurs on the opposite side of the dysplastic joint, which will show radiographic signs of subluxation/luxation.
  vi.   Diagnosis of open-mouth jaw locking is made based on history, clinical signs, and diagnostic imaging (radiographs, computed

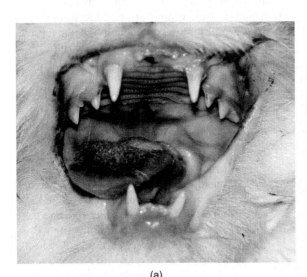

(a)

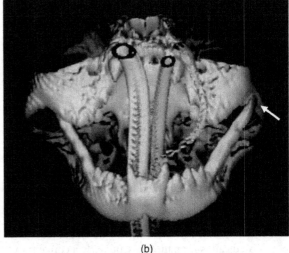

(b)

FIGURE 16.26 Cat with open-mouth jaw locking. (a) The animal presents with its mouth wide open. Contrary to temporomandibular joint luxation, there is no contact between mandibular and maxillary teeth. (b) Computed tomography imaging of the head of the same cat. Three-dimensional reconstruction reveals the coronoid process of the left mandible being locked ventrolateral to the zygomatic arch (arrow). (Reprinted with permission: Reiter AM, Symphysiotomy, symphysiectomy and intermandibular arthrodesis in a cat with open-mouth jaw locking—case report and literature review. Journal of Veterinary Dentistry 2004; 21: 147–158.)

tomography); open-mouth jaw locking may be bilateral, therefore, an attempt should be made to manually "lock" the coronoid process on the previously unaffected side by opening up the mouth and manipulating the lower jaw toward that side, as both sides may require surgery.

vii. Treatment:

1. Acute treatment—Open the jaw even further (sedation may be needed) to release the coronoid process from the lateral aspect of the zygomatic arch, and then close the mouth. Place tape muzzle until definitive surgery.

2. Definitive surgery—Partial resection of the coronoid process, partial resection of the zygomatic arch, or a combination of both techniques.

j. TMJ fracture:

i. Fractures of the mandibular condyle, coronoid process, mandibular fossa, retroarticular process, zygomatic arch, and separation of the temporal bone from the parietal bone are usually treated conservatively, as they often heal by bony union or as a pain-free but functional nonunion.

ii. Comminuted and intra-articular fractures can lead to joint arthrosis and ankylosis; they can be treated with condylectomy, though it is controversial whether to perform this surgery immediately after trauma or once healing complications become apparent; tape muzzles are contraindicated because joint immobility may promote TMJ ankylosis (particularly in young cats and dogs).

iii. Fractures of the zygomatic arch that have been allowed to heal in a depressed position can inhibit rostral movement of the coronoid process (resulting in decreased mandibular opening); treatment entails removal of the offending section of arch or rigid fixation of a fresh fracture.

k. TMJ ankylosis:

i. Causes include TMJ trauma and associated callus formation (particularly a concern in young cats and dogs, with or without fracture of the bones forming the joint) or extensive new bone formation associated with otitis media and craniomandibular osteopathy.

ii. Ankylosis results in a progressive inability to open the mouth, leading to malnutrition, weight loss, dehydration, atrophy of the muscles of mastication, and respiratory obstruction.

iii. True or intracapsular ankylosis:

1. Radiographic features include loss of joint space and mandibular condyle contour and irregular new bone formation.

2. Treatment consists of condylectomy and excision of excessive bone.

3. Prognosis is guarded due to high rate of reankylosis of cut bony surfaces.

iv. False or extracapsular ankylosis:

1. An example of extracapsular ankylosis would be fusion between a fractured zygomatic arch and coronoid process without TMJ involvement.

2. Surgical treatment depends on the nature and location of the lesion.

6. **PALATE TRAUMA**

a. Defects of the hard and soft palate can be congenital or acquired after birth.

b. Palate defects acquired after birth—Usually located in the hard palate; resulting from chronic infection (e.g., severe periodontal disease), trauma (e.g., falls from great heights, electric cord and gunshot injury, dog bites, foreign body penetration, and pressure wounds from malocclusion), neoplasia, and surgical and radiation therapy; leading to nasal discharge, sneezing, chronic rhinitis, and occasionally aspiration pneumonia:

i. Acute oronasal fistula following tooth extraction is diagnosed by direct visualization of the nasal cavity and hemorrhage at the ipsilateral nostril; chronic oronasal fistula is a common result of loss of incisive and maxillary bone associated with severe periodontal disease, typically in the area of a canine tooth.

ii. Traumatic cleft palate (Figures 16.27a and 16.27b) is a midline cleft of the hard palate usually associated with falls from heights (e.g., high-rise syndrome in cats); although some of these clefts (if they are very narrow) could heal spontaneously in 2–4 weeks with conservative management, the benefit of initial surgical management outweighs the risk of developing a persistent palate defect.

iii. Electric cord injury occurs most often in young animals, with burns often progressing deep into tissue along pathways of current flow; life-threatening complications are

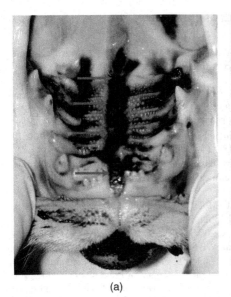
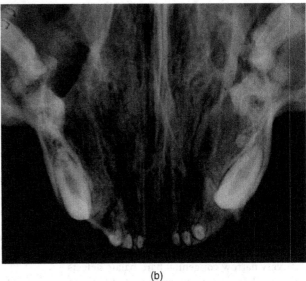

(a)   (b)

FIGURE 16.27   Cat with traumatic cleft palate. (a) Photograph; very narrow traumatic clefts may sometimes heal sponta-neously with conservative management; however, the benefit of immediate surgical repair outweighs the risk of developing a persistent palate defect. (b) Radiograph obtained with dental film, showing separation of bones of the hard palate. (Copy-right 2010 Alexander M. Reiter, University of Pennsylvania.)

usually related to neurogenic pulmonary edema or smoke inhalation; initially, the patient is managed conservatively (wound lavage and antibiotic therapy), and the injured tissues are left to necrose so that the maximum amount of tissue is retained; once the necrotic tissue is evident, conservative debridement may be initi-ated; necrosis of the hard palate is common, and oronasal defects require further surgery.

iv. Gunshot injury can be devastating, with bullets damaging tissue in three ways: lacer-ation and crushing, shock waves, and cavita-tion; shotguns impart a uniquely destructive force at close range, causing shattered bones and progressive vascular compromise of soft tissue; acute care considerations include air-way compromise and substantial hemorrhage; initial surgical treatment involves removal of necrotic hard and soft tissues and missile frag-ments; however, definitive palate repair is often delayed until viable tissues have determined themselves.

v. Palate injuries from dog bites, foreign body penetration, and maloccluding teeth are care-fully debrided prior to surgical repair.

c. The choice of surgical repair of palate defects depends on the location and size of the defect and the amount of tissue available for flap procedures:

i. Principles of palate surgery:

1. The best chance of success is with the first procedure.

2. Teeth at the surgical site and those that could traumatize flaps should be extracted.

3. Electrocoagulation for hemostasis should be avoided.

4. Flaps must be made larger than the defect they will cover.

5. Blood supply must be retained to the flaps.

6. Flaps should be handled as carefully as possible.

7. Connective tissue surfaces or cut edges should be sutured together.

8. A two-layer closure should be provided if practical.

9. Suture lines should not be located over a void if possible.

10. Closure under tension must be avoided.

ii. Techniques—Successful repair of palate defects is best performed by an experienced oral surgeon. Therefore, early referral is advised rather than making attempts at closure that could further compromise viability of available tissue:

1. Advancement flap—Usually sufficient to close an oronasal fistula in the area of an extracted or missing tooth.

2. Overlapping double flap—Preferred technique for repair of congenital primary and secondary hard palate defects; minimal tension on the suture line, which is not located directly over the defect; area of opposing connective tissue is large, which results in a stronger scar.

3. Medially positioned double flap (usually with uni- or bilateral releasing incisions along the dental arch)—May be utilized for very narrow congenital hard palate defects, soft cleft palates, or traumatic cleft palates that did not heal.

4. Modified split palatal U-flap—Useful for large caudal hard palate defects.

5. Combinations of advancement, rotation, transposition, overlapping, and axial pattern flaps, which are created from available palatal and vestibular mucosa and sutured across the defect 6–8 weeks following extraction of several teeth.

6. Tongue flap—The edges of the dorsal aspect of the tongue are excised and apposed to the debrided edges of the palatal defect; the tongue is separated from the palate several weeks later, leaving enough tongue tissue with the palate to close the defect without tension.

7. Myoperitoneal free flaps.

8. Permanent or removable silicone or acrylic obturator.

BIBLIOGRAPHY

Booth PW, Schendel SA, Hausamen J-E. *Maxillofacial Surgery*. Churchill Livingstone, Elsevier, St. Louis, 2007.

Cohen S, Burns RC. *Pathways of the Pulp*. Mosby, Philadelphia, PA, 2002.

DeForge DH, Colmery BH. *An Atlas of Veterinary Dental Radiology*. Iowa State University Press, Ames, 2000.

Degner DA, Lanz OI, Walshaw R. Myoperitoneal microvascular free flaps in dogs: an anatomical study and a clinical case report. *Veterinary Surgery* 1996; 25: 463–470.

Evans HE. *Miller's Anatomy of the Dog*. WB Saunders, Philadelphia, PA, 1993.

Fonseca RJ, Walker RV, Betts NJ. *Oral and Maxillofacial Trauma*. WB Saunders, Elsevier, Philadelphia, PA, 2005.

Gorrel C, Penman S, Emily P. *Handbook of Small Animal Oral Emergencies*. Pergamon Press, Oxford, U.K., 1993.

Harvey CE. *Veterinary Dentistry*. WB Saunders, Philadelphia, PA, 1985.

Harvey CE, Emily PP. *Small Animal Dentistry*. Mosby – Year Book, St. Louis, 1993.

Mulligan TW, Aller MS, Williams CA. *Atlas of Canine and Feline Dental Radiography*. Veterinary Learning Systems, Trenton, 1998.

Reiter AM. Symphysiotomy, symphysiectomy and intermandibular arthrodesis in a cat with open-mouth jaw locking - case report and literature review. *J Vet Dent* 2004; 21: 147–158.

Reiter AM, Lewis JR, Rawlinson JE, Gracis M. A case series study on hemisection of carnassial teeth in client-owned dogs. *Journal of Veterinary Dentistry* 2005a; 22: 216–226.

Reiter AM, Smith MM. The oral cavity and oropharynx. In: Brockman DJ, Holt DE, eds. *BSAVA Manual of Canine and Feline Head, Neck and Thoracic Surgery*. BSAVA, Gloucester, 2005b; 25–43.

Verstraete FJM. *Self-Assessment Color Review of Veterinary Dentistry*. Manson Publishing Ltd., London, 1999.

TRAUMA-ASSOCIATED SOFT TISSUE INJURY TO THE HEAD AND NECK

John R. Lewis and Alexander M. Reiter

1. INITIAL CONSIDERATIONS: AIRWAY, BREATHING, CIRCULATORY, AND BRAIN ISSUES

a. Oropharyngeal trauma may concurrently result in trauma to other important structures. Therefore, a thorough initial assessment of the entire patient is important. Before proceeding with the oral examination, ensure a patent airway and support the cardiovascular and respiratory systems to help maximize oxygen delivery to the tissues (see Chapter 1: Global Approach to the Trauma Patient). Airway trauma may be the greatest threat to life in head trauma patients, and its treatment should be prioritized.

b. Oral bleeding, if significant, may result in circulatory compromise:

1. If 20–25% of blood volume is lost within a 10-minute period, hypovolemic shock will occur. Treatment of hemorrhage involves intravenous replacement with crystalloids, colloids, and/or blood products, identification of the site of hemorrhage, and control of further hemorrhage.

2. Oral bleeding may also affect breathing if decreased mentation or improper laryngeal function allows for aspiration of blood and subsequent pneumonia. The airway should be protected by placement of a cuffed endotracheal tube until bleeding can be stopped.

c. Head trauma may result in intracranial edema or hemorrhage. Attempts to deal with oropharyngeal trauma should be delayed until the patient has proven itself to be stable, except in cases where trauma is significant enough to result in circulatory compromise or airway obstruction.

2. ANATOMY AND TERMINOLOGY

a. Terms used to describe a location or direction in reference to the head:

1. Rostral—Referring to a location toward the tip of the nose.

2. Caudal—Referring to a location toward the tail.

3. Ventral—Referring to a location toward the lower jaw.

4. Dorsal—Referring to a location toward the top of the head or muzzle.

b. Terms describing a location in reference to the teeth:

1. Mesial—Surface of the tooth closest to the midline of the dental arch, which is the most rostral crown surface of canine, premolar and molar teeth; when referring to incisors, the mesial side is the most medial surface of the crown.

2. Distal—Surface of the tooth that is farthest from the midline of the dental arch, which is the most caudal crown surface of the canine, premolar and molar teeth; when referring to the incisors, the distal side is the most lateral surface of the crown.

Manual of Trauma Management in the Dog and Cat, First Edition. Edited by Kenneth J. Drobatz, Matthew W. Beal and Rebecca S. Syring.
© 2011 John Wiley & Sons, Inc. Published 2011 by John Wiley & Sons, Inc.

3. Vestibular—Surface of the tooth facing the lips or cheek; "buccal" and "labial" are acceptable alternatives.

4. Facial—Refers to the surfaces of the rostral teeth visible from the front.

5. Lingual—Refers to the surface of mandibular teeth facing the tongue.

6. Palatal—Refers to the surface of maxillary teeth facing the palate.

7. Occlusal—Refers to the surface of the tooth facing the tooth of the opposing dental arch.

8. Proximal—Mesial and distal surfaces of a tooth that come in close contact to an adjacent tooth.

9. Interproximal—Refers to the space between adjacent teeth.

c. Terms of specific soft tissue structures of the oral cavity and pharynx:

1. Frenulum—V-shaped fold of mucosa seen most obviously at sites like the ventral tongue surface (lingual frenulum) and the vestibular surface of the mandible lateral to the canine and premolar teeth (labial frenulum).

2. Caruncle—Fleshy protuberance, most commonly seen associated with the openings of the sublingual and mandibular salivary ducts beneath the tongue.

3. Palatoglossal folds—Bilateral bands of tissue that run from the caudal aspect of the tongue to the soft palate.

4. Buccal mucosa—Mucosa of the lip and cheek, which lies against the teeth.

5. Alveolar mucosa—Mucosa covering the mandible, incisive bone and maxilla that joins the gingiva at the mucogingival junction.

6. Vestibule—Trough created by the merging of the buccal and alveolar mucosa of the upper or lower jaw.

7. Alveolar jugum—prominence associated with the root of a tooth palpable beneath the alveolar bone and mucosa.

8. Rugae—Prominent folds of palatal mucosa overlying the hard palate.

9. Commissure—caudal aspect of the lip margin where the upper and lower lips meet.

3. DIFFERENTIAL DIAGNOSES OF COMMONLY ENCOUNTERED HEAD AND NECK CONDITIONS

a. Differential diagnoses of facial swelling: tooth root abscess due to fractured or periodontally diseased teeth; neoplasia; acute masticatory myositis; inflammation or infection secondary to foreign body or bite wound; blunt trauma; jaw fracture with concurrent soft tissue swelling; calcinosis circumscripta; sialocele; frontal sinus mucocele; branchial cyst; and sialadenitis.

b. Differential diagnoses of oral hemorrhage: pathological or traumatic jaw fracture (see Chapter 16: Trauma-Associated Musculoskeletal Injury to the Head); acutely fractured teeth with pulp exposure; hematemesis; bleeding dyscrasias (von Willebrand's disease being the most common); bite wounds; osteonecrosis; severe periodontal disease; self-trauma of oral neoplastic growth; foreign body; luxation, avulsion, exfoliation or eruption of teeth; vasculitis; and stomatitis.

c. Differential diagnoses of inability or reluctance to close the mouth: temporomandibular joint luxation; open mouth jaw locking; trigeminal neurapraxia; malocclusion due to eruption or displacement of teeth; neoplasia; oropharyngeal foreign body; and bilateral mandibular fractures.

d. Differential diagnoses of inability or reluctance to open the mouth: masticatory myositis; tetanus; ocular and orbital pathology; middle ear disease; neoplasia; oropharyngeal foreign body; mandibular or maxillary fracture; and temporomandibular joint luxation/dysplasia/arthritis.

e. Differential diagnoses of ptyalism (due to overproduction of saliva or ineffective swallowing): oropharyngeal foreign body; esophageal or gastric disease; nausea; hypoglossal nerve damage; neoplasia of the tongue or orpharynx; pain associated with an acutely fractured tooth; oral or lingual ulceration; and rabies.

f. Differential diagnoses of exophthalmos: zygomatic sialadenitis; neoplasia; ocular or orbital pathology; tooth root abscess of the maxillary first or second molar; masticatory myositis; foreign body; fractures of the skull; and extraocular muscle myositis.

g. Differential diagnoses of ulceration or irregular appearance to the tongue:

1. Dorsal surface—Viral ulceration (calicivirus in cats); chemical, electrical, or thermal burns (Figure 17.1); neutropenia of any cause; uremia; eosinophilic granuloma complex (most common in cats, arctic dog breeds, and Cavalier King Charles Spaniels); lingual calcinosis circumscripta; Candidiasis; neoplasia (melanoma

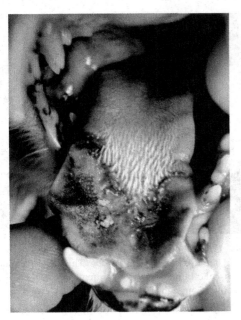

FIGURE 17.1   Lingual ulceration in a cat secondary to chewing on an electrical cord days earlier (Copyright 2010 John R. Lewis, University of Pennsylvania).

most common in dogs and squamous cell carcinoma most common in cats); nutritional deficiencies; vasculitis; hypoglossal nerve damage (wrinkled, curved appearance to tongue); *Actinomyces* infection; foreign bodies(plant, wood or other); hairy tongue.
2. Laterodorsal surface—Calcinosis circumscripta; eosinophilic granuloma; uremia; and stomatitis due to autoimmune or immune-mediated origin.

3. Sublingual or frenulum area—Tongue chewing lesions; ranula; and linear foreign body.
4. Size—bird tongue (microglossia); macroglossia.
h. Generalized ulceration or randomly scattered lesions of oral cavity and/or lips—Neutropenia; vasculitis; uremia; leptospirosis; toxic epidermal necrolysis; pemphigus vulgaris; bullous pemphigoid; systemic lupus erythematosus; and discoid lupus erythematosus.

4. **LIP AVULSION**
   a. Signalment: More common in cats than dogs.
   b. Location: Lower lip is more commonly affected than upper lip (Figure 17.2a). The most rostral extent of the lower lip is often involved, but the avulsion may extend caudally to include the lip ventral to the premolars or molars bilaterally. Unilateral lesions may occur but are rare.
   c. Etiology: Mostly in cats that have sustained vehicular trauma or have been stepped on (soft tissue of the lip becomes entrapped under foot, and the animal instinctively pulls its head away, resulting in a tear of the mucosa at its thinnest point, the mucogingival junction).
   d. Treatment:
   1. These wounds should not be allowed to heal by second intention due to contracture and long-term exposure of the underlying bone. The mouth has excellent blood supply, so closure of even chronic lip avulsions is possible after appropriate lavage and debridement.
   2. Physiologic saline or dilute chlorhexidine digluconate (0.12%) is used liberally to remove debris and minimize bacterial contamination.

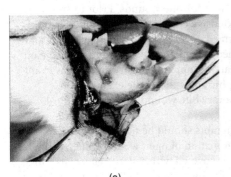

(a)

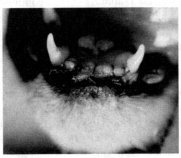

(b)

FIGURE 17.2   Avulsion of the lower lip in a cat. Subcutaneous sutures are placed that engage the intermandibular and symphyseal soft tissue to minimize dead space (a). Deep simple interrupted interdental sutures are placed (b) (Copyright 2010 John R. Lewis, University of Pennsylvania).

3. The subcutaneous tissue and the soft tissue overlying the bone are debrided with a scalpel blade or bone curette.

4. Simple interrupted or horizontal mattress subcutaneous sutures engage the periosteum, intermandibular, and symphyseal soft tissue and are placed with 2–0 to 4–0 absorbable monofilament (Figure 17.2b). These sutures are necessary to reduce dead space and minimize the likelihood of dehiscence.

5. Once the dead space is eliminated at the caudal extent of the defect, the rostral extent adjacent to the incisors is closed with 2–0 to 4–0 absorbable monofilament suture, which is often placed interdentally, circumdentally, or transosseously in a simple interrupted pattern (Figure 17.2c).

6. Some surgeons advocate using stainless steel transosseous sutures to minimize the likelihood of suture breakdown with the wires tightened extraorally. Stainless steel sutures are rarely necessary in the authors' opinion, but may be considered if first attempts with absorbable monofilament fail.

7. Relying on the alveolar mucosa alone is not recommended since its suture-holding ability is poor.

8. An Elizabethan collar is placed postoperatively to prevent self-induced trauma to the surgical site.

e. Follow-up: Teeth may have been traumatized by placement of transosseous sutures and may require future treatment. Stainless steel or nonabsorbable sutures, if used, should be removed in two weeks.

5. LACERATIONS AND BITE WOUNDS

a. Many of the tenets of bite wound and laceration treatment (see Chapter 20: Bite Wound Trauma) apply to orofacial lacerations and bite wounds, but some differences in treatment exist:

1. Lacerations and bite wounds often create full thickness penetration of the oral mucosa and skin.

2. As in other areas of the body, bite wounds may present as the "tip of the iceberg" and soft tissue trauma is often accompanied by hard tissue trauma. Dogs can generate upward of 450 psi of force with their jaws. The length of the canine teeth in dogs and cats and the strength

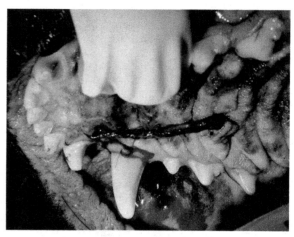

FIGURE 17.3 Puncture wound through the hard palate of a dog due to a bite by another dog. The major palatine neurovascular bundle has been traumatically transected and is bleeding (Copyright 2010 John R. Lewis, University of Pennsylvania).

of the jaws may cause jaw fractures (Figure 17.3) or intracranial trauma. Exploration and/or advanced diagnostics (CT, MRI) may be warranted.

3. If teeth are missing from the aggressor or recipient, diagnostics should be performed to ensure they are not embedded in the soft tissues, nasal passage or trachea.

b. Hemorrhage may be significant in laceration and bite wound patients, especially in cases of multiple areas of trauma resulting in internal and external hemorrhage. Assess each wound individually for the potential of life-threatening hemorrhage. Identification and treatment of hypovolemic shock (see Chapter 3: Shock in the Trauma Patient) is critical.

c. The head and neck region is one of the most common sites for bite wounds. Prior to anesthesia, an extensive cranial nerve evaluation should be performed. Concurrent neck bite wounds and subcutaneous emphysema should raise suspicion of tracheal or esophageal injury and may warrant radiographic and endoscopic examination.

d. Temporary bite wound care in the critical patient:

1. Attempts should be made to minimize the contamination of open wounds. Keep extraoral wounds covered with a sterile gauze dressing until initial assessment and lavage are performed.

2. Cultures of bite wound fluid or tissue may be submitted prior to administration of broad-spectrum antibiotics. Cultures obtained from intraoral wounds or superficial extraoral wounds are likely to result in growth of contaminants.

3. Sterile lubricant may be placed over wounds prior to clipping of hair. Clip hair around wounds if clipping is tolerated by the patient. Cleanse the skin around the wound with warm sterile saline. Perform liberal lavage of lacerations and bite wound sites with warm sterile saline if tolerated.

4. Cover extraoral wounds with a sterile gauze dressing until definitive treatment is performed.

e. Definitive treatment of lacerations and bite wounds:

1. Definitive treatment may not be performed until hours or days after wounds occur depending on the time elapsed between trauma and presentation or stability of the patient. Intraoral wounds are treated differently than skin wounds. Even older intraoral wounds may require only debridement and lavage prior to closure due to the great vascularity and immune defenses of the mouth. Closure of intraoral wounds is often desirable due to the fact that intraoral wounds left to heal by second intention will become contaminated with food, oral bacteria, and foreign material.

2. Wounds should be explored, debrided, and thoroughly lavaged with warm saline or dilute (0.12%) chlorhexidine digluconate. The viability of tissues should be assessed based on color, temperature, and presence of bleeding. In cases of older full-thickness lacerations, extraoral wounds are often left to heal by second intention whereas intraoral wounds are often closed at the time of initial debridement.

3. When superficial exploration provides evidence of significant tissue damage, a skin incision is made over the extraoral puncture site, and the site is explored and debrided. Foreign material and necrotic tissue are removed, and the incision may be partially or completely closed after appropriate drainage has been established. Complete primary closure of extraoral wounds should be reserved for those wounds with minor contamination that are dealt with within 6 hours of occurrence.

4. Drain placement is sometimes necessary if significant dead space has been created by the trauma or exploration. Small Penrose drains (C.R. Bard, Inc., Covington, GA) are often sufficient, and drainage should be directed to an extraoral opening in a location as ventral as possible. Prior to placement of a drain, care should be taken to ensure all severed vessels have been located and ligated so the drain does not act as a portal for continued bleeding. Drains should not be placed to lie directly under the suture line if at all possible. Ideally, drains should not communicate with the oral cavity to prevent contamination of subcutaneous tissue with opportunistic oral bacteria.

5. Absorbable monofilament of moderate longevity is often the suture of choice for suturing intraoral lacerations. Poliglecaprone 25 (Monocryl, Ethicon, Inc., Somerville, NJ) is most commonly used (4–0 in medium and large dogs and 5–0 in cats and small dogs).

6. Aerobic and anaerobic culture and sensitivity of infected bite wounds is warranted, with empirical antimicrobial treatment pending culture results. Appropriate antibiotics for bite wounds include those that provide broad-spectrum (aerobic and anaerobic) coverage. Intraoperative ampicillin (22 mg/kg IV) and postoperative amoxicillin/clavulanate (14 mg/kg PO q12h) may be administered while culture results are pending. Clindamycin and metronidazole may be used in concert with broad-spectrum antibiotics to provide additional anaerobic coverage. Cat bites are more likely to become infected based on deep inoculation of *Pasteurella multocida*, *Bacteroides* and *Fusobacterium* spp.

6. OROPHARYNGEAL FOREIGN BODIES

a. Signalment: Foreign bodies are more common in dogs than cats, with younger animals more commonly affected.

b. Clinical signs: Dogs may present with clinical signs of pawing at the face, swelling in the intermandibular or neck region, retching, or gagging. Occasionally, pyrexia, depression, and dehydration may be seen. Cats may present with gagging or vomiting due to a linear foreign body. Ptyalism (either clear or blood tinged saliva), decreased appetite and decreased water intake may be seen

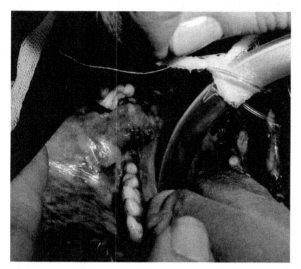

FIGURE 17.4 Sutured laceration showing a common location for lodging of oropharyngeal foreign bodies (Copyright 2010 John R. Lewis, University of Pennsylvania).

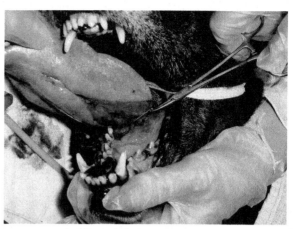

FIGURE 17.5 Linear foreign body in a 10-year-old dog presenting for dysphagia and vomiting (Copyright 2010 John R. Lewis, University of Pennsylvania).

in both species. Draining sinus tracts may be seen intraorally or extraorally.

c. Location: Dogs that chew on wooden sticks or bones may have a sharp piece lodged in the area of the palatoglossal folds, lateral to the base of the tongue and medial to the ramus or condyle of the mandible (Figure 17.4). Sticks may become lodged between the left and right maxillary fourth premolar teeth. Cats often ingest linear foreign bodies that wrap around the base of the tongue, creating sublingual edema that obscures the foreign body. Dogs may also be affected by linear foreign bodies, but less commonly (Figure 17.5).

d. Diagnostics: Since many foreign bodies (especially wood) are not radiopaque, head and neck radiographs may not allow for diagnosis of a foreign body. Advanced diagnostics such as CT scan and MRI are often more helpful in ruling out other differentials and pinpointing the exact location of a foreign body.

e. Approach:

  1. Some foreign bodies such as those lodged between the maxillary arcades may be easily removed with sedation of the patient.

  2. If a foreign body can be visualized and removed intraorally, the site may be lavaged, debrided, and often closed primarily to prevent food, hair and plaque accumulation within the wound.

  3. Sometimes, the intraoral puncture wound has healed by the time the patient presents with clinical signs. In these cases, the surgical approach is decided based on diagnostics that reveal the most direct route for retrieval of the foreign body with minimal consequences on the patient. Since small objects may be difficult to find, CT or ultrasound guided injection of methylene blue dye (0.1–0.2 mL) may allow for easier dissection and location of the foreign body. A common mistake is excessive injection of dye, which may diffuse into the surrounding area and defeat the desired purpose.

  4. The best approach to foreign bodies lodged medial to the mandibular condyle is often via an extraoral approach through the ventral neck.

f. Embedded foreign bodies that require surgical retrieval usually warrant aerobic and anaerobic culture and sensitivity of wounds, with empirical antimicrobial treatment prior to culture results. Appropriate antibiotics should provide anaerobic coverage (penicillins, clindamycin, and metronidazole) to deal with opportunistic oral organisms. Intraoperative ampicillin (22 mg/kg IV) and postoperative amoxicillin/clavulanate (14 mg/kg PO q12h) may be administered while culture results are pending.

g. Follow-up: Foreign bodies lodged between teeth may cause damage to the supporting structures of the teeth referred to as the periodontium. These teeth should be monitored for periodontal pocket formation, gingival recession, and loss of pulp vitality.

h. Client education: Clients should be made aware that oropharyngeal foreign bodies can be difficult to diagnose (especially if not radiopaque) and treat. Multiple surgeries may be necessary to resolve the problem.

7. **Projectile trauma:**

a. Human-animal interactions involving projectiles (bullets, arrows, slingshots, etc.) may occur due to malicious acts or result from mistaken identity. When this type of trauma involves the head and neck, the patient must be evaluated for life-threatening changes in airway, breathing, circulation, and mentation. Most patients do not require immediate anesthetic procedures and can be serially monitored for residual effects from trauma. However, some patients may need to be sedated or anesthetized immediately after presenting if hemorrhage is significant enough to adversely affect circulation in spite of more conservative efforts.

b. Ballistics: The kinetic energy of the projectile and its ability to transfer that energy dictates the severity of damage. Velocity is the most significant factor in determining the amount of kinetic energy and therefore the severity of the wound. Ballistic shape, diameter, and deformation upon impact also affect the degree of damage due to the fact that rapid deceleration causes increased energy transfer to the tissues. Bones, teeth, and tissues can become secondary projectiles (Figure 17.6). Low-velocity (less than 2000 feet per second) projectiles produce a predictable amount of damage along and immediately adjacent to the bullet tract. However, high-velocity projectiles are able to cause shock waves and cavitation, particularly in tissues with high water content (such as the oropharynx). Blood vessels remote from the bullet's course may be disrupted, and wide separation of fascial planes may occur. Although it is common for the entrance wound to be small and the exit wound to be devastatingly large, this does not hold true in every case. This is explained by yaw, which is deviation of the bullet from the longitudinal axis of its line of flight. Since deceleration varies as the square of the angle of yaw, a high-velocity bullet may be slowed abruptly when impacting the tissues, causing enormous energy transfer and destruction. The forces

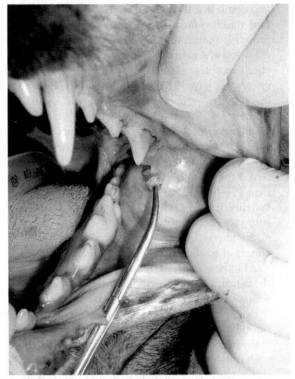

FIGURE 17.6 A hard structure was palpated emerging from the left buccal mucosa in a dog suffering a gunshot trauma to the right mandible. Exploration revealed a piece of tooth that became a secondary projectile after being hit by the bullet (Copyright 2010 John R. Lewis, University of Pennsylvania).

of spin may still be moving, and the bullet may reestablish point-on flight before exiting the body.

c. Bullets: If the bullet does not hit bone, it may exit the body without leaving shrapnel in the body. Wounds presenting on opposite sides of the body or adjacent wounds that appear aligned should raise suspicion of a bullet wound. Bullets often deform on impact, especially if they contact bone or are low-velocity projectiles, resulting in fragmentation of the bullet. Contrary to popular belief, bullets are not sterilized by the gases of combustion upon being fired. Hair, skin, bone, and tooth fragments may be dragged into the cavity and contaminate the bullet tract with bacteria. The bullet tract should be explored and the main fragments removed during exploration if removal poses no additional risk to the patient. Every small fragment does not need to be removed. Lead fragments within a joint should be removed, as this may result in arthritis, and rarely, systemic absorption of lead. Similarly, patients that have incurred projectile trauma to the head and neck should have chest and abdominal radiographs performed to check for shrapnel in the chest or abdomen. Dogs or cats that have been shot in the mouth often ingest bullet fragments, which is more likely to result in lead toxicity. Patients who have radiographic evidence of swallowed bullet fragments should be monitored for their passing via serial radiographs, and serum lead levels may be evaluated. Patients with whole blood lead levels greater than 35–40 μg/dL are suggestive of lead toxicosis. Patients that have elevated levels may be treated with succimer.

d. Shotguns: A shotgun shell contains up to 4 ounces of small round metal balls (historically, lead but now replaced by steel). These balls are contained within a plastic and metal shell casing. Shotguns cause trauma only at close range, and in cases of very close range, exploration of the wound may reveal not only metal but also pieces of the plastic shell and wadding both of which are not radiopaque. The degree of tissue damage from a close range shotgun blast may not be realized for days after the trauma. Tissue that looks healthy today may be necrotic tomorrow. Serial debridement may be necessary and reconstruction should be delayed until the full extent of the injury is known.

e. Arrows: Patients that have been shot by an arrow may present with a wound of unknown origin if the arrow breaks off below the skin (Figure 17.7) or if the arrow grazes the patient. Arrowheads designed for hunting often have three "broad" razor-sharp triangular projections that widen further from the tip. These can create a challenge during retrieval of the arrow. Blindly pulling the arrow from the entrance wound or advancing an arrow that has not fully exited is not recommend due to the potential to cause further trauma. Rather, the patient should be prepared for surgery, and surgical dissection to the level of the arrowhead should be done. Once the tip is exposed, dissection is continued to expose the barbs of the arrowhead. These barbs can be removed at the level of the shaft to prevent further injury prior to removing the rest of the arrow. A Jacobs' chuck can be tightened around the tip of the arrowhead to allow for easier manipulation during removal.

f. Projectile injuries are often clean-contaminated wounds that warrant aerobic and anaerobic culture and sensitivity of wounds, with empirical antimicrobial treatment prior to culture results. Appropriate antibiotics should provide anaerobic coverage (penicillins, clindamycin, and metronidazole) to deal with opportunistic oral organisms. Intraoperative ampicillin (22 mg/kg IV) and postoperative amoxicillin/clavulanate (14 mg/kg PO q12h) may be administered while culture results are pending.

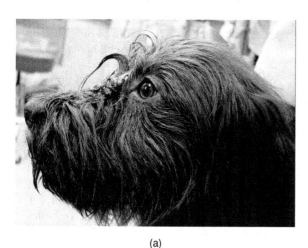

(a)

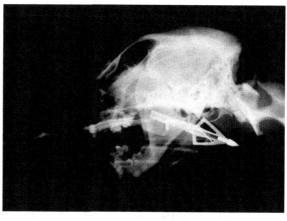

(b)

FIGURE 17.7 Patient presented with wound of unknown origin at the bridge of the nose (a). Radiograph of the head reveals a metal arrowhead and a six-inch fiberglass shaft that has broken off beneath the skin (b) (Copyright 2010 John R. Lewis, University of Pennsylvania).

g. Significant swelling is often seen with blunt or sharp trauma. Cold compresses (10–15 minutes q6h), if tolerated, may help to decrease trauma-associated swelling. These compresses should be continued until swelling has reached its peak, at which point warm compresses may be placed.

h. Client education: Clients should be made aware that the full extent of damage caused by projectile wounds may not be immediately apparent. Multiple surgeries may be necessary to remove shrapnel and reconstruct the defect. Unexpected dehiscence may occur due to tissue devitalization, especially in cases of high-velocity projectiles.

8. **Sialocele:**

a. Alternate terms: Salivary mucocele, or ranula when occurring beneath the tongue.

b. Signalment: More common in dogs (especially younger dogs) than cats.

c. Etiology: Sialoceles may arise from one of the major salivary gland–duct complexes (mandibular, sublingual, parotid, or zygomatic) or from accessory salivary tissue that is distributed throughout the mouth. Experimental attempts to produce sialoceles including duct ligation, duct laceration, and rupture of the capsule in healthy dogs are not always successful in producing the disease state, suggesting that sialoceles may have a developmental, rather than traumatic, etiology. Sialocele is not a cyst, but rather a tissue reaction to extravasation of saliva from the gland or duct. A ranula (sublingual sialocele) may be seen as a complication of rostral mandibulectomy, which usually occurs months after surgery. Ligation of the mandibular and sublingual salivary gland ducts with long-lasting absorbable or nonabsorbable suture may help to prevent iatrogenic ranula after mandibulectomy. A "pseudoranula", a swelling identical in appearance to that of a ranula, may occur within hours of sublingual or mandibular surgery. This edematous condition usually resolves on its own within days.

d. Clinical presentation: Painless, fluctuant swelling may be seen in the neck or intermandibular area. Intraoral examination may reveal a smooth, diffuse swelling beneath the tongue or in the area of the palatoglossal fold. Decreased tongue function due to swelling may result in drooling or reluctance to eat or drink. Masticatory trauma to the mucosa covering a ranula may result in blood-tinged saliva.

e. Diagnostics: When the cervical swelling appears to be on midline, the patient may be placed in perfect dorsal recumbency to determine if the sialocele arises from the left or right side. Gravity will cause the swelling to shift to the affected side. Fine needle aspiration of the swelling reveals a clear or blood-tinged and usually viscous fluid. Pseudo-ranulas may occur after oral surgery due to edema, which develops sublingually. Unlike a true ranula, fine needle aspiration will not produce fluid. A sialogram (cannulation of the salivary duct with a blunt metal or plastic cannula and infusion of a radiopaque iodine contrast agent) is rarely performed but may provide additional information (Figure 17.8). More commonly, CT scan or MRI are employed with the help of intravenous contrast agents, which helps to rule out other differentials such as swelling due to inflammation or neoplasia.

f. Treatment:

1. "Pseudoranulas" resolve after a few days without treatment. Ranulas that arise after mandibulectomy may also resolve with time, but this usually takes weeks to months, and sometimes they may not fully resolve.

2. Ranulas that are large enough to suffer from masticatory trauma should be treated surgically as soon as possible:

1. Marsupialization is a treatment that creates a window in the mucosa overly-

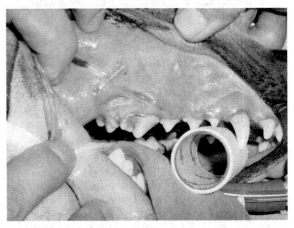

FIGURE 17.8 Cannulation of the parotid duct and injection of iodinated contrast agent allow contrast studies of salivary glands by means of radiography or CT imaging (Copyright 2010 John R. Lewis, University of Pennsylvania).

ing the swelling, allowing for intraoral drainage. This technique is not considered to be as effective as removal of the affected gland–duct complex since granulation tissue may result in closure of the created window.

3. Most cervical, pharyngeal, or sublingual sialoceles arise from either the mandibular or sublingual salivary gland or duct. Since these two glands share a capsule and are intimately associated with each other, removal of both glands should be performed.

g. Follow-up: Intraoperative or postoperative antibiotics are not always necessary for sialoceles that show no evidence of secondary infection. Monitor surgical site for signs of seroma formation. If a drain was placed, instruct client of proper drain care and removal in 2–4 days.

9. SIALADENITIS

a. Alternate or related terms: Necrotizing sialometaplasia, sialadenosis, hypersialosis, salivary gland necrosis, and salivary gland infarction.

b. Signalment: Most common in middle-aged dogs with no apparent sex predilection; the disease has occasionally been documented in cats.

c. Clinical signs: Difficulty eating, decreased appetite, ptyalism, pain, swelling, exophthalmos (with zygomatic salivary gland involvement), lip smacking, frequent swallowing, gagging, and vomiting.

d. Etiology: Unknown. In humans, necrotizing sialometaplasia is a self-limiting disease affecting minor salivary gland tissue, most commonly salivary tissue located within the palatal mucosa. In contrast, the disease seen in dogs and cats usually affects one of the major salivary glands (mandibular, sublingual, parotid or zygomatic) and is often a life-threatening condition. Esophageal disease is often seen concurrently in affected animals, which has raised suspicion of neurogenic pathogenesis associated with abnormalities of the vagal nerve. When esophageal disease is successfully treated, salivary gland disease seems to resolve.

e. Diagnosis: Biopsy provides definitive diagnosis and allows for exclusion of other diseases such as neoplasia. Due to the difficulty associated with biopsy of some of the salivary glands (especially the zygomatic gland), aspirates may be obtained for cytology, which often show inflammation and metaplasia. CT scan or MRI may help provide a

diagnosis in conjunction with intravenous contrast agents. Aspirates may be more productive when guided by CT imaging.

f. Treatment: Surgical removal of the affected glands produces minimal if any improvement of clinical signs. Antibiotics, nonsteroidal anti-inflammatory drugs, or anti-inflammatory doses of prednisone have resulted in favorable responses in some cases. Phenobarbital administration (2 mg/kg q12h PO, which may be able to be weaned after several months) has resulted in dramatic improvement within days of administration in some cases, providing more support for a neural pathogenesis. Electroencephalogram performed on one affected dog showed changes consistent with canine limbic epilepsy, a partial epilepsy of varying symptoms, depending on the part of the brain from which the epileptogenic focus arises. One case that relapsed after eight months of phenobarbital therapy normalized after addition of oral potassium bromide.

10. SOFT-TISSUE TRAUMA OF DENTAL ORIGIN

a. Definition: Malocclusion of various origins can result in trauma of the adjacent soft tissue structures.

b. Signalment: Usually young dogs or cats, associated with eruption of deciduous or permanent teeth in an abnormal location or at an abnormal angle.

c. Mandibular distoclusion (previously referred to as mandibular brachygnathism): Present when the mandible is significantly shorter than the maxilla, resulting in palatal trauma. The mandibular canine teeth and/or incisor teeth place pressure on the soft tissue structures of the hard palate when the mouth is closed. Left untreated, chronic trauma to the palatal mucosa and underlying bone and concurrent inflammation and infection may result in long-term development of an oronasal fistula (Figure 17.9).

d. Treatment of mandibular distoclusion: If mild but significant enough to cause trauma, an orthodontic appliance may be placed to allow the teeth to be moved to an area where no soft tissue trauma occurs. If the degree of mandibular distoclusion is moderate or severe (i.e., when the mandibular canine teeth are at the same level as the maxillary canine teeth rostrocaudally), orthodontic movement of these teeth is very difficult. Partial crown reduction, partial pulpectomy, pulp

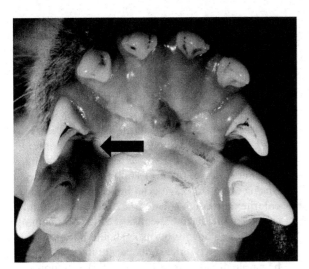

FIGURE 17.9   Palatal trauma associated with a malpositioned right mandibular canine tooth in a dog (Copyright 2010 John R. Lewis, University of Pennsylvania).

dressing and restoration of the mandibular canine teeth should be considered in these cases to the height of the adjacent third incisor to prevent continued trauma.

e. Mandibular mesioclusion (previously referred to as maxillary brachygnathism): Considered a breed standard in brachycephalic dogs and cats. Soft tissue trauma to the mucosa caudal to the mandibular incisors may result from the maxillary incisors. Also, the maxillary incisors may impinge upon the mandibular canine, second incisor, or third incisor teeth, resulting in severe attrition of the lingual surface of these teeth.

f. Base-narrow or linguoverted canines: Base-narrow is the term used to describe mandibular canine teeth that are causing occlusal trauma due to a shorter distance between the base of the crowns of the right and left mandibular canine teeth. The term linguoversion describes a tooth that is in its anatomically correct position in the dental arch, but which is abnormally angled in a lingual direction, resulting in trauma. Both of these situations can usually be resolved with orthodontic movement.

g. Loss of the maxillary canine tooth allows the upper lip to be positioned more medially, which may result in soft tissue trauma from the opposing mandibular canine tooth. This phenomenon is especially common in cats due to the sharpness of their canine tooth cusps, and an ulcerated, recessed puncture may be seen at the mucocutaneous junction of the upper lip. Extraction of the maxillary canine tooth in cats warrants preemptive odontoplasty (minimal smoothing of the sharp cusp without invading the pulp) of the mandibular canine tooth.

h. Tongue-chewing lesions: Normal tissue beneath the tongue can become trapped between the cheek teeth, resulting in thickening and fibrosis of the sublingual mucosa. The lesions are seen most commonly in middle-aged and older small breed dogs and manifest as thickened redundant tissues beneath the tongue. Some degree of ulceration may also be seen depending on the most recent episode of trauma. This condition is often bilaterally symmetrical. If severe or chronically ulcerated, excision of the lesions should be considered. If the lesions are not symmetrical, consider submission of tissue for histopathological evaluation.

i. Cheek-chewing lesions: Similar signalment and etiology as described above. Large lesions may mimic or obscure a neoplastic process. Oral squamous cell carcinoma and fibrosarcoma can occasionally be seen arising from the area of cheek chewing lesions raising speculation of the prolonged effects of chronic trauma in these areas. If severe or chronically ulcerated, excision of the lesions and submission for histopathology should be considered.

j. Iatrogenic trauma may occur during extraction of teeth:

1. Ocular and brain trauma has been documented as a complication of extraction of maxillary molars in dogs and cats. Sublingual trauma during extraction of mandibular teeth (due to slippage of hand instruments or entrapment of soft tissue into high- or low-speed equipment) may occasionally result in edema or ranula formation.

2. Mandibular fractures may occur during elevation of periodontally diseased first molars, especially in small breed dogs where the roots extend to the ventral cortex of the mandible. Even careful attempts at extraction of firmly-rooted mandibular canine teeth in dogs and cats may result in iatrogenic fracture of the rostral mandible.

3. Extraction of maxillary canine teeth may result in epistaxis due to creating or exposing a preexisting oronasal fistula. Closure of the extraction site with a well-designed mucope-riosteal flap will prevent formation of a long-term oronasal fistula (see Chapter 16: Trauma-Associated Musculoskeletal Injury to the Head).

11. CHEMICAL, ELECTRICAL, AND THERMAL BURNS

a. Clinical signs: Oropharyngeal burns may present with a known history of exposure, but oral bleeding, ptyalism, decreased appetite, lethargy, and malodor are often the first signs noticed by the client. Thermal burns are often painful, hyper-emic, and exudative. Electrical burns are often nonpainful and pale yellow. Chemical burns tend to be painful, pruritic, and erythematous.

b. Signalment: Chemical and electrical burns may occur more often in young, curious dogs and cats that ingest caustic chemicals (such as potpourri oil, alkaline cleaning products, etc.) or chew on electrical cords. Oropharyngeal thermal burns are rare but occur most commonly when clients heat food excessively (particularly in microwave ovens) prior to feeding it to pets.

c. Prognosis: Variable, depending on surface area, depth and importance of structures affected by burns. In humans, the head and neck are considered to account for approximately 9% of the body surface area. Patients with burns that involve greater than 20% of the body surface area may develop life-threatening metabolic complications.

d. Treatment of thermal burns: Due to the difficulty in initially assessing the long-term vitality of tissue, reconstructive efforts should be delayed until the tissues declare themselves. Tissues that appear healthy on presentation may become rapidly devitalized in the days to follow. Staged debridement may be necessary. If the patient shows signs of self-mutilation at the burn site due to pruritus or nerve damage, efforts should be taken to prevent further damage, such as placement of Elizabethan collars. Fluid therapy is considered for patients with greater than 20% of body surface area involvement and for those patients where oropharyngeal involvement makes drinking difficult. Fluid loss from burn patients is a result of increased capillary permeability especially during the first 24 hours, resulting in loss of plasma protein and electrolytes. Colloids may be necessary depending on serum protein levels. Nutritional support (total parenteral nutrition, esophagostomy, or gastrostomy tube feeding) is often necessary due to decreased appetite and inability to prehend and swallow food appropriately when the oropharynx is involved. Pain medication is of paramount importance including frequent administration or constant rate infusions of opioids (see Chapter 5: Anesthesia and Analgesia in the Trauma Patient). Systemic antibiotics should be considered in the case of severe burns, sepsis or if other debilitating systemic illness is present. Topical antibacterial rinsing of the oral cavity can be accomplished with chlorhexidine digluconate (0.12%). Although topical silver sulfadiazine is considered the ointment of choice for cutaneous burns, it should not be used in the oral cavity since it may result in hepatic or hematologic side effects if ingested. Use of topical local anesthetic sprays containing benzocaine should be discouraged, since its use in dogs, cats, and humans has resulted in methemoglobinemia.

e. Treatment of electrical burns: Most commonly seen as a result of chewing on electrical cords. Electrical burns may result in widespread thrombosis and delayed tissue destruction since electrical resistance is low within vessels. Assess the patient for cardiac or respiratory side effects such as neurogenic pulmonary edema. Local treatment is similar to that of thermal burns, and staged debridement and reconstruction are often necessary since it may take two to three weeks to appreciate the full extent of the soft tissue injury. Oral chlorhexidine digluconate rinse (0.12%) may be used q8-12h. Fluid and nutritional support may be necessary as for thermal burns.

f. Treatment of chemical burns: Remove offending chemical from the exposed surface of the patient (consider shaving or washing the animal's fur, particularly in cats with chemical burns on their tongues). Acids, bases, and most household solutions may be rinsed with water. Solvents and petroleum products are more challenging to deal with since volatilization of fumes may cause damage to the lungs. If pruritus is severe, Elizabethan collars, sedation, and/or administration of anti-inflammatory medications may be necessary. Oral chlorhexidine digluconate rinse (0.12%) may be used q8-12h. Depending on the severity of the lesions, surgical debridement may or may not be necessary. Fluid and nutritional support may be necessary as for thermal burns.

12. IDIOPATHIC TRIGEMINAL NEURAPRAXIA

a. Alternate terms: Mandibular neurapraxia, trigeminal neuritis, trigeminal neuropathy. Neurapraxia may be the most appropriate term for the condition seen in dogs, which refers to a transient episode of motor paralysis with little or no sensory or autonomic dysfunction. Neurapraxia describes nerve damage in which there is no physical disruption of the nerve or nerve sheath, and the injury is followed by a complete recovery.

b. Description: Trigeminal neurapraxia is a disease of the mandibular branch of the trigeminal nerve, which results in flaccid paralysis or paresis of the muscles innervated by this branch. Unlike the maxillary or ophthalmic branches of the trigeminal nerve, the mandibular branch contains both sensory and motor fibers. Therefore, sensory and motor deficits are possible, but sensory deficits alone are rarely recognized in dogs.

c. Signalment: Middle-aged dogs, with a breed predilection seen in Golden retrievers. No sex predilection has been observed.

d. Etiology: Idiopathic trigeminal neurapraxia has been postulated to occur due to concussive or stretching injuries of the nerve. Immune-mediated mechanisms have also been implicated. Mandibular motor nerve dysfunction may also result from nonidiopathic causes such as neoplastic (e.g., lymphosarcoma, myelomonocytic leukemia) or infectious diseases (e.g., rabies, *N. caninum*).

e. Clinical signs: The patient presents with a "dropped lower jaw" appearance and is not able to close its mouth due to mandibular paralysis. On physical examination, there is no physical impedance of closing the mouth, and the examiner can assist the patient to close the mouth without occlusal abnormalities. Other possible signs include drooling, difficulty prehending food and drinking, anorexia, and weight loss. Concurrent neurologic diseases such as Horner's syndrome and facial nerve paralysis have been documented to occur with mandibular neurapraxia.

f. Differential diagnoses: Other diseases that can cause inability or reluctance to close the mouth include temporomandibular dislocation, open mouth jaw locking (coronoid process of the mandibular ramus locks ventral or lateral to the zygoma (see Chapter 16: Trauma-Associated Musculoskeletal Injury to the Head), middle ear disease, neoplasia, and foreign bodies.

g. Diagnosis: Idiopathic mandibular neurapraxia is a diagnosis of exclusion. Mandibular neurapraxia can be distinguished from other differentials during physical examination based on the flaccid paralysis or paresis of the lower jaw in the absence of paralysis elsewhere.

h. Treatment: No specific medications are indicated. Supportive care is important. Though these patients have normal tongue and swallowing function, swallowing can be a challenge since normal deglutition requires the mouth to be nearly closed. Loose tape muzzles help to keep the lower jaw in a more normal position and allow for easier swallowing. Feedings can be supplemented by placing balls of canned food in the caudal oropharynx and closing the mouth to facilitate swallowing. Patients may require water by syringe or other means to maintain hydration. Administration of corticosteroids does not seem to shorten the duration of clinical signs. Mean time to resolution is usually two to three weeks.

BIBLIOGRAPHY

Archibald J, Holt JC, Sokolovsky V. Head and neck injuries. In: Catcott EJ, ed. *Management of Trauma in Dogs and Cats*. American Veterinary Publications, Santa Barbara, CA, 1981; 53–112.

Brooks DG, Hottinger HA, Dunstan RW. Canine necrotizing sialometaplasia: a case report and review of the literature. *J Am Anim Hosp Assoc* 1995; 31 (1): 21–25.

Gorrel C, Penman S, Emily PP. Soft tissue trauma. In: Gorrel C, Penman S, Emily PP, eds. *Small Animal Oral Emergencies*. Pergamon Press, Oxford, England, 1993; 17–23.

Harvey CE, Emily PP. Oral lesions of soft tissue and bone: differential diagnosis. In: Harvey CE, Emily PP, eds. *Small Animal Dentistry*. Mosby, St. Louis, MO, 1993; 42–88.

Mayhew PD, Bush WW, Glass EN. Trigeminal neuropathy in dogs: a retrospective study of 29 cases (1991–2000). *J Am Anim Hosp Assoc* 2002; 38 (3): 262–270.

Morgan RV. *Manual of Small Animal Emergencies*. Churchill Livingstone, New York, NY, 1985; 119–157.

Pavletic MM. *Bite Wound Management in Small Animals*. American Animal Hospital Association Professional Library Series, Lakewood, CO., 1995.

Pavletic MM, Trout NJ. Bullet, bite, and burn wounds in dogs and cats. *Vet Clin North Am Small Anim Pract* 2006; 36 (4): 873–893.

Pope ER. Head and facial wounds in dogs and cats. *Vet Clin North Am Small Anim Pract* 2006; 36 (4): 793–817.

Rawlinson JE, Reiter AM. Ballistics-understanding and managing maxillofacial gunshot wounds. In: Proceedings of the 20th Annual Veterinary Dental Forum, 2006; 41–45.

Schroeder H, Berry WL. Salivary gland necrosis in dogs: a retrospective study of 19 cases. *J Small Anim Pract* 1998; 39 (3): 121–125.

Slatter DH. *Pocket Companion to Textbook of Small Animal Surgery*. 1st edition. WB Saunders, Philadelphia, PA, 1995; 146–150.

Smith MM, Smith EM, La Croix N, Mould J. Orbital penetration associated with tooth extraction. *J Vet Dent* 2003; 20: 8–17.

Smith MM, Davidson Domnick EB. Salivary mucocele. In: Cote E, ed. *Clinical Veterinary Advisor: Dogs and Cats*. Mosby, St. Louis, MO, 2007; 713–714.

Stonehewer J, Mackin AJ, *et al.* Idiopathic Phenobarbital-resonsive hypersialosis in the dog: an unusual form of limbic epilepsy? *J Small Anim Pract* 2000; 41: 416–421.

Verstraete FJM. Dental pathology and microbiology. In: Slatter DH, ed. *Textbook of Small Animal Surgery*. 3rd edition. WB Saunders, Philadelphia, PA, 2003; 2324–2325.

Waldron DR, Smith MM. Salivary mucoceles. *Probl Vet Med* 1991; 3 (2): 270–276.

Walshaw R. Oral foreign body. In: Cote E, ed. *Clinical Veterinary Advisor: Dogs and Cats*. Mosby, St. Louis, MO, 2007; 405–406.

Wiggs RB, Lobprise HB. Domestic feline oral and dental disease. In: Wiggs RB, Lobprise HB, eds. *Veterinary Dentistry: Principles and Practice*. Lippincott-Raven, Philadelphia, PA, 1997; 482–517.

CHAPTER 18

TRAUMA-ASSOCIATED MUSCULOSKELETAL INJURY TO THE APPENDICULAR SKELETON

Stephen J. Mehler

1. EXTERNAL COAPTATION-PRINCIPLES OF BANDAGES, SPLINTS, AND SLINGS

a. Principles of external coaptation:

   i. Padding:

      1. Comfortable.

      2. Too much padding allows movement of fracture.

      3. Too little padding allows for soft tissue injury (cast disease).

   ii. Functions of a bandage/splint:

      1. Protection of wounds

      2. Absorption of draining material

      3. Compression of soft tissue:

        a. Limits dead space

        b. Limits fluid accumulation (seroma, hematoma)

      4. Stabilization of fractures or underlying soft tissue injuries

   iii. Forces that can be neutralized with a bandage/splint:

      1. Bending

      2. Rotation

      3. Shear

      4. Tension (as occurs with avulsion fractures such as fractures of the olecranon, greater trochanter, and tibial tuberosity) is poorly neutralized by external coaptation:

        a. Internal fixation and a postoperative non-weight-bearing sling is best for these fractures.

   iv. Reduction of the fracture:

      1. Fracture reduction must be achieved before application of cast or splint.

      2. General anesthesia is needed for fracture reduction.

      3. Reduction is sufficient when cortical overlap of at least 50% is achieved and documented with radiographs:

        a. Perfect reduction should always be the goal.

        b. If acceptable reduction cannot be achieved and maintained, then open reduction and internal fixation is required.

   v. Alignment of the fracture:

      1. Perfect alignment of the limb must be achieved with closed reduction and external coaptation.

      2. Complications of imperfect alignment of the limb include:

        a. Malunion:

          1. Rotational

          2. Angular

        b. Gait abnormalities

        c. Lameness

        d. Secondary osteoarthritis

Manual of Trauma Management in the Dog and Cat, First Edition. Edited by Kenneth J. Drobatz, Matthew W. Beal and Rebecca S. Syring.
© 2011 John Wiley & Sons, Inc. Published 2011 by John Wiley & Sons, Inc.

vi. Bandages, splints, and cast should be applied with the limb in a normal standing, weight-bearing position.

vii. The joint above and below the fracture must be immobilized when a bandage, splint, or cast is used:

1. Conventional casts and splints should only be used for fractures below the elbow and stifle.

2. Fractures of the humerus or femur should never be coaptated with routine bandages or splints.

3. Only a spica splint can immobilize the shoulder or hip and the distal joints of the limb:

   a. A spica splint provides preoperative immobilization of humeral and femoral fractures.

   b. Most humeral and femoral fractures require internal fixation.

viii. Soft bandages:

1. Provide moderate weight-bearing.

2. Provide moderate joint mobility.

3. Best used for management of dead space induced by surgical wounding, protection of wounds, and management of limb edema secondary to surgery, inflammation, and lymphatic obstruction.

ix. Casts and splints:

1. Allow for weight-bearing.

2. Immobilize joints more so than a soft bandage.

3. Casts provide rigid immobilization of the limb and superior stability compared to splints and soft bandages.

x. Factors that influence success of external coaptation include the following:

1. Owner compliance.

2. Patient compliance.

3. Patient temperament.

4. Failure to restrict the affected animals activity, failure to maintain a clean and dry bandage, and failure to return for follow up bandage changes may lead to catastrophic complications.

xi. Complications of external coaptation (Figures 18.1a–c):

1. Swelling

2. Skin abrasion

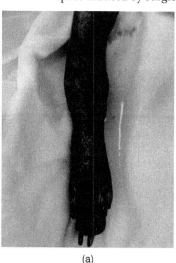 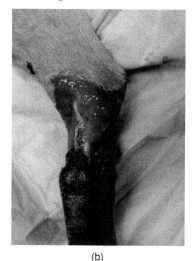 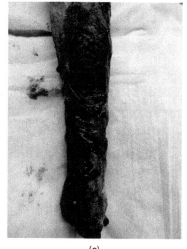

(a)　　　　　　　　(b)　　　　　　　　(c)

FIGURE 18.1 (a) Antebrachium of 2-year-old Maltese that was managed in a splint for a closed radius and ulna fracture. The owners did not bring the dog in for its weekly splint rechecks. At three weeks post splinting the dog presented to the emergency room for malodorous discharge from the splint, anorexia, and lethargy. The toes are swollen, there is severe vascular injury to the limb. Notice the black coloration of the skin. The limb had no sensation, was cold, and did not bleed when cut with a scalpel blade. The limb required amputation as a result of poor splint care. (b) Same dog as in (a). The bandage had slipped distally and acted as a tourniquet at the elbow. There was full thickness erosion down to the ulna. (c) Moist dermatitis in a young Jack Russell Terrier. The bandage had become wet 4 days earlier and appeared to have dried externally. The dog presented to the emergency room for acute lameness of the bandaged limb.

3. Moist dermatitis

4. Vascular compromise

5. Compression of peripheral nerves leading to temporary or permanent dysfunction

6. Limb necrosis

7. Self mutilation

8. Muscle contracture

9. Loss of joint mobility and range of motion

b. Types of bandages, splints, and slings:

   i. Bandages:

      1. Robert–Jones (Figures 18.2a and 18.2b):

a. Bulk provides support.

b. Mild compression reduces swelling.

c. Excellent temporary support:

   1. Preoperative to provide comfort, reduce swelling, and decrease the risk for further tissue damage.

   2. Postoperative to limit damage to the surgical site and to limit seroma formation.

d. Inadequate for primary stabilization:

   1. Cotton padding loosens rapidly after application.

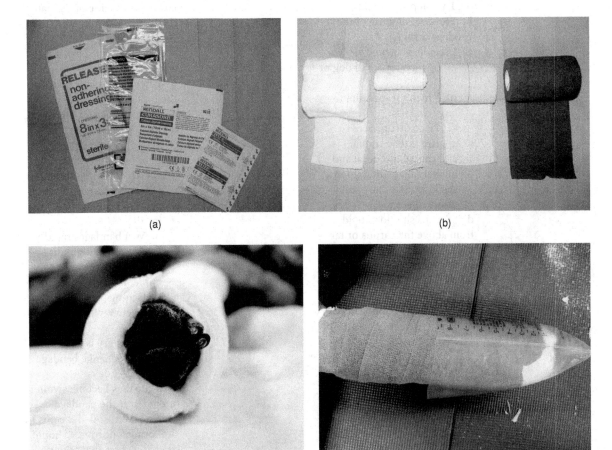

(a)   (b)

(c)   (d)

FIGURE 18.2 (a) Examples of nonadherent dressings (primary layers) for placement directly over wounds and incisions to be placed within a bandage. (b) Materials used for most bandages. From left to right; cast padding, elastic gauze, elastic tape, and flexible self-adherent wrap. (c) The two middle toes should be exposed after applying most bandages, splints, and casts. This allows for evaluation of the toes for swelling. (d) An inexpensive and effective means of protecting a bandage from becoming wet or soiled while the patient is outside is to place an used and dry fluid bag over the bandage.

2. Loosening results in instability at the fracture site.

e. Uses include the following:

1. Fractures below the elbow and stifle.

2. Dislocations at or below the elbow or stifle.

f. Application principles:

1. Extends from mid-humerus/femur to toes.

2. Open wounds are covered with a nonadherent dressing after appropriate wound care.

3. Tape stirrups are applied:

  a. This step is mandatory.

  b. Prevents slipping of the bandage distally.

  c. Use adhesive tape:

    a. $1/2$ inch for small dog or cat

    b. 1 inch for medium to large dog

    c. Two stirrups are applied either cranial and caudal or lateral and medial, depending upon the location of any soft tissue injuries.

  d. Stirrups should extend from above the carpus or tarsus to 6 inches beyond the toes

4. 12-inch roll cotton is unrolled:

  a. Discard the paper insert.

  b. Reroll the cotton.

  c. Divide the roll into six inch halves.

5. Always begin at the toes when wrapping the limb.

6. Roll the cotton from the toes to the axilla or inguinal region.

7. Overlap the roll cotton 50% on itself as you proceed up the limb.

8. Leave the nails of the two middle toes exposed for evaluation (Figure 18.2c).

9. Apply elastic gauze over the cotton:

a. Start with the toes and work proximally.

b. Apply with strong and even pressure.

c. Apply 2–3 layers.

d. If sufficiently compressed, the bandage should sound like a "ripe melon" when struck with a finger.

e. Invert the tape stirrups and apply them to the outside of the elastic gauze.

f. Apply elastic tape or flexible self-adherent wrap to cover the outside of the bandage.

10. Bandage care:

a. Observe toes for swelling at least twice a day.

b. Check the temperature of the toes.

c. Observe toes for abrasions.

d. Keep the bandage dry:

  a. Apply a waterproof boot or plastic sheet (Figure 18.2d) when the pet is taken outside and remove it when brought back inside.

  b. Wet bandages rapidly lead to moist dermatitis and should be changed immediately.

e. Loosening:

  a. Occurs within hours to days.

  b. If surgery is to be delayed, change bandage every 2–3 days.

f. If the toes become swollen or cold or if the bandage becomes wet, soiled, begins to slip, or malodorous it should be changed by a veterinarian immediately.

g. Every patient sent home with a bandage, splint, cast, or sling is discharged with a bandage care information sheet (see Table 18.1).

TABLE 18.1
AN EXAMPLE OF A BANDAGE CARE INFORMATION SHEET. IT IS REQUIRED TO BE SIGNED BY THE OWNER BEFORE THE PET LEAVES THE HOSPITAL.

Take Home Instructions for Bandages, Splints, and Casts

Please follow those instructions checked or circled below:

Exercise: To allow proper healing_____ activity should be restricted as indicated below.

Patient's name

_____Cage rest for_____weeks
_____Keep indoors and allow leash walks only for _____ weeks/months
_____Then gradually increase activity for next _____ weeks until full activity is achieved

Bandage Information:

_____The bandage, splint, cast, or sling should stay on for___days/weeks. It should be kept clean and dry at all times. Put a plastic bag on when walking outside and remove the bag when back inside.

Check your pet's toes twice daily for swelling or coldness.

If the bandage, splint, cast, or sling gets wet, dirty, has an odor, begins to slip, or the toes become swollen or cold, the bandage, splint, cast, or sling should be immediately evaluated and changed by your local veterinarian or referral veterinarian.

Incision:

_____Check the incision(s) TWICE daily for redness, swelling, or drainage. If any of these occur, please call your local veterinarian
_____Do not let your pet lick the incision(s). An E-collar has been sent home with your pet and we recommend that the pet wears this collar at all times.

Medications:

_____

_____

_____

_____

_____

Diet:
_____Normal.
_____Your pet should lose approximately_____ pounds over the next ____ days/weeks/months.
This can be accomplished by_____

_____   _____

_____   _____

_____

Follow-up Instructions:

_____See veterinarian in _____ days/weeks for bandage, splint, cast, or sling removal.

_____See veterinarian in _____ days/weeks for suture removal.

_____   _____

Printed Owner's Name   Owner's Signature

2. Modified Robert–Jones (Figures 18.3a–e):

    a. Application is similar to Robert–Jones:

        1. Less cotton is used.

        2. Or use cast padding.

    b. Provides less immobilization than Robert–Jones.

    c. Contraindicated for temporary preoperative fracture support.

    d. Best used after internal fixation to reduce swelling without rigid joint immobilization.

    e. Most commonly used bandage for soft tissue wounds occurring on the limbs.

ii. Splints:

  1. Reinforced modified Robert–Jones:

    a. Enhance immobilization of joints.

    b. Improve stability of coaptation.

    c. Best uses:

        1. Temporary preoperative stabilization of fractures.

        2. Postoperative external coaptation to protect an internal repair of bone or joint.

    d. Reinforcing material is applied superficial to the cast padding and elastic gauze but deep to the outer layer.

    e. Materials:

        1. Preformed spoon splints (Figure 18.4a):

            a. Plastic or metal

            b. Forelimb:

                a. Will not immobilize the elbow.

                b. Do not use for injuries above the carpus.

            c. Hind limb:

                a. Does not extend above the tarsus.

                b. Do not use for injuries above the tarsus.

        d. Preformed full limb splints (Figure 18.4b)

        e. Advantages include time saving application and there are many sizes and materials to choose from.

        f. Disadvantages include that they are not always a good fit for each patient and are difficult to adapt to changes in the underlying bandage.

  2. Moldable splint material (Figure 18.4c and 18.4d):

    a. Aluminum rods (Figure 18.4e):

        a. Bend to conform to the lateral aspect of the limb.

    b. Fiberglass casting tape (Figure 18.4f):

        a. Refer to casting section for use and application.

        b. Use 3–6 layers.

        c. Apply to the lateral or caudal surface of the limb.

        d. Apply adhesive tape over the fiberglass.

        e. Advantages include a "made for each patient" fit and are adaptable to changes in the bandage.

        f. Disadvantages include some materials being expensive and takes longer to construct.

    c. Orthoplast (Johnson & Johnson, New Brunswick, NJ):

        a. After a thin modified Robert–Jones bandage is placed the orthoplast material is placed in a warm water bath.

        b. Once the material has softened, it is molded to the limb.

        c. Sharp corners are cut or rounded and once the material has hardened a layer of self-adhesive tape is applied over the splint.

2. Spica Splint (Figure 18.5):

    a. Immobilizes the hip or shoulder joint as well as the distal limb.

    b. Temporary preoperative coaptation of humeral and femoral fractures should be applied in the following situations:

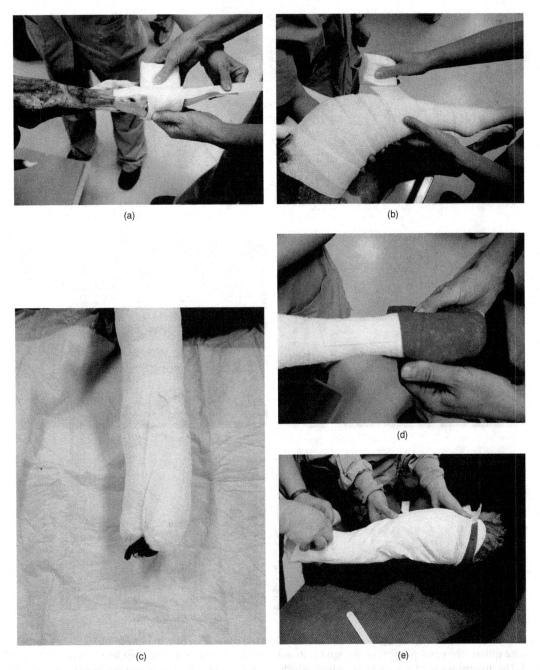

FIGURE 18.3   (a) A modified Robert–Jones is being applied to the limb of this dog after having a tibial plateau leveling osteotomy (TPLO) to help reduce early post operative swelling. Tape stirrups are a necessary component of these bandages by preventing slipping. The first layer of cast padding is applied after tape stirrups are adhered to the foot. Bandage application always starts at the toes and moves proximal. (b) Multiple layers of cast padding is used. Notice the 50% overlap. The cast padding should extend above the joint to be immobilized. (c) After the cast padding and elastic gauze are applied the tape stirrups are inverted and adhered to the bandage. (d) Flexible self-adherent wrap is applied as the third layer of the bandage. Each layer is started at the level of the toes and is applied in a proximal direction. Elastic tape could also be used be for this layer. (e) A self-absorbing pad may be applied to the completed bandage for temporary water resistant protection.

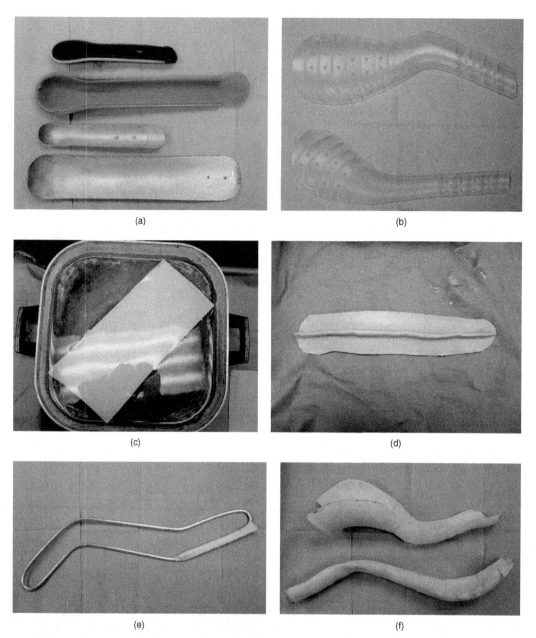

FIGURE 18.4 (a) Preformed spoon splints for the antebrachium. Plastic and metal splints are available. (b) Preformed full limb plastic splints. The upper image is for the hind limb and the bottom image is for the front limb. (c) Orthoplast splint material. The material is placed in a warm water bath, which softens the material and makes it moldable to the limb. It should be assessed frequently for softening. If the material becomes too soft it is difficult to work with and will thin too much to provide adequate support. (d) After being heated the material is molded to fit the limb. The ridge in the material is created to help increase the strength and stiffness of the material. (e) An aluminum rod has been bent to conform to the lateral aspect of the hind limb to supplement and reinforce a modified Robert–Jones. The rod should be placed on the limb between the elastic gauze and outer layer (elastic tape or self-adherent wrap) of the bandage. (f) Fiberglass casting tape molded to the limb to reinforce a modified Robert–Jones bandage. The top image is for the caudal aspect of the hind limb and the bottom image is for the caudal aspect of the front limb.

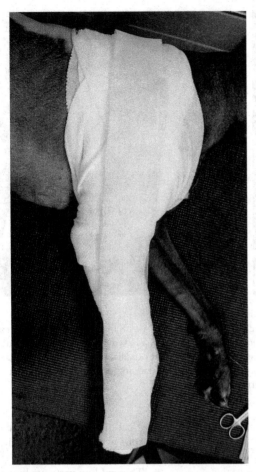

FIGURE 18.5   A spica splint is being applied. Cast padding and elastic gauze layers are applied around the limb and wrapped around the torso caudal to the contralateral limb and alternating caudal and cranial to injured limb. Then, a reinforcing material is applied to the lateral aspect of the limb and should extend to dorsal midline of the shoulder or hip. In this image, fiberglass casting tape has been used as a reinforcing material.

  1. A delay is expected before surgery.
  2. Long-distance transport to a referral center.
  3. To cover a wound in an animal with a humeral or femoral fracture.
  4. When open humeral or femoral fractures are present.
 c. Most femur and humerus fractures can be managed with cage rest and

analgesics while awaiting surgery, as Spica splints may not be well tolerated by some patients due to the extent of patient immobility.
  d. Internal fixation is still required in most cases:
   1. Exceptions:
     a. Humeral or femoral green-stick fractures in young animals.
  e. Application principles:
   1. Begins like a modified Robert–Jones:
     a. Stirrups are not needed.
   2. At the inguinal or axillary region:
     a. Roll cotton or cast padding is wrapped around the torso:
       a. Caudal to the contralateral front limb or cranial to the contralateral hind limb.
       b. Alternating caudal and cranial to injured limb.
   3. Elastic gauze follows the same pattern over the cotton or cast padding.
   4. Add reinforcing material:
     a. Aluminum rod:
       a. Begins at lateral toes and ends at dorsal midline.
     b. Fiberglass casting tape:
       a. Begins at lateral toes and ends at dorsal midline.
       b. Use 6–8 layers.
   5. Elastic tape or flexible self-adherent wrap is applied over the bandage and reinforcing material.
  f. Bandage care:
   1. Same as other bandages.
   2. If applied correctly, this bandage will not slip.
   3. Abrasion development:
     a. Inguinal region
     b. Axillary region
   4. Avoid compression of the thorax.
 iii. Slings:
   1. Velpeau (Figures 18.6a and 18.6b):
     a. Non-weight-bearing sling
     b. Applied to the forelimb only

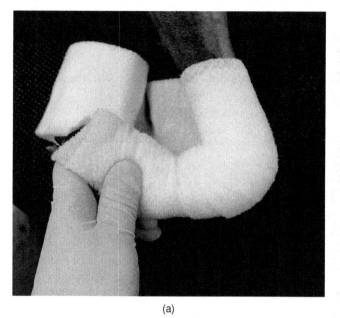

(a)

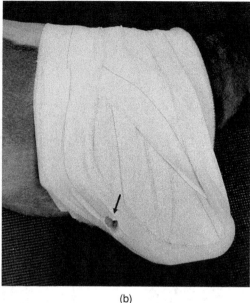

(b)

FIGURE 18.6 (a) Placement of a Velpeau sling. Cast padding encircles the paw and carpus with the joint in moderate flexion to prevent hyperflexion of the carpus. (b) The carpus, elbow, and shoulder are held in a flexed position as the padding is wrapped around the torso and covers the flexed limb completely. The padding is wrapped caudal and, if necessary, cranial to the contralateral limb. Elastic gauze and tape are then used sequentially to cover the cast padding. A small window is cut in the bandage over the lateral paw to assess the toes and foot (black arrow).

   c. Maintains the shoulder, elbow, and carpus in flexion
   d. Common uses:
      1. Shoulder luxation:
        a. Is only indicated for traumatic medial luxations:
          a. Will not work for congenital medial luxations.
        b. Contraindicated with lateral luxations as this sling promotes lateral translation of the proximal humerus.
        c. This splint should be applied after closed reduction of a traumatic medial luxation.
      2. Conservative management of scapular fractures.
   e. Application:
      1. Ideally, applied in the awake and standing patient.
      2. Can be placed in the anesthetized patient in lateral recumbency with the affected limb up.

   3. Cast padding encircles the paw and carpus with the joint in moderate flexion:
      a. The padding prevents hyperflexion of the carpus.
   4. The carpus, elbow, and shoulder are held in a flexed position as the padding is wrapped around the torso and covers the flexed limb completely.
   5. Wrap the padding caudal to the contralateral limb.
   6. If the patient is active it may be necessary to wrap the padding cranial and caudal to the contralateral limb.
   7. Elastic gauze and flexible self-adherent wrap are then used sequentially to cover the cast padding.
   8. A small window is cut in the bandage over the lateral paw to assess the toes and foot.

f. Bandage care:
1. Abrasions of the contralateral axilla are common.
2. Do not overly compress the thorax.
3. Do not overly compress the paw and carpus.
4. Recheck the patient every 2–4 days while the bandage is in place.

2. Ehmer sling (Figures 18.7a–d).
a. Non-weight-bearing sling.
b. Applied to the hind limb only.
c. Maintains mild internal rotation of the hip.
d. Maintains abduction of the limb.
e. Uses:
1. Applied after closed reduction of craniodorsal hip luxation.
2. Contraindicated in ventrocaudal luxation:
a. Promotes ventral and caudal translation of the femoral head.
3. Applied after open reduction of craniodorsal hip luxation.
4. Postoperative internal repair of some acetabular and femoral fractures.
f. Application:
1. Cast padding is wrapped around the metatarsus:
a. Prevents abrasions and skin necrosis.
2. Elastic gauze is wrapped around the metatarsus and continued around the medial aspect of the stifle joint:
a. The stifle and tarsus are maintained in a flexed position.
3. The gauze is continued over the cranial and lateral aspect of the stifle joint:
a. The gauze is placed as proximal as possible over the thigh.
4. Continue the gauze distally toward the hock, going behind the hock to the medial aspect of the tarsus, then dorsally back over the metatarsals.

5. Several layers of gauze are applied on the same manner until sufficient bulk is established.
6. Elastic tape is placed over the gauze and overlaps onto the skin:
a. This helps keep the bandage in place.
7. If placed properly, there are no circumferential bands of material on the limb.
g. Bandage care:
1. Can be safely maintained for 2 weeks, and if often recommended to be maintained for 7–10 days following closed reduction of a cranial dorsal hip luxation.
2. Frequent (every 4 days) observation of the sling is performed while in place.
3. Abrasions and pressure necrosis may develop over the cranial thigh and medial tarsus.
4. Check the toes daily for swelling.
5. Slippage of the sling from the stifle is the most common complication:
a. Very common in cats
6. Slipping of the bandage can be counteracted by extending the gauze and tape around the torso.

3. Carpal flexion bandage (Figures 18.6a and 18.8):
a. Non-weight-bearing sling
b. Moderate flexion of the carpus
c. Uses:
1. Relieves tension of the flexor tendons.
2. Most commonly used to protect flexor tendon repair.
3. Prevent weight-bearing after orthopedic repair.
d. Application:
1. Flex the carpus 90–100° and wrap with cast padding and elastic gauze.
2. Elastic tape is wrapped in a circular pattern from the digits and paw to the distal radius.
e. Bandage care:

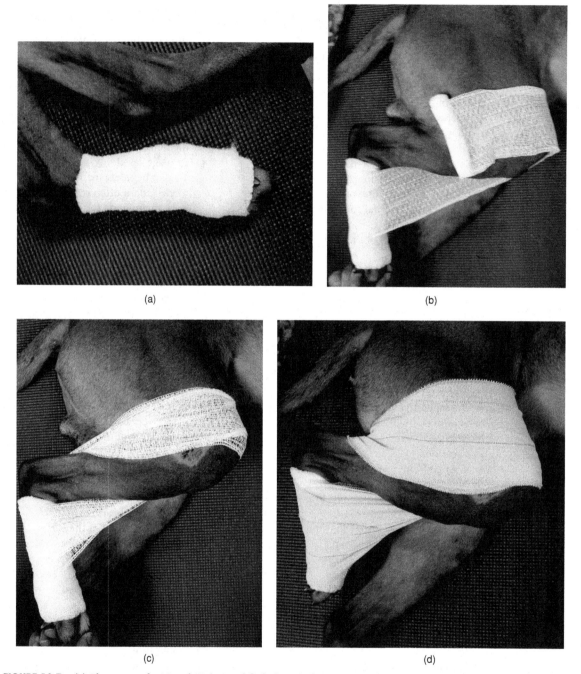

(a) (b)

(c) (d)

FIGURE 18.7 (a) Placement of a 90 and 90 (or modified Ehmer) sling. Cast padding is wrapped around the metatarsus to prevent abrasions and skin necrosis. (b) Elastic gauze is wrapped around the metatarsus and continued around the medial aspect of the stifle joint. The stifle and tarsus are maintained in a flexed position at 90 degrees and the gauze is continued over the cranial and lateral aspect of the stifle joint. (c) The gauze is continued medially back to the tarsus and dorsally back over the metatarsals. Several layers of gauze are applied on the same manner until sufficient bulk is established. (d) Elastic tape is placed over the gauze and overlaps onto the skin to help keep the bandage in place. If placed properly, there are no circumferential bands of material on the limb.

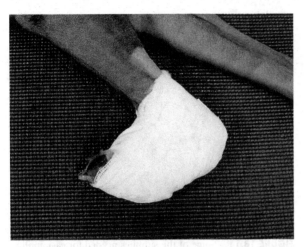

FIGURE 18.8 Placement of a carpal flexion bandage. The initial part of the bandage is started as shown in Figure 18.6a. Then, elastic tape is wrapped in a circular pattern from the digits and paw to the distal radius. A second band of tape can be placed perpendicular to the original bandage to help prevent the bandage from slipping.

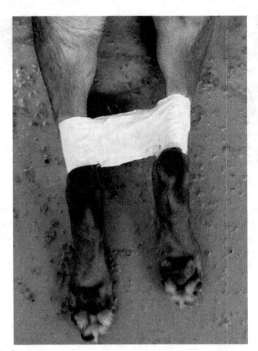

FIGURE 18.9 Hock hobbles are placed just proximal to the tarsus. Double over a piece of adhesive tape of sufficient length to wrap around both hocks. The strip is wrapped around both hindlimbs proximal to the tarsus. The strip should be loose enough to allow ambulation but prevent abduction. The strip is secured to itself with tape.

    1. Excessive flexion or duration of flexion (as little as 10–14 days) can lead to contracture of the carpus and flexor tendons.
    2. Assess the toes daily for swelling.
  4. Hobbles:
    a. Allows weight-bearing and walking while placed on the hind limbs.
    b. Prevents abduction of the hind limbs.
    c. Hock hobbles (Figure 18.9):
      1. Placed just proximal to the tarsus.
      2. Often used in animals recovering from pelvic trauma and following acetabular fracture repair.
      3. Application:
        a. Double over a piece of adhesive tape of sufficient length to wrap around both hocks.
        b. No adhesive surface should be exposed.
        c. The strip of tape is wrapped around both hind limbs proximal to the tarsus.

        d. The strip should be loose enough to allow ambulation but prevent abduction.
        e. The strip is secured to itself with tape.
    d. Stifle hobbles (Figure 18.10):
      1. Placed just proximal to stifle joints.
      2. Best used following closed reduction of caudoventral coxofemoral luxation.
      3. Application:
        a. Similar application to hock hobbles.
        b. Modification is mandatory to prevent slipping:
          a. A second strip of doubled over tape is made with no adhesive surface exposed.

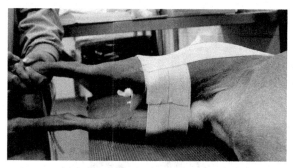

FIGURE 18.10 Stifle hobbles are placed just proximal to the stifle. Similar application to hock hobbles except a second strip of doubled over tape is made and is secured to the first strip at its lateral and cranial surface. The second strip runs dorsally over the back of the dog, cranial to the pelvis, and is secured to the opposite craniolateral aspect of the hobble.

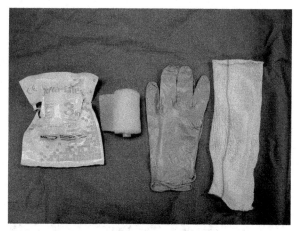

FIGURE 18.11 Some of the supplies needed for cast application. From left to right; fiberglass tape in package, fiberglass tape removed from package, gloves should be worn to protect hands, and cast stockinet.

   b. This strip is secured to the first strip at its lateral and cranial surface.
   c. The second strip runs dorsally over the back of the dog, cranial to the pelvis, and is secured to the opposite craniolateral aspect of the hobble.
  iv. Casts:
   1. Cylindrical cast (Figure 18.11):
    a. Resists bending and rotational forces:
      1. Must be able to immobilize a joint above and below the injury.
    b. Minimal neutralization of shear and compressive forces.
    c. Completely encloses the limb from the toes to the midshaft of the humerus or femur.
    d. Uses:
      1. Fractures or joint conditions below the elbow or stifle only.
      2. Postoperative protection of an internal repair.
      3. Most effective for definitive repair in the following:
        a. Young, rapidly healing patients
        b. Minimally displaced fractures

     c. Radius, ulna, tibia, and fibula fractures
   4. Do not use over open wounds or on limbs with extensive soft tissue swelling:
    a. Small windows can be cut into the cast over a wound.
    b. Large defects in the cast will lead to inefficient stability of the coaptation.
  e. Materials:
   1. Plaster:
    a. Advantages:
      a. Inexpensive
      b. Strong
    b. Disadvantages:
      a. Weakens when wet
      b. Does not dry easily
      c. Radiopaque
      d. Heavy
   2. Fiberglass:
    a. Advantages:
      a. Lightweight
      b. Strong
      c. Impact resistant
      d. Radiolucent
      e. No loss of strength when wet
      f. Easy to dry

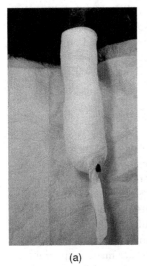 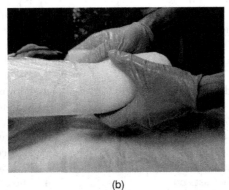 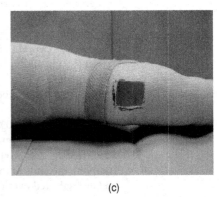

(a)   (b)   (c)

FIGURE 18.12 (a) Application of a fiberglass cast. Tape stirrups are applied. Then, a one-layer thick cast stockinet is placed on the limb. Cast padding is applied to the limb with no more than two layers are applied. The padding is overlapped by 50%. (b) Gloves are worn for application of casting tape. Immerse the tape in cold water and squeeze the roll a few times. Quickly apply the casting tape to the limb. The cast encloses the toes but the end of the cast is left open to evaluate the toes. Apply with moderate pressure and tension, with 50% overlap and avoid wrinkles in the tape. (c) Small windows can be cut into the cast over a wound. Large defects in the cast will lead to inefficient stability of the coaptation.

    b. Disadvantages:
        a. Expensive (5–10 times more than plaster)
        b. Less then ideal handling
  f. Application (Figures 18.12a–c):
    1. General anesthesia.
    2. Distraction of the fracture and digital manipulation are used for reduction.
    3. Radiographs are made to assess reduction before cast application.
    4. Apply tape stirrups as previously described.
    5. Apply a one layer thick cast stockinet:
        a. The length should exceed above and below the cast margins by 1–2 inches.
    6. Pressure doughnuts are made out of cast padding to cover pressure points:
        a. Forelimb:
            a. Accessory carpal bone
        b. Olecranon

        b. Hind limb:
            a. Calcaneus
  7. Cast padding is applied to the limb as previously described:
        a. Doughnuts are placed under the cast padding.
        b. No more than two layers are applied.
        c. Overlap padding by 50%.
  8. Gloves are worn for application of casting tape:
  9. Casting tape:
        a. 2 inch for small dogs and cats
        b. 3 inch for medium to large dogs
  10. Immerse the tape in cold water and squeeze the roll a few times:
  11. Quickly apply the casting tape to the limb:
        a. Fiberglass sets in 5–10 minutes

b. Wrap the tape around the toes several times.

c. The cast will encircle the digits but the end of the cast should be left open to evaluate the toes.

d. The cast padding should extend beyond the casting tape at the top and bottom of the bandage.

e. Apply with moderate pressure and tension.

f. Apply with 50% overlap.

g. Avoid wrinkles in the tape.

12. After the first layer of tape is complete the ends of the stockinet are reflected over the cast and the tape stirrups are inverted and adhered to the casting tape.

13. A second layer of casting tape is applied over the first with 50% overlap.

14. Use 2 full layers (with 50% overlap) for most dogs and cats.

15. Use 3 full layers for large dogs.

g. Cast care:

1. Keep clean and dry.

2. If lameness or odor develop during the casted period the cast should be changed under general anesthesia.

3. Monitor the toes for swelling and abrasions.

4. Can be maintained on an adult for 4 weeks.

5. If placed on a growing animal, the cast must be changed every 2 weeks.

h. Cast removal (Figures 18.13a and 18.13b):

1. Oscillating cast saw must be used for removal of fiberglass casts.

2. Sedation or tranquilization is required.

3. The cuts are made on two sides:

a. Medial and lateral

b. Cranial and caudal

4. The cuts are made with an up and down motion of the saw and not by running the saw from side to side up and down the cast.

2. Modification of casts:

a. Bivalve (Figures 18.14a–c):

1. Advantages:

a. Allows frequent cast changes to deal with underlying wounds.

b. Assess soft tissues during the casting period.

2. Disadvantages:

a. May lead to excessive motion of the fracture resulting in:

a. Delayed union

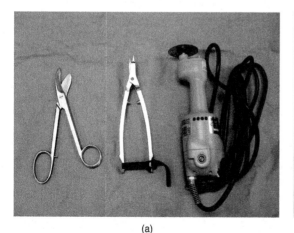

(a)

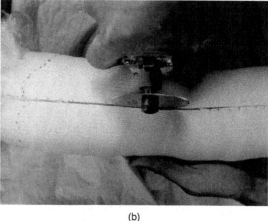

(b)

FIGURE 18.13   (a) Materials used for cast removal. From left to right; cast scissors, cast spreader, and oscillating cast saw. (b) An oscillating cast saw must be used for fiberglass cast removal. Sedation or tranquilization is required. Cuts are made on two sides of the cast by moving the saw up and down, not side to side.

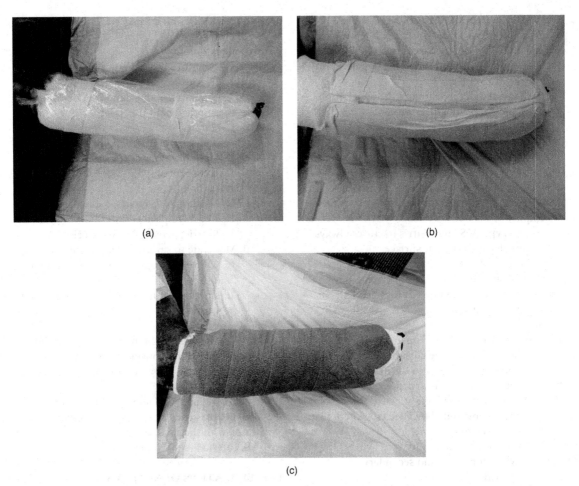

FIGURE 18.14 (a) Preparation for a bivalve cast. A plastic bag can be temporarily applied to the limb to prevent the fiberglass casting tape from sticking to the bandage. (b) An oscillating saw is used to cut the cast tape along the medial and lateral sides. (c) The bivalved cast is covered and held together with elastic tape or flexible self-adherent wrap.

 b. Malunion
 c. Nonunion
3. Application:
 a. Tape stirrups and stockinet are not incorporated into the cast but are taped to the outside of the cast.
 b. An oscillating saw is used to cut the cast tape along the medial and lateral sides after the tape has been applied and dried.
 c. Trim any sharp edges of the cast.

 d. The bivalved cast is covered and held together with elastic tape or flexible self-adherent wrap.
 b. Half cast:
  1. Shorter than full cast
  2. Stays below the elbow or stifle
  3. Uses:
   a. Minimally displaced metacarpal and metatarsal fractures
   b. Immobilize carpal and tarsal joints

2. SALTER–HARRIS CLASSIFICATION SYSTEM

a. This classification system can only be applied to young animals with an open physis:

 i. Type I: fracture through the hypertrophic zone (physis).

 ii. Type II: fracture through the hypertrophic zone and part of the metaphysis.

 iii. Type III: fracture through the hypertrophic zone and part of the epiphysis:

  1. Type III Salter–Harris fractures always involve the articular surface.

 iv. Type IV: fracture through the hypertrophic zone, part of the metaphysis, and part of the epiphysis:

  1. Type IV Salter–Harris fractures always involve the articular surface.

 v. Type V: Crushing injury to the physis.

b. Salter–Harris fractures III and IV may have a worse long-term prognosis as they are articular fractures and secondary osteoarthritis will ensue.

c. Damage to an active and open physis can result in complete or incomplete closure of the growth plate. Secondary pathology to the developing long bone and associated joints depends on the location of the growth plate, the bone affected, the percentage of growth contributed by affected growth plate, the age and breed of dog:

 i. Angular limb deformity

 ii. Joint incongruity and secondary osteoarthritis

 iii. Chronic pain and abnormal gait

d. A patient with suspicion of damage to an active growth plate should be referred to an orthopedic surgeon as soon as possible. Secondary pathologic changes occur rapidly in actively growing animals:

 i. The location of the injury, the chronicity of the injury, the degree of secondary pathology, the type of fracture, and the age of the animal will determine the best surgical intervention and may include the following:

  1. Corrective osteotomies with internal fixation or external skeletal fixation.

  2. Corrective osteotomies with distraction osteogenesis.

  3. Physectomy and internal or external fixation.

  4. Complete surgical closure of an incompletely closed physis.

3. FRACTURE OF THE SCAPULA

a. Characterization:

 i. Location:

  1. Fractures of the body and spine

  2. Fractures of the neck

  3. Fractures of the glenoid cavity, including the supraglenoid tuberosity

 ii. Function:

  1. Stable extra-articular

  2. Unstable extra-articular

  3. Intra-articular

b. Scapular body:

 i. Minimal displacement:

  1. Apply Velpeau sling

  2. Restrict activity for 3–4 weeks

 ii. Moderate to severe displacement:

  1. will require open reduction and internal fixation;

  2. supplement internal fixation with a support bandage or Velpeau sling.

c. Acromion:

 i. Origin of deltoid muscles; therefore, this process is under constant tension.

 ii. Fractures of the acromion require internal fixation.

d. Neck, glenoid, and supraglenoid tuberosity:

 i. There is usually severe displacement associated with these fractures.

 ii. Internal fixation required.

4. DISLOCATION OF SCAPULA

a. Serratus ventralis provides the majority of the muscle support for the scapula and limb:

 i. Dislocation of the scapula typically results from avulsion of this muscle from the medial aspect of the scapula.

 ii. Clinical signs of dislocation include a high riding scapula with weight bearing and increased mobility of the scapula.

b. Cats and small dogs with acute dislocation:

 i. Closed reduction.

 ii. Velpeau sling.

 iii. Surgical repair is almost always required for functional and cosmetic result.

c. Medium- and large-breed dogs:

 i. Internal fixation, Velpeau sling, or spica splint for 2–3 weeks, and restricted activity is ideal and provides for the best outcome.

 ii. Velpeau sling or spica splint for 3 weeks and restricted activity for 4–6 weeks without surgery provides a less favorable outcome and frequently fails.

5. LUXATION OF THE SHOULDER JOINT
   a. Congenital:
      i.   Capsular laxity
      ii. Glenoid dysplasia
      iii. Small breed dogs
      iv. Medial instability
   b. Traumatic:
      i. Usually results in a lateral luxation of the humeral head; however, medial luxations are possible.
      ii. Disruption of lateral support structures.
   c. Lateral luxation:
      i.   Trauma
      ii. Large-breed dogs
      iii. Requires disruption of soft tissues:
           1. Lateral joint capsule
           2. Lateral glenohumeral ligament
           3. Infraspinatus tendon
      iv. Treatment for acute luxation:
           1. Closed reduction and conservative treatment:
              a. Reduction should occur under heavy sedation or general anesthesia.
              b. The limb is distracted and abducted.
              c. Do not use a Velpeau sling in lateral shoulder luxation.
              d. Use a spica splint or non-weight-bearing sling, such as a carpal flexion bandage for 10–14 days.
      v.   Treatment for failed conservative management or chronic luxation:
           1. Open reduction
           2. Internal fixation
   d. Medial luxation:
      i.   Most common
      ii. Often congenital in small breeds
      iii. Mostly due to trauma in large breeds
      iv. Treatment:
           1. Closed reduction:
              a. For luxations secondary to trauma only.
              b. Manual reduction should be attempted under general anesthesia.
              c. Post reduction radiographs are made for confirmation.
              d. Velpeau sling is ideal for 14 days.

           2. Open reduction and internal fixation should be considered for the following:
              a. Chronic luxations.
              b. Congenital luxations.
              c. Those that fail conservative management.
   e. Cranial and caudal luxation:
      i. Rare
      ii. Require open reduction and internal fixation

6. FRACTURE OF THE HUMERUS
   a. Concurrent injuries are often present when the humerus is fractured:
      i.   Spinal trauma such as fractures, luxations, traumatic disk protrusion, or hemorrhage/inflammation (see Chapter 9: Traumatic Spinal Injury).
      ii. Brachial plexus injuries (see Chapter 8: Trauma-Associated Peripheral Nerve Injury).
      iii. Peripheral nerve injuries (see Chapter 8: Trauma-Associated Peripheral Nerve Injury):
           1. Radial nerve neuropraxia is characterized by inability to extend the carpus and elbow. Animals with radial nerve damage often walk on the dorsum of the paw.
           2. Sensory deficits may be noted on the lateral aspect of 5th digit (ulnar nerve injury) and dorsal paw (radial nerve injury) (see Figure 8.3 in Chapter 8: Trauma-Associated Peripheral nerve injury).
           3. This injury usually resolves after fracture stabilization.
   b. Temporary preoperative fracture stabilization:
      i.   Bandage must immobilize a joint above and below fracture.
      ii. Robert Jones, modified Robert Jones, and antebrachial splints are contraindicated:
           1. These bandages may increase instability of fracture.
           2. It is best to leave injured leg without bandage rather than placing one of the aforementioned bandages/splints.
      iii. Spica splints are appropriate for humeral fractures.
   c. Proximal fractures:
      i.   Greater tubercle:
           1. More common in immature animals

2. Tend to be avulsion fractures
ii. Fracture-separation of proximal epiphysis:
   1. Salter–Harris I
   2. Salter–Harris II
iii. Humeral head, neck, and proximal meta-physeal fractures:
   1. Uncommon fractures
   2. Require internal fixation
d. Midshaft:
   i. Most common type of humeral fracture seen.
   ii. Midshaft humeral fractures have a high risk for concurrent radial nerve damage.
e. Distal:
   i. Classification:
      1. Distal shaft
      2. Supracondylar:
         a. Involve supracondylar foramen.
         b. Does not extend into condyle.
      3. Unicondylar:
         a. Capitulum:
            1. This refers to the lateral aspect of condyle.
            2. Articulates with head of radius.
            3. More commonly injured:
               a. Often seen associated with minor trauma in young animals as a result of jumps or falls.
            4. Spaniels at increased risk:
               a. Male cocker.
               b. Middle-aged.
               c. Can be bilateral (radiographs and/or CT contralateral limb).
               d. Secondary to incomplete ossification.
         b. Trochlea:
            1. This refers to the medial aspect of condyle.
            2. Articulates with trochlear notch of ulna.
         c. All condylar fractures are articular.
      4. Dicondylar:
         a. Common in dogs
         b. Low incidence in cats (lack supratrochlear foramen)
         c. Associated with major trauma
         d. T fracture and Y fractures:
            1. Salter–Harris III and IV fractures of the condyle
            2. Repair with transcondylar screw and pins or plate and screws

7. **LUXATION OF THE ELBOW JOINT**
a. Congenital:
   i. Humeroulnar articulation:
      1. Most common.
      2. Seen in small breed dogs.
      3. Frequently bilateral.
      4. Results in severe limb deformity and dysfunction.
   ii. Caudolateral radial head dislocation:
      1. Results in mild deformity and dysfunction.
   iii. Polyarthrodysplasia, a congenital condition in animals causing multiple joint abnormalities including ectrodactyly (split-hand deformity), can be associated with congenital elbow luxation.
b. Acquired:
   i. Traumatic (Figure 18.15):
      1. Dog fights
      2. Vehicular trauma
      3. Associated with training or agility
   ii. Uncommon injury.
   iii. Usually results in a lateral luxation of the radius and ulna.
   iv. Many injuries are associated with rupture of both collateral ligaments.
   v. Characteristic physical findings:
      1. Non-weight-bearing lameness
      2. Limb abducted
      3. External rotation
      4. Slight flexion
      5. Swelling of the elbow
      6. Pain on palpation
      7. Decreased range of motion
      8. Indistinct lateral humeral epicondyle
      9. Radial head and olecranon positioned laterally
   vi. Early closed reduction often has excellent results (Figure 18.15):
      1. General anesthesia is required.
      2. Distraction of limb for muscle fatigue.
      3. Hook anconeus into olecranon:
         a. Flex the limb greater than 90°.
         b. Internally rotate antebrachium.
         c. Simultaneous abduction of the limb.
         d. Internally rotate the antebrachium.
         e. Apply pressure to the radial head to force it medially.
   vii. Open reduction and internal stabilization is required if external reduction is unsuccessful.

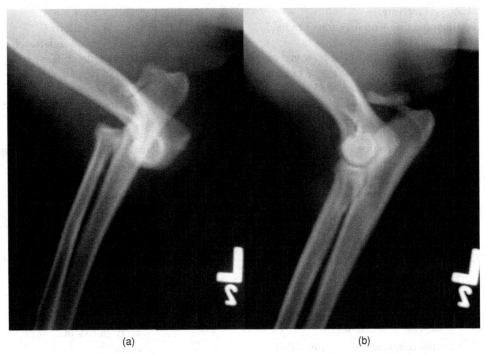

(a)   (b)

FIGURE 18.15   Lateral radiograph of a lateral elbow luxation in a dog (a) The pull of the triceps has displaced the antebrachium in a proximal direction. After closed reduction, (b) the lateral radiograph of the same dog's elbow. Notice the fracture fragment from the olecranon and anconeal process.

    viii. After care:
      1. Soft padded bandage or spica splint for 7–10 days
      2. Restrict activity for 4–6 weeks
      3. Physical therapy and passive range of motion after bandage removal
    ix. Prognosis:
      1. Good for acute luxation with closed reduction
      2. Less favorable with chronic luxations or those requiring open reduction

8. FRACTURES OF THE ANTEBRACHIUM
  a. Radius:
    i. Radial head:
      1. Rare:
        a. Often intra-articular, slab fractures
        b. Open repair necessary
    ii. Radial shaft:
      1. Ulna intact—the ulna can act as an internal splint when intact, making the fracture more stable.

      2. Minimal displacement of the radius is often noted when the ulna is intact.
      3. Definitive treatment with external coaptation:
        a. Modified Robert–Jones with caudal splint.
        b. Full cast.
        c. Bivalve cast.
        d. Surgery is usually not required for radius fractures that have an intact ulna.
    iii. Radial styloid process:
      1. Intra-articular fracture.
      2. Avulsion of medial collateral ligament, which inserts on the radial styloid process.
      3. Results in medial joint instability.
      4. Open repair needed.
  b. Ulna:
    i. Olecranon:
      1. Fractures of the olecranon can be extra-articular or intra-articular.
      2. Fragment displaces proximally due to the upward pull of triceps muscle.
      3. Internal fixation is necessary.

ii. Monteggia fracture:
1. Ulnar fracture with luxation of radial head:
   a. Type I: Fracture of the proximal or middle third of the ulna with a cranial dislocation of the radial head.
   b. Type II: Fracture of the proximal or middle third of the ulna with caudal dislocation of the radial head.
   c. Type III: Fracture of the ulnar metaphysic with a lateral dislocation of the radial head.
   d. Type IV: Fracture of the proximal or middle third of the ulna and radius with cranial dislocation of the radial head.
2. These fractures result in the disruption of annular and interosseous ligament.
3. Closed reduction and external coaptation is rarely successful.
4. Internal repair is often indicated.

iii. Ulnar shaft fractures with an intact radial head:
1. External coaptation is recommended.

iv. Ulnar styloid process:
1. Intra-articular fracture.
2. Avulsion of lateral collateral ligament, which inserts on the ulnar styloid process.
3. Results in joint instability.
4. Open repair needed.

c. Radius and ulna fracture (Figures 18.16 and 18.17):
i. Diaphyseal:
1. External coaptation can be attempted with these fractures. External coaptation is best for simple oblique fractures:
   a. Cylindrical or bivalve casts:
      1. Resists bending
      2. Resists rotation if incorporates joints above and below
      3. Axial compression not neutralized
      4. Attain at least 50% of bone overlap
      5. Maintain alignment
      6. Minimize angulation
      7. Small-breed dogs:
         a. High risk of delayed and nonunion

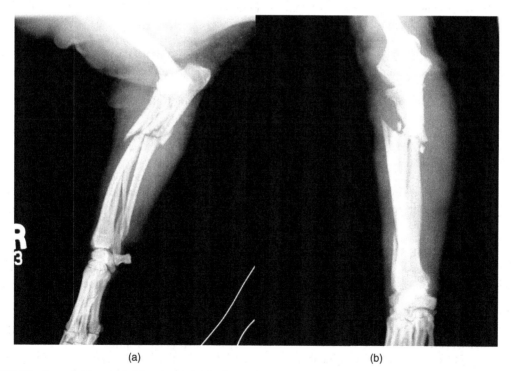

(a)   (b)

FIGURE 18.16   Lateral (a) and AP (b) radiograph of a dog with a severely comminuted radius and ulna fracture after being hit by a car.

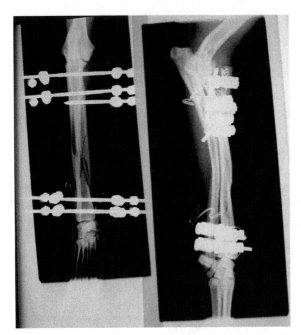

FIGURE 18.17 Postoperative radiographs of the dog demonstrating stabilization of the antebrachium with a type II external skeletal fixation device.

    b. Diminished antebrachial blood supply

    c. Internal or external fixation is recommended

2. Internal fixation or external skeletal fixation (ESF) are typically the preferred option for definitive repair unless there are financial concerns or if coexisting disease is present that precludes anesthesia and surgery. This is especially true for small/toy breed dogs:

    a. ESF provides a limited approach concept that helps to preserve the internal environment of the fracture and causes less trauma to the soft tissues that are needed for fracture fragment blood supply during bone healing.

    b. ESF is the preferred treatment for open fractures.

  ii. Epiphyseal:

    1. External fixation

    2. Internal fixation

9. FRACTURES OF THE BONES OF THE CARPUS

  a. Radial carpal bone:

    i. Rare

    ii. Occurs more frequently in working dogs

    iii. External coaptation is appropriate for nondisplaced fractures:

      1. Cast

      2. Mason metasplint

    iv. Surgical intervention for displaced fractures

  b. Accessory carpal bone:

    i. Documented to occur most often in racing greyhounds.

    ii. Due to the direction of racing the right leg is often affected.

    iii. Most are avulsion fractures.

    iv. External coaptation is usually not successful.

    v. Surgical intervention is recommended.

10. LIGAMENTOUS INJURIES OF THE CARPUS

  a. Collateral ligaments:

    i. Radial (medial) collateral injured more commonly than ulnar (lateral) collateral:

      1. Primary repair of the ligament can be attempted for acute injuries.

      2. Synthetic implant repair may be needed when the injury is chronic or when there is significant loss of ligament length.

      3. Partial or complete carpal arthrodesis should be considered if large or giant breed dog or if significant loss of ligament is present.

    ii. Palmar ligament injury:

      1. Injury occurs as a result of carpal hyperextension.

      2. Common injury as a result of jumps or falls..

      3. External coaptation is often unsuccessful.

      4. Partial or panarthrodesis of the carpus is often required for successful outcome.

    iii. Flexor tendon lacerations:

      1. Lacerations to the palmar surface of the carpus result in partial or complete laceration of the flexor tendons.

      2. Animals with these injuries often present for severe hemorrhage as a result of concurrent vessel laceration.

      3. Physical examination findings include; hyperextension of distal interphalangeal joint, elevation of the 3rd phalanx and nail while weight bearing, and plantigrade position of one or more digits.

4. Primary repair of tendon ends:
   a. Locking loop pattern (Figures 18.18a–h)
   b. Three-loop pulley pattern (Figures 18.19a–e)
   c. Splint with carpus straight or in partial flexion
iv. Chronic lacerations or failed tenorrhaphy:
   1. Fusion podoplasty involves extensive removal of interdigital skin and suturing or fusion of remainder of skin, once healed, this prevents spreading apart of toes during weight bearing.
   2. Tendon lengthening with fascia lata grafts.
   3. Post operative cast or padded cranial splint for 6 weeks is required for chronic laceration repairs and failed tenorrhaphy.

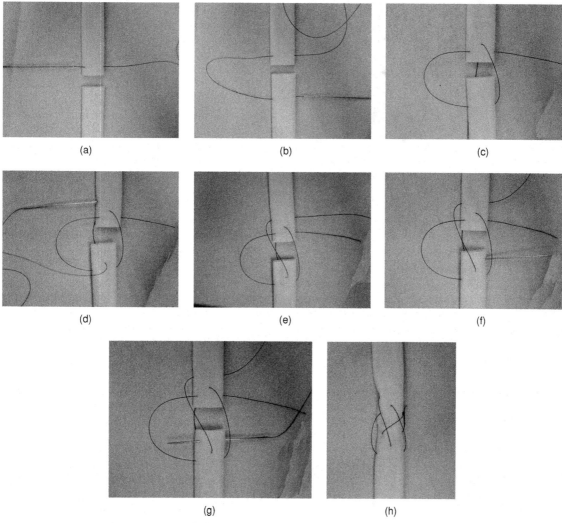

(a)   (b)   (c)
(d)   (e)   (f)
(g)   (h)

FIGURE 18.18   (a–h) Three-loop pulley suture pattern for repair of lacerated tendons and ligaments. Suture passes on either side of the rupture three times at 120° intervals with near-far, middle-middle, and far-near bites. (a) and (b) Illustrate the first set of bites in the first plane using a near-far technique. (c) and (d) Illustrate the second set of bites in the second plane using a middle-middle technique. (e–g) Illustrate the final set of bites in the third plane using a far-near technique. (h) The two ends of suture are tied with a square knot.

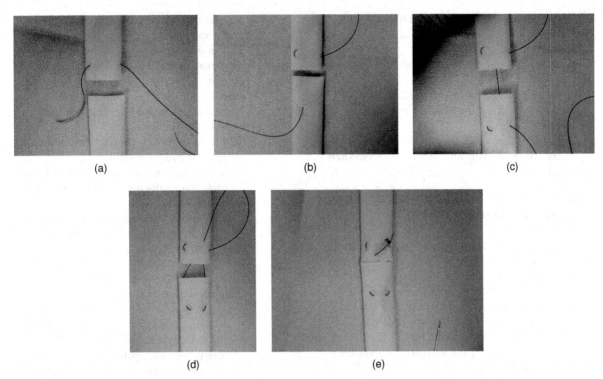

(a)　　　　　　　　(b)　　　　　　　　(c)

(d)　　　　　　　　(e)

FIGURE 18.19 (a–e) Locking loop suture pattern for repair of tendons and ligaments. The longitudinal suture passes deep to the transverse suture to lock the suture around the fibers of the tendon/ligament. (a) The first set of bites run in a transverse plane in the proximal tendon unit from outside the tendon to in and from in to out. (b) The second set of bites run in a longitudinal plane just proximal to the first bite. This suture line runs deep to the transverse suture line and passes from outside to inside passing across the tendon gap and then inside to outside in the distal tendon unit. (c) The third set of bites run in a transverse plane in the distal tendon unit with the bites passing from outside to inside and inside to outside in a transverse plane in the distal tendon unit. The suture line runs superficial to the longitudinal suture line. (d) The final set of bites run in a longitudinal plane just distal to the third bite. This suture line runs deep to the transverse suture line and passes from outside to inside passing across the tendon gap and then inside to outside in the proximal tendon unit. (e) The two ends of suture are tied together with a square knot.

11. FRACTURES OF THE METACARPAL AND METATARSAL BONES

a. Often causes a non-weight-bearing lameness.

b. Metacarpal bone fractures are more common than metatarsal fractures.

c. External coaptation can be used for the following:

   i. Stress fractures.

   ii. Fractures of one or two metacarpal/tarsal bones.

   iii. Fractures that have minimum displacement.

   iv. One of the main weight-bearing bones (metacarpal/tarsal 3 and 4) should be intact.

   v. The articular surface should not be involved.

   vi. The fractures should not be comminuted.

d. Acceptable forms of external coaptation include the following:

   i. Mason metasplint

   ii. Cast

   iii. Modified Robert–Jones and palmar or plantar splint and metal walking bar

e. Internal fixation should be considered if:

   i. More than two bones are fractured.

   ii. Both major weight-bearing bones are fractured (the third and fourth metacarpals/tarsals).

   iii. If severe displacement is present.

   iv. If there are comminuted fractures.

   v. If the fracture involves the articular surface.

12. FRACTURES AND DISLOCATION OF THE DIGITS

a. Uncommon.

b. Reduction and external coaptation is appropriate for most cases.

c. Rarely, internal fixation is needed.

d. If severely comminuted, digit amputation can be performed:

    i. Digits 3 and 4 are responsible for 80% of initial weight-bearing and should be saved when possible.

13. COXOFEMORAL LUXATION

a. Craniodorsal:

    i. Most common direction for hip luxation secondary to trauma

    ii. Physical examination findings:

        1. Affected limb appears shorter.

        2. Adduction and external rotation (due to the pull of the iliopsoas on the lesser trochanter) of affected limb.

        3. Swelling, pain, and crepitus over the luxated hip.

        4. The distance between the greater trochanter and ipsilateral tuber ischium is increased on affected side compared to contralateral side.

    iii. Radiographs are needed for a definitive diagnosis:

        1. Evaluate for concurrent fractures in the pelvis and limb.

        2. Evaluate for evidence of underlying hip dysplasia and osteoarthritis in the coxofemoral joint.

b. Caudoventral:

    i. Most commonly occurs secondary to severe and acute abduction of the limb.

    ii. Physical examination findings:

        1. Affected limb appears longer.

        2. Abduction and internal rotation of affected limb.

        3. Swelling, pain, and crepitus over the luxated hip.

        4. Femoral head lodges in obturator foramen.

        5. Greater trochanter is displaced medially on affected side.

    iii. Radiographs are needed for a definitive diagnosis (Figure 18.20):

        1. Evaluate for concurrent fractures in the pelvis and limb.

        2. Evaluate for evidence of underlying hip dysplasia and osteoarthritis in the coxofemoral joint.

c. Treatment:

    i. Normal coxofemoral joints (absence of fractures or hip dysplasia):

        1. Closed reduction should be attempted as soon as the patient is stable:

            a. External reduction becomes increasingly more difficult 24–48 hours after injury.

            b. Often unsuccessful after 4–5 days:

                1. Progression of inflammation

                2. Fibrosis

                3. Contraction of muscles

            c. Craniodorsal luxation

        2. Open reduction is needed if closed reduction fails:

            a. Other options include femoral head and neck ostectomy, total hip arthroplasty, and triple pelvic osteotomy but are rarely, if ever, indicated in a luxated hip without evidence of fractures or hip dysplasia.

    ii. Abnormal joints or normal joints with unsuccessful closed reduction:

        1. Open reduction and internal fixation.

        2. Femoral head and neck excision.

        3. Total hip arthroplasty is the most expensive but probably the best option for dogs with luxation secondary to hip dysplasia.

    iii. Closed reduction of craniodorsal luxations (normal joints) (Figure 18.21):

        1. General anesthesia or sedation and epidural is necessary.

        2. Lateral recumbency with affected limb up.

        3. Apply traction and external rotation to the limb for several minutes.

        4. Counter traction is applied with a towel or sling in the inguinal area with one end of the towel in front of the affected limb and the other end behind the affected limb.

        5. The greater trochanter is identified and used for leverage to move the femur caudally and distally over the lip of the acetabulum.

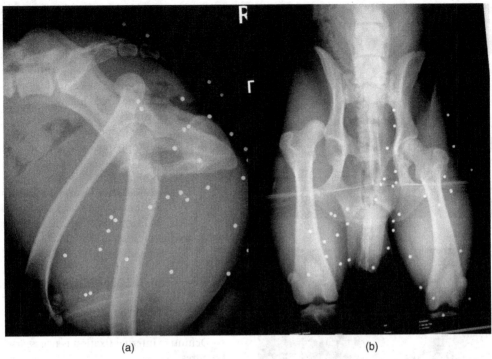

FIGURE 18.20 Lateral (a) and ventrodorsal (b) radiograph of a dog with a craniodorsal coxofemoral luxation. This dog has excellent hips and is a good candidate for closed reduction attempts. The diffuse buck shot is not associated with this dogs recent trauma history and the owners were unaware of the dog being shot.

6. Steps 3–5 are performed simultaneously.

7. Once the femoral head is over the acetabulum, internal rotation is applied to the limb.

8. When reduced assess stability:
    a. Apply pressure to greater trochanter and take the hip through range of motion.
    b. Excessive limb extension and external rotation will lead to reluxation.

9. Ehmer flexion sling placement (see page 303 earlier in chapter):
    a. Non-weight-bearing sling.
    b. This sling provides joint flexion, abduction, and internal rotation of the limb, which directs the femoral head into acetabulum.
    c. Can be removed in 7–10 days.
    d. Recheck patient every 3 days while Ehmer sling in place for complications:
        1. Ulcerations
        2. Pressure necrosis
        3. Sling loosening or displacement
        4. Vascular constriction
    e. Cats do not tolerate an Ehmer sling well and routinely get out of them. Therefore, surgical repair may be more likely to be needed in cats.

10. Radiographs are should be taken after the sling is placed to document reduction.

11. A fair to good prognosis for successful closed reduction and function.

iv. Closed reduction of caudoventral luxations: (Figure 18.22)
    1. General anesthesia or sedation and epidural is necessary.
    2. Lateral recumbency with affected limb up.
    3. Apply traction to the limb at the level of the stifle.

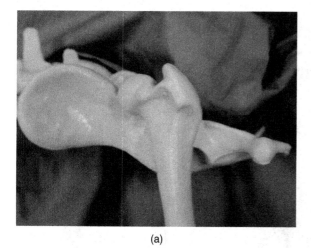

(a)

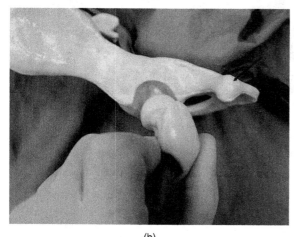

(b)

FIGURE 18.21 Closed reduction of craniodorsal hip luxation (a) Apply traction and external rotation to the limb. Countertraction is applied with a towel or sling in the inguinal area. The greater trochanter is identified and used for leverage to move the proximal femur caudally and distally. Once the femoral head is over the acetabulum, internal rotation is applied to the limb (b).

4. Counter traction is applied to the ipsilateral tuber ischium.
5. Disengage the femoral head from the obturator foramen:
    a. Adduction of the limb
    b. Traction of the limb
6. The proximal aspect of the limb is lifted laterally and cranially until it is seated in the acetabulum.

7. Hobbles are placed at the level of the hock or stifle for 3–5 days (see Figures 9 and 10).
8. An Ehmer sling is contraindicated as it inherently predisposes to reluxation.
9. Conversion of a caudoventral luxation into a craniodorsal luxation is not necessary or indicated.
10. When reduced assess stability:
    a. Apply pressure to greater trochanter and take the hip through range of motion.
    b. Excessive limb abduction and internal rotation will lead to reluxation.
11. Radiographs are made to document reduction.
12. A good prognosis for successful closed reduction and return to normal function if no evidence of hip dysplasia is present.

14. FRACTURES OF THE FEMUR
  a. Definitive internal fixation is necessary for most fractures.
  b. Concurrent injuries are common:
    i. Musculoskeletal
    ii. Neurologic:
      1. Spine (see Chapter 9: Traumatic Spinal Injury)
      2. Head trauma (see Chapter 7: Traumatic Brain Injury)
      3. Peripheral nerve injury (see Chapter 8: Trauma-Associated Peripheral Nerve Injury):
        a. Assess deep pain perception in the affected limb:
          1. Lateral digits (sciatic nerve)
          2. Medial digits (femoral nerve)
    iii. Abdominal viscera (see Chapter 11: Trauma-Associated Parenchymal Organ Injury)
    iv. Thoracic cavity (see Chapter 6: Trauma-Associated Thoracic Injury)
    v. Body wall (see Chapter 13: Trauma-Associated Body Wall and Torso Injury)
    vi. Compartment syndrome of the upper limb and thigh
  c. Classification:
    i. Proximal:
      1. Epiphyseal
      2. Physeal

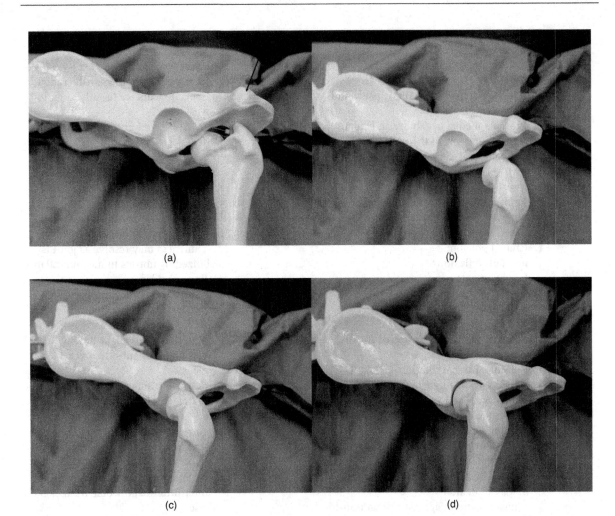

FIGURE 18.22   Closed reduction of caudoventral hip luxation (a) Apply traction to the limb at the level of the stifle. Countertraction is applied to the ipsilateral tuber ischium (black arrow). Disengage the femoral head from the obturator foramen (b) Apply adduction and traction of the limb. The proximal aspect of the limb is lifted laterally and cranially (c) until it is seated in the acetabulum (d).

    3. Neck
    4. Greater trochanter avulsion
  ii. Midshaft (diaphyseal)
  iii. Distal
  iv. Metaphyseal
  v. Physeal
  vi. Condylar
d. Preoperative external coaptation:
  i. Often not necessary:
    1. Cage rest
    2. Analgesia
    3. Sedation

  ii. If placing a bandage use a Spica splint (see page 298 above).

15. **STIFLE JOINT**
  a. Stifle disorders are a frequent cause of hind limb lameness.
  b. Structure and function:
    i. Lateral and medial meniscus:
      1. Energy absorption.
      2. Stabilize the joint.
      3. Lubricate the joint.

    4. Prevent synovial impingement during weight bearing.

ii. Medial collateral (femorotibial) ligament:

    1. Strong attachment to joint capsule and medial meniscus.

    2. Prevents medial instability and valgus and medial opening of the joint.

iii. Lateral collateral (femorotibial) ligament:

    1. Inserts on the fibular head.

    2. Limits varus and lateral opening of the joint.

iv. Caudal cruciate ligament:

    1. Cranial portion:

        a. Taut in flexion

        b. Lax in extension

    2. Caudal portion:

        a. Taut in extension

        b. Lax in flexion

    3. Prevents caudal translation of the tibia relative to the femur.

    4. Prevents internal rotation.

    5. Protects against hyperextension.

    6. Limits varus and valgus.

v. Cranial cruciate ligament:

    1. Craniomedial band:

        a. Taut in extension and flexion

    2. Caudaolateral band:

        a. Taut in extension

        b. Lax in flexion

    3. Primary restraint against cranial translocation of the tibia.

    4. Primary restraint against hyperextension.

    5. Limits internal rotation.

    6. Prevents excessive varus and valgus.

c. Common stifle injuries:

i. Cranial cruciate injury:

    1. The most common cause of hind limb lameness in dogs:

        a. Acute:

            1. Traumatic:

                a. Uncommon

                b. Young dogs (<4-year-old)

                c. Usually an avulsion fracture of the tibial insertion site and not an actual ligament tear

            2. Acute tear of a chronically diseased and injured ligament:

                a. More common in large breed.

                b. Most common in 5–7-year-old dogs.

                c. Small-breed dogs with cranial cruciate tears are usually older (>7 years).

                d. More common in spayed females.

                e. Commonly associated with chronic degenerative joint disease (radiographically).

    b. Chronic:

        1. Intermittent chronic lameness and degenerative joint disease.

        2. Lameness may resolve as joint is stabilized by fibrous tissue and inflammation subsides.

    c. Clinical signs and diagnosis:

        1. Acute tears:

            a. Severe lameness early on.

            b. Often non-weight-bearing.

            c. Lameness subsides over 3–5 weeks.

            d. No obvious evidence of degenerative joint disease.

            e. Often have joint effusion.

        2. Chronic tears:

            a. More insidious onset of lameness.

            b. History of lameness is often intermittent and worse from exercise.

            c. Thickened joint with joint effusion.

            d. Medial buttress:

                a. Periarticular thickening around the medial collateral ligament

            e. Radiographic evidence of degenerative joint disease.

            f. Often a bilateral disease.

    d. Physical examination findings:

        1. Observe at rest.

        2. Observe at walk.

        3. Observe at trot.

        4. Patients with bilateral cranial cruciate ligament rupture may present nonambulatory:

            a. This can be confusing and misleading.

b. Nonambulatory is not synonymous with paralysis.

c. Be sure to complete a thorough orthopedic and neurologic examination to rule out primary or concurrent spinal cord disease.

5. All joints of all limbs are evaluated for pain, instability, or other abnormalities:

   a. Leave the affected limb for last.

   b. Often a bilateral disease.

6. Palpate affected limb and reference contralateral limb:

   a. Symmetry of alignment

   b. Symmetry of muscle mass

   c. Palpation pain of long bones or joints

7. Palpate for joint effusion:

   a. The normal patellar ligament should be readily palpated and feel like a taut band of tissue or a pencil.

   b. Fluid in the stifle joint makes the patellar ligament more difficult to palpate.

8. Range of motion:

   a. Document range of motion:

      a. Increased

      b. Decreased

   b. Crepitus

   c. Clicking:

      a. May indicate meniscal damage.

   d. Pain:

      a. Be sure to keep manipulations of the stifle joint isolated.

      b. Concurrent stressing of other joints with disease may be confusing and misleading.

   e. Pain on hyperextension of the knee will often be found in a patient with a cranial cruciate ligament rupture.

   f. Cranial drawer:

      a. Direct:

         i. Standing or in lateral recumbency.

         ii. To be done by placing fingers on very specific bony landmarks.

         iii. Femur landmarks include the patella and lateral fabella.

         iv. Tibial landmarks include the tibial tuberosity and fibular head.

         v. Keep femur stable while moving the tibia in a cranial and caudal direction.

         vi. Moving the femur or internally rotating the tibia will confound results.

         vii. Drawer should be assessed in extension and flexion to rule out partial tears.

         viii. Because of increased muscle tone, stress, pain, or anxiety, some patient may need to be sedated before performing this test.

         ix. Cranial drawer with an abrupt stop in observed normally in young dogs (puppy drawer).

         x. Direct drawer may be painful in dogs with cruciate disease but also in normal dogs.

      b. Indirect (Cranial tibial thrust):

         i. Standing or in lateral recumbency.

         ii. Mimics normal loading of tibia that generates tibial thrust.

         iii. Keep the stifle joint in slight flexion.

         iv. Flex and extend the hock with one hand while the other hand is palpating the tibial tuberosity for cranial subluxation.

   e. Imaging:

      1. Radiographic evaluation:

         a. Assess and document joint effusion.

         b. Assess and document degenerative joint disease.

c. Rule out other stifle, distal femur, or proximal tibial sources of pain.

d. Include both stifle joints for comparison:

   a. Often a bilateral disease

e. May observe cranial dislocation of proximal tibia relative to femur.

f. May observe distal displacement of popliteal sesmoid.

g. May observe subchondral bone cysts.

2. Stifle ultrasound

3. MRI

f. Arthroscopy

g. Joint fluid analysis and cytology:

   1. Often mimics results of degenerative joint disease:

      a. Cell counts are typically $<5000/mm^3$.

      b. Protein consistent with a modified transudate.

h. Treatments:

   1. Medical:

      a. Initial rest followed by physical therapy:

         a. Controlled leash walks

         b. Controlled stair climbing

         c. Swimming

         d. Low impact physical activity

      b. Nonsteroidal anti-inflammatory (NSAID):

         a. To be used in dogs with no evidence of gastrointestinal, hepatic, or renal disease.

         b. Do not mix an NSAID with any other NSAID, including aspirin.

         c. Do not mix NSAIDs with corticosteroids.

      c. Weight loss:

         a. Obesity is most likely to be the number one cause of exacerbating clinical signs of osteoarthritis.

      d. Chondroprotectants

      e. Acupuncture

   2. Surgical:

      a. Intracapsular repair:

         a. Primary repair of ligament

         b. Screw or pin and wire for avulsion fractures

         c. Grafts:

            i. Natural

            ii. Synthetic

      b. Extracapsular.

      c. Osteotomies.

      d. Regardless of surgical method used all medical therapies should also be pursued pre and postoperatively.

2. Caudal cruciate:

   a. Uncommon

   b. Large-breed dogs

   c. Severe trauma:

      1. Large force applied to the proximal tibia forcing it in a caudal direction relative to the femur.

      2. Up to half of cases with bony avulsion:

         a. Mostly from femur origin site

   d. Clinical signs and diagnosis:

      1. Lameness.

      2. Pain on palpation of joint.

      3. Direct drawer will be present but be careful to differentiate cranial drawer from caudal drawer:

         a. Use the tibial tuberosity as a landmark for caudal displacement.

         b. Use the contralateral limb for reference.

      4. Imaging:

         a. Radiographs:

            a. Fractures

            b. Joint effusion

            c. Degenerative joint disease

         b. Ultrasound

         c. MRI

      5. Arthroscopy

      6. Treatment:

         a. Medical (as above for cranial cruciate ligament rupture):

            a. Recommended in cases of caudal cruciate ligament rupture for at least one month.

            b. Most patients do very well with medical management.

         b. Surgical:

            a. Intra-articular

           i. Screw or wire avulsion
           fracture
      b. Extra-articular

3. Medial meniscus:
    a. C-shaped cartilage structure.
    b. Up to 80% of meniscal injuries are associated with cranial cruciate ligament injury.
    c. Occurs because of the firm attachments of medial meniscus to the tibial plateau that "traps" the meniscus between the femur and tibia during cranial tibial translocation.
    d. Bucket handle tears are common, which can "snap" back and forth under the femoral condyle and generate the "clicking" sound sometimes heard during weight bearing.
    e. Clinical signs and diagnosis:
      1. Clicking during weight bearing may be heard:
        a. The lack of audible sounds during range of motion does not rule out meniscal injury.
        b. Usually acute non-weight-bearing to partial weight-bearing lameness.
        c. Ultrasound or MRI may be useful.
        d. Arthroscopy.
    f. Treatments:
      1. Controversial
      2. Primary repair
      3. Partial menisectomy
      4. Complete menisectomy
      5. Meniscal release
      6. Meniscal replacement

4. Lateral and medial collateral ligament:
    a. Rare to have as isolated injury.
    b. More commonly associated with deranged stifle.
    c. Clinical signs and diagnosis:
      1. History of acute trauma
      2. Mild to moderate lameness
      3. Painful joint on palpation
      4. Valgus stress test:
        a. Used to diagnose medial collateral ligament injury
        b. Use opposite limb for comparison
      5. Varus stress test:
        a. Used to diagnose lateral collateral ligament injury
        b. Use opposite limb for comparison
      6. Radiographs:
        a. Avulsion fractures
        b. Other injuries
        c. Varus and valgus stress radiographs
      7. Treatments:
        a. Primary repair of torn ligament or internal fixation of avulsed bone fragment with attached ligament
        b. External coaptation for 2–4 weeks after internal repair

16. LUXATIONS/DERANGEMENT OF THE STIFLE JOINT

    a. Physical examination findings may include severe lameness, stifle swelling, excessive medial and/or lateral angulation of the tibia and fibula, cranial and caudal drawer.
    b. Rupture of supporting structures:
      i. Ligaments:
        1. Cranial cruciate
        2. Caudal cruciate
        3. Collaterals
      ii. Joint capsule.
      iii. Menisci.
      iv. Frequently clinically significant injuries involve rupture both cruciates and one collateral ligament.
    c. Usually associated with severe trauma.
    d. Thorough assessment for concurrent trauma.
    e. Preoperative external coaptation:
      i. Robert–Jones
      ii. Modified Robert–Jones
    f. Open reduction and reconstruction of the joint is necessary.

17. PATELLAR LUXATION

    a. Femoropatellar instability is a common cause of lameness in dogs.
    b. Traumatic or developmental:
      i. Developmental medial luxation is most common
      ii. Lateral luxation in large-breed dogs secondary to genu valgum
      iii. Acute traumatic patellar luxation:

1. Medial or lateral
2. Non-weight-bearing lame
3. Pain on joint manipulation

c. Physical examination findings:
   i. Rule out cranial cruciate ligament rupture and other causes of stifle pain.
   ii. Place one hand over the patella and use the other hand to elevate the tibia and place the stifle in flexion and extension.
   iii. Note the presence of spontaneous luxation.
   iv. Isolate the patella between thumb and finger and with the stifle in extension try to luxate the patella medial and lateral.

d. Radiographs:
   i. To document luxation.
   ii. To identify concurrent injury or abnormality.
   iii. Skyline views are useful to evaluate the trochlea of the femur.

e. Treatment for acute traumatic patellar luxation:
   i. Internal fixation by suturing the fascial defect that allowed the patella to luxate.
   ii. External coaptation for 10–14 days to protect the soft tissue repair.
   iii. Physical therapy to preserve long-term range of motion.

18. PATELLAR FRACTURES

a. Uncommon.
b. Caused from a direct blow to the patella.
c. Patella is a crucial structure and provides extra extensor force for the stifle.
d. Treatment:
   i. Very small displaced pieces can be removed.
   ii. Tension band and cerclage wire that encircles the patella to overcome quadriceps tension forces.
   iii. Conservative management is not recommended for clinical patients as nonunion and chronic lameness is likely.

19. FRACTURES OF THE TIBIA AND FIBULA

a. Common.
b. High incidence of open fractures (compared to other long bone fractures):
   i. Minimal soft tissue covering
c. High incidence of osteomyelitis (compared to other long bone fractures):
   i. Minimal extra-osseous blood supply

d. Classification:
   i. Fractures isolated to the tibia or fibula:
      1. Fibular head:
         a. Insertion point for lateral collateral ligament.
         b. Results in stifle joint instability.
         c. Internal fixation is required.
      2. Fibular shaft:
         a. Soft padded bandage for 5–7 days.
         b. External coaptation is often not required.
      3. Tibial tuberosity (Figure 18.23):
         a. Avulsion fracture.
         b. Internal fixation is often required.
         c. If not displaced:
            1. External coaptation, such as a lateral splint, caudal splint, bivalve cast, or full cast
            2. Strict cage rest for 6–8 weeks
      4. Tibial shaft:
         a. Intact fibula acts as an internal splint
         b. External coaptation
            1. Modified Robert–Jones:
               a. Add a cranial or plantar splint.
               b. Add a walking bar.
            2. Fiberglass cast
            3. Bivalve cast
      5. Malleolus:
         a. Lateral or Medial.
         b. Intra-articular fracture.
         c. Avulsion fractures of the collateral ligaments of the tarsocrural joint.
         d. Internal fixation is required.
         e. Preoperative external coaptation:
            1. Modified Robert–Jones:
               a. Add a cranial or plantar splint.
               b. Add a walking bar.
   ii. Fractures of the tibia and fibula:
      1. Shaft (diaphyseal):
         a. Most common tibial and fibular fracture
         b. Treatment:
            1. External coaptation may be performed in some cases:
               a. Requirements:
                  a. Two-piece fracture
                  b. Transverse or short oblique
                  c. Distant from either joint
            b. External coaptation (cylindrical casts) mechanics:

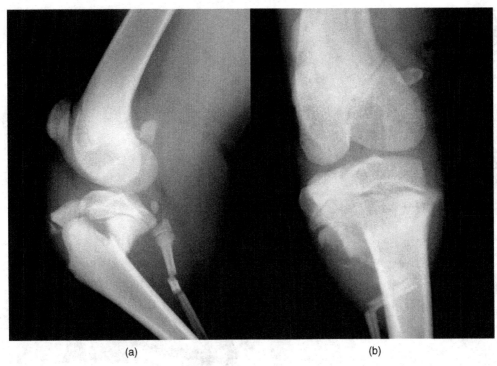

(a)   (b)

FIGURE 18.23 Lateral (a) and orthogonal (b) radiographs of a puppy with a Salter–Harris II fracture of the proximal tibia, tibial tuberosity avulsion, and comminuted fracture of the proximal fibula.

    a. Resists bending.
    b. Resists rotation if incorporates joints above and below.
    c. Axial compression is not neutralized.
    d. Attain at least 50% of bone overlap.
    e. Maintain alignment.
    f. Minimize angulation.
2. Internal fixation or external skeletal fixation (ESF) are typically the preferred option for definitive repair unless there are financial concerns or if coexisting disease is present that precludes anesthesia and surgery:
    a. ESF provides a limited approach concept that helps to preserve the internal environment of the fracture and causes less trauma to the soft tissues that are needed for fracture fragment blood supply during bone healing.

    b. ESF is the preferred treatment for open fractures.
2. Shaft (epiphyseal):
    a. Internal fixation
3. Physeal (see Salter–Harris classification):
    a. Closed reduction and external coaptation is often unsuccessful.
    b. Internal fixation is usually indicated.

20. FRACTURES/LUXATIONS OF THE TARSUS
  a. Fractures of the calcaneus:
    i. Disruption of the common calcaneal tendon
    ii. Avulsion fracture
    iii. Plantigrade stance
    iv. Common in racing greyhounds
    v. Early internal fixation is recommended
  b. Avulsion of the gastrocnemius tendon (Figures 18.24a and 18.24b):
    i. Anatomy of calcanean tendon:
      1. Gastrocnemius tendon
      2. Common tendon of biceps femoris, semi-tendinosus, and gracilis muscles

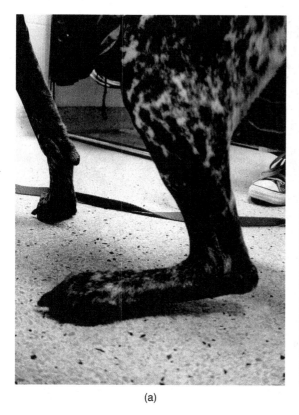
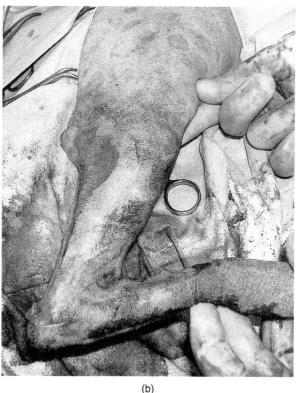

(a)   (b)

FIGURE 18.24   (a) Partial calcanean tendon rupture in a dog. Notice the plantigrade stance and curling of the toes occurring because the superficial digital flexor tendon remains intact. (b) Intraoperative image of the lateral aspect of the right leg of a dog with an acute traumatic calcanean tendon laceration. The blue wrap is over the dog's foot. The surgeon's right hand is on the proximal and cranial aspect of the tibia and the left hand is on the plantar surface of the foot. Notice the hyperflexion of the tarsal joint while the stifle is in extension.

    3. Tendon of the superficial digital flexor muscle
  ii. Physical examination findings:
    1. Swelling at the tip of the calcaneus, extension of the stifle, flexion of the tarsus, and flexion of the digits:
      a. Dropped hock and crab-like appearance of the affected foot:
        1. Occurs because the superficial digital flexor tendon is still intact.
      b. Painful swelling of the gastrocnemius muscle bellies at the level of the proximal and caudal tibia.
  iii. Internal fixation:
    1. Locking loop suture pattern (see page 316 and Figures 18.19a–e above).

    2. Three loop pulley suture pattern (see page 316 and Figures 18.18a–h above).
    3. Use bone tunnels (tunnels are made in the bone with an IM pin or fine drill bit and are used to anchor suture) with either suture pattern.
    4. Postoperative external coaptation is recommended:
      a. Modified Robert–Jones with lateral splint for 6 weeks.
  c. Laceration of the common calcanean tendon (Figures 18.24a and 18.24b):
    i. Associated with acute trauma
    ii. If wound is fresh and considered to be contaminated:
      1. Debride wound and edges of tendon
      2. Copious lavage

3. Locking loop or three loop pulley suture pattern

4. Postoperative external coaptation is recommended:

    a. Modified Robert–Jones with lateral splint for 6 weeks

iii. If wound is greater than 4–6 hours or assumed to be dirty/infected:

    1. Initial aggressive surgical debridement.

    2. Utilize mechanical debridement for 24–48 hours.

    3. Locking loop or three loop pulley suture pattern.

    4. Postoperative external coaptation is recommended using a Modified Robert–Jones bandage containing a lateral splint for 6 weeks.

d. Fractures of the talus, central tarsal bone, second, third, and fourth tarsal bone:

    i. Most are articular fractures.

    ii. Nondisplaced and nonavulsion fractures can be treated conservatively with splints or casts.

    iii. Displaced or avulsion fractures require internal fixation.

    iv. Small fragments may be removed surgically.

e. Luxation of the tarsocrural joint:

    i. Malleolar fractures

    ii. Collateral ligament injuries

    iii. Treatment options:

        1. Internal fixation.

        2. Acute injuries:

            a. Tendon reconstruction

        3. Pantarsal arthrodesis.

        4. Postoperative external coaptation is recommended:

            a. Modified Robert–Jones with lateral splint for 6 weeks

f. Injury of the short collateral ligaments:

    i. Physical examination findings may include lameness, instability of the medial and/or lateral aspect of the hock joint, and swelling of the tarsus.

    ii. Internal fixation is recommended:

        1. In small dogs and cats, primary ligament repair and imbrication of soft tissue may be successful.

        2. In large dogs primary repair of the ligaments is often not possible and screws and washers with wire or suture is often required.

3. Postoperative external coaptation is recommended with a modified Robert–Jones with lateral splint for 6 weeks.

g. Plantar and dorsal intertarsal subluxation:

    i. Physical examination may include moderate to severe lameness, increased opening or closing angle of the hock during flexion and extension, and pain on palpation of the tarsal bones.

    ii. Bilateral injuries are common.

    iii. Initial repair with external coaptation, in non athletic dogs, can be attempted but is often unsuccessful.

    iv. Internal fixation or arthrodesis (partial or full) is often required.

h. Tarsometatarsal joint subluxation:

    i. Concomitant fractures are common:

        1. Fourth tarsal bone

        2. Proximal metatarsal bones

    ii. External coaptation is unsuccessful.

    iii. Arthrodesis of the tarsometatarsal joint is recommended.

i. Luxation of the superficial digital flexor tendon:

    i. Physical examination findings include moderate lameness, swelling over the proximal aspect of the calcaneus, and palpation of the tendon slipping off of the proximal calcaneus with flexion and extension of the hock. In most cases, the tendon can be manually displaced and reduced.

    ii. Shetland sheepdogs and collies.

    iii. Lateral luxation.

    iv. Conservative treatment is often unsuccessful.

    v. Internal fixation is required.

21. TENDON INJURIES

a. Most commonly injured tendons:

    i. Calcanean tendon

    ii. Triceps tendon

    iii. Deep gluteal tendon

b. Goals of repair:

    1. Resist gap formation

    2. Promote primary healing

    3. Decrease adhesions

    4. Maintain blood supply

c. Three-loop pulley (Figures 18.18a–h):

    i. Suture passes on either side of the rupture three times at 120° intervals.

    ii. Near-far, middle-middle, far-near.

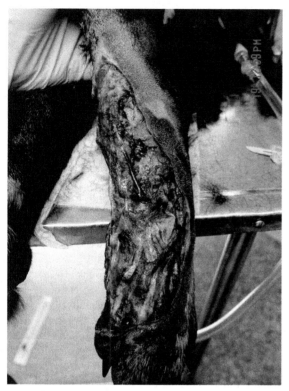

FIGURE 18.25 Dorsal and lateral shearing injury to the hind limb of a dog. This is a severe injury with loss of soft tissue and bone and major neurovascular compromise. The limb was amputated.

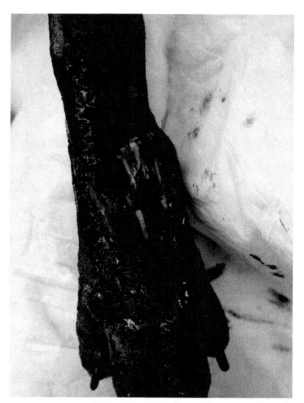

FIGURE 18.26 Dorsal and lateral shearing injury to the hind limb of a dog. The metatarsal bones are exposed and fractured. There is loss of soft tissue, bone, and collateral ligaments of the tarsus but the limb was spared by arthrodesing the hock and applying a free skin graft to the dorsal metatarsal region.

    iii. Strong, inelastic, and nonabsorbable suture material is used.

  d. Looking loop (Figures 18.19a–e):
    i. Best used on sheathed tendons.
    ii. The longitudinal suture passes deep to the transverse suture.

22. SHEARING INJURIES (Figures 18.25 and 18.26)

  a. Damage to the medial or lateral aspect of the carpus or tarsus:
    i. Medial injury is most common.
  b. Abrasion injury involving:
    i. Skin.
    ii. Tendons.
    iii. Ligaments.
    iv. Muscles.
    v. Bone.
    vi. Surprisingly, severe and debilitating neurologic injury is not a common component of

these injuries; however, it does occur in some cases and neurologic status should be evaluated on presentation.
  c. Most injuries with involvement of bone and joint.
  d. Many with joint instability.
  e. Assess neurologic and vascular integrity of distal limb:
    i. Some cases may require partial foot amputation and reconstruction or limb amputation.
  f. Radiographs are necessary:
    i. Make varus and valgus stress radiographs to assess instability.
    ii. Assess loss of bone and concurrent fractures.
  g. Primary closure of the wound is avoided:
    i. Contaminated
    ii. Dirty and infected

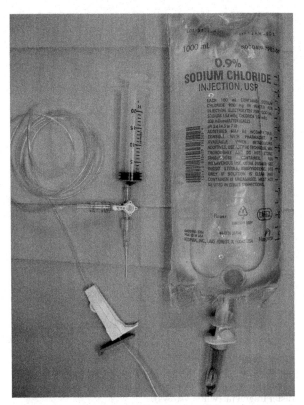

FIGURE 18.27   Set up for a simple wound lavage system. Intravenous infusion set tubing, 20–60 cc syringe, 18 gauge intravenous catheter, three-way stopcock, and a 1 L bag of NaCl.

3. As the saline dries from the gauze, wound fluid and exudate is drawn into the gauze and dries there (to dry).

4. The bandage should be changed at least once every 24 hours and sometimes more frequently (if strikethrough present).

5. Wet-to-dry and dry-to-dry bandages are considered adhesives and are damaging to granulation tissue. Their use is limited to early debridement of wounds and should not be a replacement for initial aggressive surgical debridement and lavage.

6. Discontinue the use of wet-to-dry bandages once a granulation bed begins to form.

7. Dry-to-dry bandages use dry sterile gauze in direct contact with a wound and are reserved very effusive wounds. They go on dry and come off dry.

vii. Granulation tissue should begin to cover the wound in 5–7 days (Figure 18.28).

viii. When the wound is completely covered by granulation tissue definitive repair of the joint is performed:

    1. Synthetic ligaments

    2. External skeletal fixation

    3. Arthrodesis

ix. In some cases, wound contracture and scar tissue provide enough stabilization to avoid definitive surgery:

h. Immediate lavage and debridement:

    i. Remove all devitalized tissue.

    ii. Remove all foreign material.

    iii. Copious lavage (Figure 18.27).

    iv. Tissue culture of the wound.

    v. Sterile dressing is applied and covered by a bandage:

        1. Robert–Jones

        2. Modified Robert–Jones

         a. Splint

    vi. Daily sterile bandage changes initially:

        1. Wet-to-dry (or dry-to-dry) bandages are used initially for grossly contaminated wounds and wounds with devitalized tissue.

        2. Sterile gauze is moistened (wet) with sterile saline and placed in direct contact with the wound.

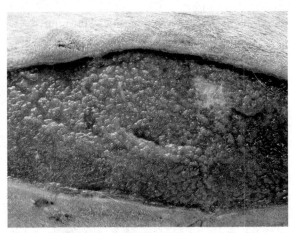

FIGURE 18.28   Eleven-day-old shearing injury of the front limb of a dog. The entire wound has been covered in a healthy granulation bed and is ready for definitive repair.

1. Many referral hospitals are beginning to use vacuum-assisted wound closure devices that rely on intermittent suctioning of wounds to improve the wound environment and expedite definitive wound closure (Guille et al., 2007). For more information about these devices, visit http://www.kci1.com/35.asp.

23. OPEN FRACTURES

a. Goals of open fracture management:
  i. Identifying and treating concurrent life-threatening injuries.
  ii. Aggressive debridement and lavage of affected tissues.
  iii. Procuring tissue and wound cultures.
  iv. Application of protective bandages. The following assumes previous stabilization of the patient and focuses on treating the injury to the limb.
  v. Orthopedic and soft tissue injuries are treated as soon as the patient is stable:
    1. Prolonged delays in temporary or definitive stabilization of the fracture are associated with a poorer functional outcome.
    2. Sedation and analgesia is recommended for evaluation of the limb, manipulation, radiographs, and wound care.
    3. The injured limb is examined for hemorrhage, devitalized tissue, nerve damage and sensation, and obvious deformity or fractures.
    4. Radiographs are made of the injured limb and of the contralateral limb if needed:
      a. If air is identified on radiographs within the soft tissues or closely associated with the fracture site an open fracture is confirmed.
      b. Air is not always observed in an open fracture.

b. Fracture classification:
  i. Type I (first degree)—soft tissue wound less than 1 cm long, minimal soft tissue damage, caused by low energy forces, usually a simple or two piece fracture. (Figure 18.29).
  ii. Type II (second degree)—soft tissue wound larger than 1 cm long that communicates with

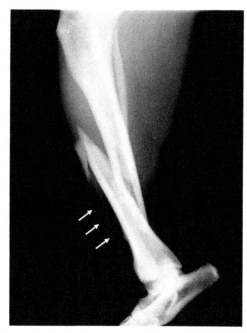

FIGURE 18.29 Lateral radiograph of the tibia of a dog after sustaining unknown trauma. There is a midshaft, spiral, comminuted, grade I open fracture. Notice the small amount of gas in the soft tissues associated with the sharp tip of the distal fragment (white arrows).

the fracture, moderate soft tissue damage, caused by high energy forces.
  iii. Type III (third degree)—high energy trauma and severe soft tissue damage, often with loss of soft tissue and bone:
    1. Type IIIa—the bone can be covered and the tissues reconstructed without skin flaps or grafts.
    2. Type IIIb—require major reconstructive techniques to close the wound.
    3. Type IIIc—major arterial injury that requires repair.
  iv. Type IV (fourth degree)—amputation or near amputation, severe soft tissue damage, and neurovascular injury are present.

c. Treatment of the wound:
  i. Decide if limb preservation and long-term function are possible.
  ii. All open fractures are contaminated and are considered infected if greater than 8 hours old.

iii. Contamination continues as long as the wound remains open.

iv. Sterile and nonadherent dressings are placed on the wound as soon as possible to reduce further contamination and hemorrhage.

v. Caps, masks, gowns, sterile gloves, and instruments are used every time the wound is uncovered for debridement and bandage changes.

vi. Initial wound therapy is divided into preparation, irrigation, and decontamination:

1. Apply sterile lubricant jelly to the wound and cover with sterile gauze during clipping and cleaning with an antiseptic agent.

2. After liberal fur removal, the wound and limb, the jelly, debris, and clipped fur are removed with a sterile lavage solution.

3. Warm isotonic saline or a buffered electrolyte solution (such as LRS) is used for copious lavage of the wound, 0.05% diluted chlorhexidine can also be used but iodine solutions and hydrogen peroxide should be avoided as they are toxic to fibroblasts and other cells involved in early wound healing.

4. A sterile bandage is applied after each debridement and bandage change.

5. Repair of lacerated tendons is performed with recommended suture techniques and without tension.

6. Large syringes (60 cc) and an 18 gauge catheter or pulsating jet-type devices can be used to achieve 8–9 psi, which is efficient for removing bacteria and debris.

7. Devitalized and contaminated tissue will delay soft tissue and bone healing and must be completely debrided.

8. Wound closure is delayed until the tissues are viable and the risk of infection is minimal.

vii. Bacterial culture and sensitivity are performed immediately before wound closure or after aggressive surgical debridement and lavage.

viii. Continued daily debridement can be surgical, mechanical, enzymatic, or a combination of therapies:

1. Mechanical debridement is performed with nonadherent, semi-occlusive wet-to-dry, or for effusive wounds, dry-to-dry dressings.

2. A secondary layer of absorptive cotton is applied over the primary sterile bandage to draw exudate and wound fluid away from the wound surface, this is covered with stretch or conforming gauze.

3. For fractures below the elbow or stifle, lateral or caudal splints made out of fiberglass or other materials are applied on top of the secondary layer for added support.

4. The third or outer layer is composed of elastic adhesive tape.

ix. Systemic therapies include broad-spectrum antibiotics and analgesics should be considered. Antibiotics should be chosen based upon for bacterial culture and sensitivity results.

x. Antibiotic therapy alone without aggressive surgical debridement, fracture stabilization, and proper wound care will lead to osteomyelitis, bacteremia, and possibly death.

d. General guidelines for open fracture fixation are dependent on the amount of soft tissue damage, blood supply, and level of contamination:

i. Most grade I open fractures can be treated as closed fractures.

ii. Grade II and III fractures are stabilized by external fixation techniques after closed reduction.

24. INJURIES OF THE FOOTPAD

a. Anatomy:

i. Carpal/tarsal pad

ii. Metacarpal/metatarsal pad

iii. Digital pads

b. Function of the footpad:

i. Absorb compression during standing and ambulation

ii. Sustain daily wear

iii. Provide thermal insulation

c. Types of injuries:

i. Lacerations:

1. Standing and walking forces flatten and spread the pad:

a. These forces must be overcome during healing.

b. If not, chronic nonhealing wounds may develop.

2. Treatment:

a. Debride

b. Lavage

c. Tissue culture and sensitivity

d. Suture:

　1. Appose deep layers with simple interrupted absorbable monofilament suture.

　2. Appose epithelial edges with simple interrupted, vertical mattress, or far-near-near-far suture pattern.

　3. Epithelial sutures are generally left in place for 21 days.

e. Bandage:

　1. Nonadherent bandage and spoon splint

　2. Splint for 3–4 weeks

　3. Soft bandage for additional 1 week

　4. Restrict activity while in bandage

f. Empirical antibiotic therapy pending culture results

ii. Degloving wounds should be treated as open fractures are treated.

iii. Abrasions:

　1. Superficial:

　　a. Heal by second intention

　　b. External coaptation:

　　　1. Spoon splint.

　　　2. Keep splinted until re-epithelialization occurs.

　　　3. Limit activity during healing.

　　c. Topical wound therapies:

　　　1. Acemannan (an extract of aloe vera) can be applied twice daily until epithelialization begins; it is thought to increase wound-healing rate.

　　　2. Aloe vera is thought to increase wound-healing rate and decreases

inflammation. It can be applied twice daily until epithelialization begins.

　　　3. Tripeptide copper complex may help to stimulate collagen synthesis. It can be applied 1–2 times daily until a granulation bed covers the entire wound.

　2. Full-thickness:

　　a. Loss of function

　　b. Treatment:

　　　1. Phalangeal fillet—this technique removes all three phalanges and the nail from a digit but preserves the skin and digital pad, which are used to reconstruct a foot pad defect.

　　　2. Full-thickness pad grafts.

　　　3. Full-thickness pad flaps.

　　　4. Microvascular pad transfer.

BIBLIOGRAPHY

Guille AE, Tseng LW, Orsher RJ. Use of vacuum-assisted closure for management of a large skin wound in a cat. *JAVMA* 2007; 230: 1669–1673.

Piermattei DL, Flo GL. *Handbook of Small Animal Orthopedics and Fracture Repair*. 3rd edition. WB Saunders, Philadelphia, PA, 1983.

Piermattei DL, Flo GL. *Handbook of Small Animal Orthopedics and Fracture Repair*. 4th edition. Elsevier Science, Philadelphia, PA, 2006.

Slatter DH. *Textbook of Small Animal Surgery*. 3rd edition. Elsevier Science, Philadelphia, PA, 2003; Chapters 19, 127, 130, 134–137, 139–142, 146, 149, 150, 158.

TRAUMA-ASSOCIATED MUSCULOSKELETAL INJURY TO THE PELVIS, SACRUM, AND TAIL

CHAPTER 19

Lauren May and Stephen J. Mehler

1. INTRODUCTION TO PELVIC TRAUMA

a. Trauma in the veterinary patient is one of the most common presentations to veterinary hospitals.

b. Traumatic injury can occur to the skin, muscle, bone, peripheral and central nervous system, and internal organ systems.

c. The greater the force associated with the traumatic event the more damage that is caused to the body.

d. Motor vehicle accidents and falling from heights are the most common cause of pelvic fractures in dogs and cats:

    i. Fractures are common in small animal patients with pelvic fractures accounting for 20–30% of the fractures seen in veterinary practice.

    ii. Pelvic fractures are often associated with severe muscular injury and bruising, neurovascular trauma, and abdominal and thoracic injury.

e. Because most patients with pelvic fractures have sustained a high force injury it is important to consider both concurrent systemic injuries and other musculoskeletal derangement. Many patients for example, will present in shock, have head trauma, and pulmonary contusions, all of which will need to be addressed prior to definitively treating the pelvic fractures.

2. ANATOMY AND FUNCTION (Figure 19.1)

a. The pelvis is a rectangular box-like structure formed by the ossa coxarum or pelvic girdle, sacrum and first caudal vertebra.

b. Each os coxae, also termed hemipelvises, are composed of the ilium, ischium, pubis, and the acetabular bone.

c. The femoral head fits into the acetabulum and weight transfer from the hind limb occurs at this joint.

d. The medial surface of the ilial body, also called the sacropelvic surface, articulates with the sacrum by way of the sacroiliac joint:

    i. The sacroiliac joint consists of a crescent-shaped synovial joint and fibrocartilaginous synchondrosis.

    ii. This articulation allows primary weight transfer to the vertebral column.

e. The ischium is an irregularly shaped bone that forms the caudal aspect of the os coxae:

    i. The caudolateral aspect of this bone is termed the ischiatic tuberosity.

    ii. The sacrotuberous ligament, biceps femoris, semitendinosus and semimembranosus muscles have origins in this region.

f. The prepubic tendon, which is composed of the tendinous sheaths of most of the abdominal musculature, attaches on a small eminence on the cranial and ventral aspect of the pubis, called the pubic tubercle.

Manual of Trauma Management in the Dog and Cat, First Edition. Edited by Kenneth J. Drobatz, Matthew W. Beal and Rebecca S. Syring.
© 2011 John Wiley & Sons, Inc. Published 2011 by John Wiley & Sons, Inc.

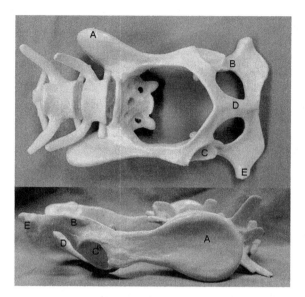

FIGURE 19.1   Anatomy of the pelvis. A. Ilium, B. Ischium, C. Acetabulum, D. Pubis, E. Ischiatic tuberosity, F. Obturator foramen

g. The axis of the canine pelvis is not parallel to the spine; it has approximately a 45° angle of inclination. This is important when assessing pelvic fracture radiographs and attempting to realign sacroiliac fractures and dislocations.

h. The pelvis is closely associated with many vessels and nerves that can sustain injury during pelvic trauma or during pelvic fracture repair:

i.   The lumbosacral nerve trunk courses caudally on the medial aspect of the ilial body. It then crosses over the dorsal border of the ilium at the greater ischiatic notch, at which level the distal continuation of the lumbosacral trunk is termed the sciatic nerve.

ii.   The cranial and caudal gluteal, pelvic, pudendal, and hypogastric nerves are anatomically associated with the pelvis.

iii.   The internal iliac, caudal and cranial gluteal, and femoral vessels are intimate with the pelvis.

i.   The pelvis encircles part of the urogenital tract.

j.   The most aboral aspect of the gastrointestinal tract is completely contained within the pelvic cavity.

3. CLASSIFICATION AND COMBINATIONS OF PELVIC FRACTURES

a. Injuries of the pelvis can be grouped into many categories, all which can be separated into two groups:

i. Fractures involving the weight-bearing axis of the pelvis should be repaired. (Figure 19.2):

a. Sacroiliac fracture/luxations

b. Ilial body fractures

c. Most acetabular fractures

ii. Fractures involving the non weight-bearing axis of the pelvis are treated conservatively:

a. Ilial wing fractures.

b. Ischial fractures.

c. Pelvic floor fractures.

d. Exception: fractures involving the non weight-bearing surface of the caudal acetabulum should be repaired.

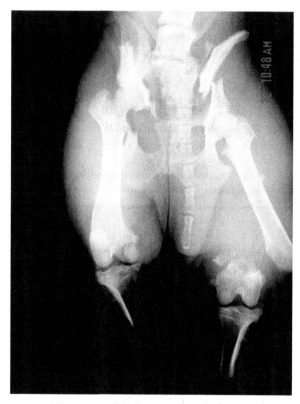

FIGURE 19.2   Ventrodorsal radiograph of a dog after being hit by a car. There are bilateral ilial fractures, right ischial, acetabular, and pubic fractures, right sacral body fracture, and a left supracondylar femur fracture. The ilial, acetabular, sacral, and femur fracture should be repaired.

b. The pelvis is a rectangular structure; therefore, there must be at least two disruptions of the pelvis (fracture or luxation) for displacement of pelvic fractures to occur.

c. Almost all cats and dogs with pelvic fractures have multiple pelvic fractures.

4. **CONCURRENT SOFT TISSUE INJURIES**

a. Depending upon the extent of trauma, injuries can range from minimal to severe, and most need to be addressed prior to addressing the pelvic fractures.

b. There is a high incidence of thoracic injury concurrent to pelvic trauma (see Chapter 6: Trauma-Associated Thoracic Injury).

c. Urinary tract trauma is often seen concurrent with pelvic trauma (see Chapter 10: Trauma-Associated Urinary Tract Injury):

  i. Clear colored urine or the ability to urinate does not rule out urinary tract trauma or rupture:

  a. Most animals with pelvic trauma will not be able to posture to urinate and may have damage to the nerves of the lower urinary system:

  1. Urinary catheters should be placed in a sterile fashion and connected to a closed collection system.

  2. If defects in the urinary tract are identified, they should be dealt with either surgically or with temporary urinary diversion followed by surgery, before the pelvic fractures are addressed.

d. Peripheral nerve injuries occur with pelvic fractures (see Chapter 8: Trauma-Associated Peripheral Nerve Injury):

  i. Sciatic nerve (including lumbosacral trunk):

  a. This is the most common nerve deficit noted in association with pelvic fractures.

  b. Sciatic nerve dysfunction in cats and dogs is reported to occur most frequently in association with ilial body fractures.

  c. Affected animals will drag the toes of the injured leg and be unable to flex or extend the hock and flex the stifle. Muscle atrophy may be evident in the gastrocnemius, cranial tibial, and thigh muscles.

  ii. Peroneal nerve (distal branch of sciatic):

  a. May see deficits in cranial tibial muscle reflex.

  b. May see decreased or loss of sensation over the dorsal aspect of the paw on the hindlimb.

  iii. Pudendal nerve:

  a. Somatic nerve to external anal sphincter and urethral sphincter.

  b. Injury may result in urinary and fecal incontinence.

  iv. Caudal nerve:

  a. May see loss of tail sensation and function.

  v. Pelvic nerve:

  a. Provides parasympathetic innervation to the bladder, external genitalia, and anus.

  b. May see changes in micturation, sensation to genitalia and anus.

  vi. Avulsion of nerve roots:

  a. May see lower motor neuron signs to the hind limbs (decreased muscle tone, hyporeflexia), urinary and fecal incontinence, loss of anal tone, and loss of tail tone and function.

  vii. Peripheral nerve entrapment:

  a. Can result in severe pain and altered or loss of function.

e. Gastrointestinal tract trauma (see Chapter 14: Trauma-Associated Gastrointestinal Injury):

  i. Small intestinal laceration:

  a. Jejunum

  b. Ileum

  ii. Rectal or colonic perforation:

  iii. Intestinal entrapment within a body wall defect or between fracture fragments

f. Vascular injury:

  i. Comminuted pelvic fractures can result in lacerations of the internal iliac artery or vein.

  ii. Laceration or fragmentation of the kidney, spleen or liver can occur concurrent to pelvic fractures (see Chapter 11: Trauma-Associated Abdominal Parenchymal Organ Injury).

  iii. Severe swelling and bruising of the inguinal region, thigh, and gravity-dependent portion of the affected limb may be evident with vascular trauma. Affected patients may have pale mucus membranes, tachycardia, hypotension, and hypothermia associated with acute blood loss.

g. Extrahepatic biliary tract rupture (see Chapter 12: Trauma-Associated Biliary Tract Injury):

   i. Hepatic duct

   ii. Common bile duct

   iii. Cystic duct

   iv. Rupture of the gallbladder (rare)

   v. Additional comments:

      a. Clinical signs of biliary tract rupture are not always observed immediately after the trauma.

      b. These patients are often discharged from the hospital and return a few days to weeks later with clinical signs.

h. Herniation of the abdominal wall and avulsion of the prepubic tendon (see Chapter 13: Trauma-Associated Body Wall and Torso Injury):

   i. Abdominal viscera may herniate through the tear.

   ii. Incarceration or strangulation of bowel or urinary bladder may occur.

   iii. These injuries must be dealt with before definitive fracture repair.

i. Crush, burn, abrasion, and slough injuries (Figure 19.3):

   i. Skin over the back and rear end is often injured.

   ii. These injuries can lead to excessive loss of total body fluid and protein with secondary volume shifts, dehydration, infection, and hypoproteinemia.

j. Common concurrent musculoskeletal injuries:

   i. Sacral body fractures

   ii. Coxofemoral joint injuries

   iii. Femoral diaphyseal fractures

   iv. Femoral head fractures

   v. Femoral shaft fractures

   vi. Spinal fractures

5. SIGNS ASSOCIATED WITH PELVIC TRAUMA

   a. Gait:

      i. Weight-bearing gait abnormities

      ii. Non weight-bearing

      iii. Partial weight-bearing

   b. Crepitus:

   c. Alteration of bony landmarks:

      i. Wings of the ilium

      ii. Greater trochanter

      iii. Ischiatic tuberosity

   d. Pain with manipulation:

      i. Hip extension and flexion

      ii. Direct palpation

      iii. Tail extension and flexion

   e. Neurologic abnormalities:

      i. Nerves affected:

         a. Sciatic:

            a. Loss of function of affected limb

            b. Absence withdrawal reflex

         b. Obturator:

            a. When standing on a smooth surface, the affected limb may slide laterally.

         c. Femoral:

            a. Loss of quadriceps function and stifle extension.

         d. Pudendal:

            a. See above.

         e. Pelvic:

            a. See above.

         f. Caudal:

            a. See above.

      ii. Clinical signs indicating neurologic abnormalities:

         a. Dragging the paw.

         b. Lack of withdrawal reflex.

         c. No limb adduction.

         d. Lack of patellar reflex or stifle extension.

         e. Lack of motor function to the tail and/or signs of urinary or fecal incontinence and loss of anal tone.

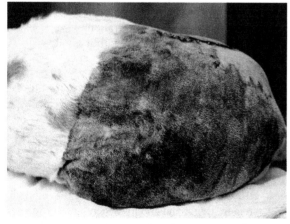

FIGURE 19.3 Severe crushing injury to the dorsum of a dog after being hit by a car. This dog has sustained severely comminuted pelvic fractures. There is a clear demarcation between dead skin and healthy skin. The black skin is firm to the touch and does not bleed when cut.

f. *Note*: Reflexes can be altered (both exacerbated and diminished) by pain, catecholamine release, shock, and administration of analgesics.

6. PHYSICAL EXAMINATION
a. Systematic examination
b. Neurologic examination
c. Rectal examination:
  i. Should be performed in all trauma cases.
  ii. Assess the degree of medial displacement of fracture fragments.
  iii. Assess rectal wall integrity.
  iv. Assess narrowing of pelvic canal.
  v. Assess anal sphincter tone.

7. DIAGNOSIS OF PELVIC FRACTURES
a. Physical examination
b. Radiographs (Figure 19.2):
  i. Ventrodorsal:
    a. Frog-legged to avoid pain associated with hip extension.
    b. Hip extended with heavy sedation or general anesthesia.
  ii. Lateral:
    a. Affected side down
    b. Dependent (down-side) hip flexed
    c. Upper hip extended and slightly oblique
  iii. True oblique views may be needed to adequately assess acetabular fractures
c. Computed tomography (Figure 19.4):
  i. Helps in identifying subtle lesions and for surgical planning of complicated and comminuted fractures.
d. Magnetic resonance imaging:
  i. Helps in assessment of soft tissue injury associated with pelvic trauma, including injury to major nerves and vessels.

8. CONSERVATIVE MANAGEMENT OF PELVIC FRACTURE
a. Justifications for conservative management:
  i. Types of fractures:
    a. Nondisplaced ilial body fractures
    b. Sacroiliac fractures/luxations:
      1. Without contralateral ilial or sacroiliac fracture or luxation
      2. Minimal displacement
    c. Most pubic, ilial wing and ischial fractures
  ii. Financial limitations of the client
  iii. Pelvic fracture/luxation that is chronic (greater than 2 weeks)
b. Conservative treatment is multifactorial:
  i. Cage confinement—this area should be well padded to prevent pressure sore formation and provide comfort. Depending on the fracture location and severity, confinement should last at least 4–6 weeks.
  ii. Restricted, controlled, and monitored activity for at least 4–6 weeks.
  iii. Sling assisted ambulation.
  iv. Adequate pain management.
  v. Monitoring of urination and defecation:
    a. Manual bladder expression if the patient is not urinating.
    b. Cleaning the animal if they are soiled with urine or stool.
  vi. Frequent turning of the patient to prevent decubital ulcers.
  vii. Rehabilitative therapy:
    a. Passive range of motion of the joints
    b. Muscle massage

9. DEFINITIVE OR INTERNAL FIXATION OF PELVIC FRACTURES
a. Justification for internal fixation:
  i. Acetabular fractures
  ii. Unilateral or bilateral instability of the weight-bearing axis of the pelvis
  iii. Fractures resulting in narrowing of the pelvic canal
  iv. Fractures in working dogs or breeding females
  v. Fractures causing nerve entrapment
  vi. Ischial tuberosity fractures causing pain and lameness
  vii. Pubic fractures in association with soft tissue herniation
b. Numerous fixation techniques are described for pelvic fractures:
  i. Bone screws
  ii. Plates
  iii. Cerclage wire
  iv. K-wires
  v. Intramedullary pins
  vi. Bone cement
  vii. Combinations of the above

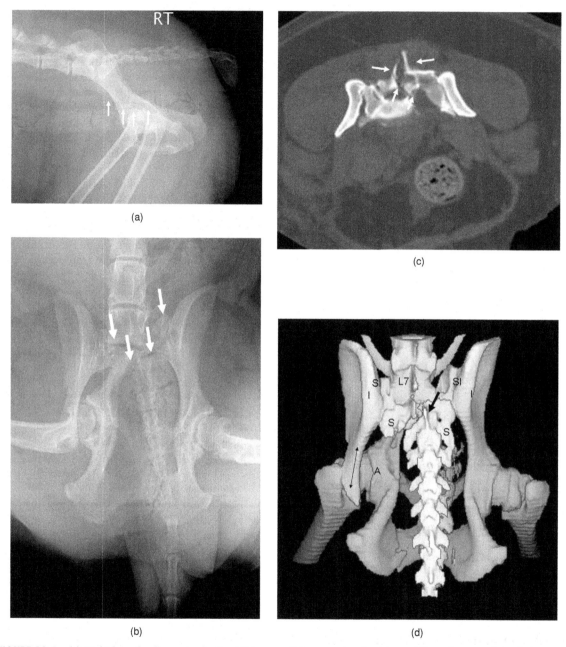

FIGURE 19.4 (a) Right lateral radiograph of a dog hit by a car 5 days previously. A long oblique fracture of the ilial wing is present (white arrow). (b) Ventrodorsal radiographic view of the same dog. There is marked medial and cranial displacement of the ilial fracture. The sacrum is fractured and displaced laterally and cranially (white arrows). There is no evidence of sacroiliac joint involvement. The tail is still attached to the sacrum and is displaced with the caudal segment. Attempts to surgically repair this fracture without a CT scan could be disastrous. (c) CT scan of the pelvis and sacrum of the same dog. The CT images demonstrate severe comminution of the sacrum with both axial and abaxial fractures (white arrows). Attempts to repair this fracture would likely lead to worsening of neurologic signs and futile attempts at adequate fracture stabilization. (d) 3-D reconstruction images of the CT scan. Displaced and comminuted sacral fracture (black arrow), L7 is the seventh lumbar vertebra, I is the ilium, SI is the sacroiliac joint. S is the sacrum, A is the acetabulum, distal aspect of the proximal ilial fracture is denoted by the double-headed black arrow.

10. COMPLICATIONS OF PELVIC FRACTURES AND REPAIR

a. Most complications involve the surrounding soft tissue:

    i. Primary (from the initial trauma)

    ii. Secondary (from the fracture fragments)

    iii. Iatrogenic (surgical manipulation and implants)

b. Complications associated with conservative treatment of pelvic fractures:

    i. Persistent lameness of one or both pelvic limbs

    ii. Osteoarthritis of the hips (when an acetabular fracture was present)

    iii. Stenosis of the pelvic canal:

        a. Obstipation and megacolon

        b. Dystocia

        c. Dysuria

c. Postoperative complications associated with fracture repair:

    i. Degenerative joint disease

    ii. Implant failure

    iii. Fracture malunion or nonunion

    iv. Sciatic nerve injury

    v. Pelvic plexus injury:

        a. Urinary incontinence

        b. Fecal incontinence

11. PROGNOSIS

a. The prognosis for animals with fractures of the flat bones of the pelvis, including the ilium, ischium, and pubis, is excellent for return to normal function.

b. The prognosis for acetabular fractures is good to excellent if reduction is anatomical and stabilization is rigid.

c. If good fracture alignment is not achieved, results range from poor to good:

    i. Patients with acetabular fractures have an increased potential to develop osteoarthritis.

    ii. Poor reduction will likely result in worse osteoarthritis later in life.

d. The prognosis for sciatic nerve dysfunction depends on many factors:

    i. Underlying cause (iatrogenic inflammation or stretch injury has a better prognosis than a traumatic severing of the nerve).

    ii. Severity of injury:

        a. Neuropraxia: Interruption of conduction down the nerve; can be associated with focal demyelination. Least severe lesion and often associated with return to normal to function.

        b. Axonotmesis: Disruption of the neuronal axon but the surrounding supporting tissue remains intact. More severe lesion but some patients can recover.

        c. Neurotmesis: Disruption of the neuronal axon and surrounding supportive tissue. Most severe lesion and recovery of function is unlikely.

    iii. Location of injury (example: injury to proximal sciatic nerve may be devastating to the function of the leg but injury to one of its distal branches may allow for continued function of the limb).

    iv. Severity of dysfunction (paresis versus paralysis versus loss of deep pain perception versus loss of withdrawal).

SACRAL FRACTURE AND SACROCOCCYGEAL FRACTURES/LUXATIONS (FIGURES 19.4A–D)

1. ANATOMY AND FUNCTION (Figure 19.5)

a. The sacrum is formed by fusion of the three sacral vertebrae.

b. Located between the ilial wings.

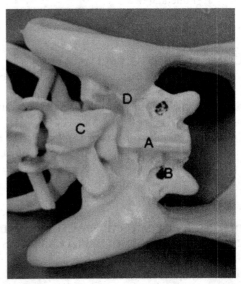

FIGURE 19.5 Anatomy of the dorsal sacrum. A. Median crest, B. Sacral foramina, C. Seventh lumbar vertebral body, D. Wing of the sacrum

c. The transverse processes from all three sacral vertebrae are fused.

d. The sacrum articulates with last lumbar vertebrae and first caudal vertebrae.

e. The sacral and coccygeal nerves, part of the caudal equina, run through the sacral canal (Figure 19.6).

f. The sacrum serves to transfers weight from each hemipelvis to the lumbar vertebrae.

2. **CLASSIFICATION**
   a. Sacral fractures (Figure 19.7):
      i. Abaxial (fractures lateral to the sacral foramina)
      ii. Axial (fractures medial to the sacral foramina)
   b. Sacrococcygeal separations:
      i.   More common in cats
      ii. Traction injuries
      iii. Bite wounds
      iv. Vehicular injuries
   c. Combination fracture and luxation

3. **CONCURRENT INJURIES**
   a. Other pelvic injuries
   b. Systemic and other injuries (see Concurrent injuries for pelvic fractures)
   c. Neurologic injury:
      i. Most common with axial fracture:
         1. Pudendal nerve
         2. Caudal nerves
         3. Pelvic nerves

4. **CLINICAL SIGNS AT PRESENTATION**
   a. Hyperpathia on palpation of the tail head or sacrum.
   b. Dysfunction of the pudendal, pelvic, and caudal nerves:
      i.   Tail may appear flaccid or piloerect.
      ii. Decreased sensation of the perineal area.
      iii. Decreased anal tone.
      iv. Absence of tail tone.
      v.   Lower motor neuron bladder.

5. **DIAGNOSIS OF SACRAL FRACTURES AND SACROCOCCYGEAL FRACTURES/LUXATIONS**
   a. Physical examination
   b. Radiographs
   c. Computed tomography:
      i. Best utilized to define the extent of fractures and define repair options.

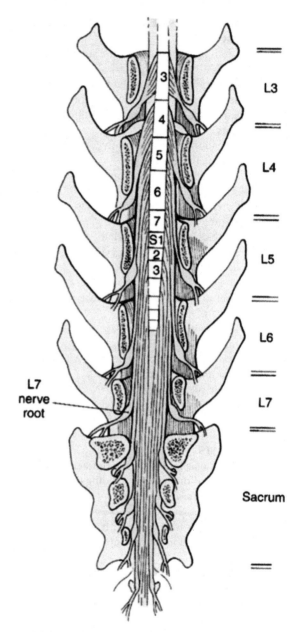

FIGURE 19.6 Nerves of the caudal equina. Note that the spinal cord ends at the fifth or sixth lumbar vertebra and the remaining neural tissue in the spinal canal are individual nerve roots of the sacrum and tail. (Reprinted with permission: Fossum TW, et al. Small Animal Surgery, 3rd edition, Copyright Elsevier, 2007)

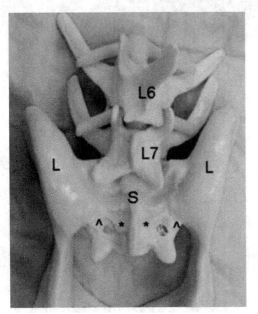

FIGURE 19.7   Anatomic demonstration of axial and abaxial fractures of the sacrum. L6 is the sixth lumbar vertebra, L7 is the seventh lumbar vertebra, L is the ilium, S is the sacrum, ˆ represents the location of an abaxial fracture and is lateral to the sacral foramen, and * represents the location of axial fractures.

    d. Magnetic resonance imaging (Figures 19.8 and 19.9):
      i. Best utilized to define nerve entrapment, injury, and avulsion.

6. **COMPLICATIONS**
    a. See pelvic fracture complications.
    b. Self-mutilation of tail.
    c. Urine scalding from lower motor neuron urinary incontinence.
    d. Fecal incontinence.
    e. Avascular necrosis of tail tip.

7. **TREATMENT**
    a. Sacral fractures:
      i. Conservative management is acceptable for nondisplaced fractures and fractures not compressing nerve roots.
      ii. Internal fixation is recommended for displaced fractures or for fractures compressing nerve roots.
    b. Sacrococcygeal fractures or luxations:

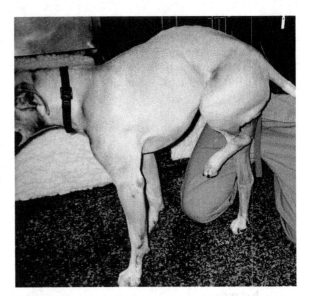

FIGURE 19.8   Root signature sign in the hind limb of a dog after being hit by a car. The dog has pelvic and sacral fractures on radiographs. An MRI was performed to better evaluate the caudal lumbar and sacral nerve roots.

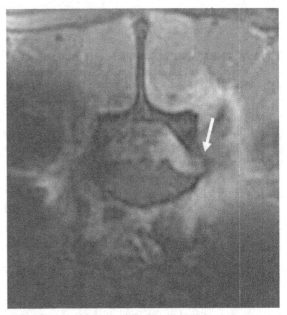

FIGURE 19.9   MRI (T2 weighted image) of the dog. The arrow is pointing at a nerve root that is severely compressed and edematous from the displaced sacral fractures. Surgical decompression of the nerve root and stabilization of the fractures resolved the neurologic derangements. No other imaging modality would have accurately diagnosed the problem and enabled a surgical therapeutic plan.

i. Conservative management is appropriate for minor and nondisplaced fractures of the coccygeal vertebrae.

ii. Tail amputation is recommended for severe fractures, avulsions, and luxations of the tail.

8. PROGNOSIS

a. The prognosis of abaxial sacral fractures in dogs is considered good.

b. The presence of fecal and/or urinary incontinence at the time of presentation or during the perioperative period is unlikely to return regardless of the treatment provided.

c. Axial sacral fractures are associated with worse prognosis.

d. Prognosis is worse if neurologic dysfunction is present:

i. Prognosis depends upon the severity of dysfunction.

e. A flaccid tail and lack of anal tone holds a poor prognosis.

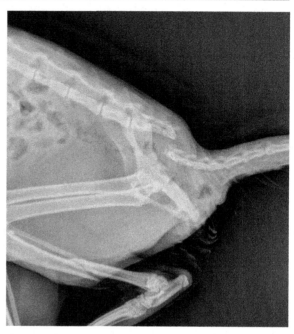

FIGURE 19.10 Lateral radiograph of a cat after sustaining unknown trauma. There is a fracture and luxation of the second caudal vertebrae and a complete midshaft fracture of the tibia and fibula.

TAIL TRAUMA

1. FRACTURE AND LUXATION (Figure 19.10)

a. Fractures of the caudal (coccygeal) vertebrae are dealt with as soon as possible because the weight of the tail may lead to further distraction of nerve roots and exacerbate neurologic dysfunction.

b. Tail amputation should be considered as soon as possible to alleviate discomfort and prevent further traction on nerve roots:

i. Procedure for proximal tail amputation (Figure 19.11):

1. The tail, caudal thigh, perineal, and caudal dorsal fur is clipped and prepped.

2. A temporary purse string suture is placed in the anus.

3. An elliptical incision is made around the base of the tail.

4. Muscle attachments to the caudal vertebrae are severed at the level of the vertebrae and saved for wound closure.

5. The tail is disarticulated at the level of the second or third caudal vertebral body.

6. There are seven arteries of the tail that should be identified and ligated (especially in large dogs). In smaller dogs and cats, only the medial and lateral caudal arteries and veins require ligation.

7. Appose the previously transected muscle bellies, subcutaneous tissue, and skin with monofilament absorbable suture material.

ii. Procedure for more distal tail amputation (Figure 19.11):

1. The level of the tail amputation is determined. This level should be based on the reason for the amputation and where the lesion is located.

2. The entire tail should be clipped and if the aspect of the tail being amputated contains a wound or open lesion, the distal aspect of the tail is covered by a plastic glove or towel, which is held in place with tape.

3. The patient is positioned in sternal recumbency. A perineal stand may be used if available.

4. The clipped region of the tail is aseptically prepped for surgery.

5. A tourniquet can be applied to the tail proximal to the amputation site.

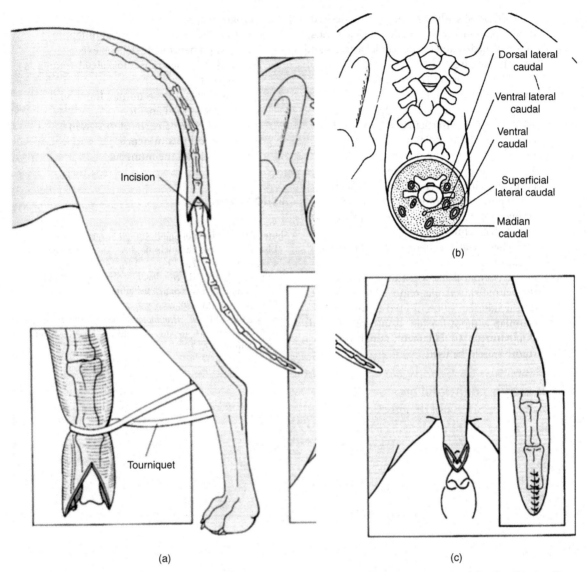

FIGURE 19.11 The procedure for a distal tail amputation. (A) Two V-shaped incisions are made in the skin distal to the coccygeal vertebrate to be removed. The skin is reflected proximally to expose the underlying musculature and bone. Note the vasculature of the tail (B)—there are seven arteries and veins of the tail that should be identified and ligated (especially in large dogs). The soft tissue surrounding the tail distal to the planned disarticulation site is transected and the tail is diarticulated between two vertebral bodies. (C) The coccygeal muscle, subcutaneous tissue and skin is closed over the distal aspect of the exposed vertebra. (Reprinted with permission: Fossum TW, et al. Small Animal Surgery, 3rd edition, Copyright Elsevier, 2007.)

6.   Two V-shaped or semilunar skin incisions are made on the dorsal and ventral aspect of the tail, distal to the predetermined site of disarticulation for the amputation ensuring that enough skin will remain to

completely close over the remaining caudal vertebrae.

7.   The skin is retracted proximally.

8.   There are seven arteries of the tail that should be located and ligated (especially in

large dogs), slightly proximal to the desired disarticulation site. In smaller dogs and cats, only the medial and lateral caudal arteries and veins require ligation.

9. The soft tissue (coccygeal muscle) surrounding the tail, just distal to the planned disarticulation site, is transected.

10. The tail is disarticulated between two caudal vertebral bodies using a scalpel blade.

11. The coccygeal muscle and subcutaneous tissue are closed over the distal aspect of the exposed vertebra using a simple appositional suture pattern with a monofilament absorbable suture.

12. The dorsal V-shaped or semilunar flap of skin is positioned over the exposed end of the tail and if needed, further skin from the ventral skin flap is removed to allow the dorsal skin flap to be sutured to the ventral skin flap without tension, using appositional skin sutures. Monofilament, nonabsorbable suture should be used.

c. Prognosis:
  a. Good for return to normal function:
    i. If no neurologic deficits exist.
    ii. If no other musculoskeletal trauma is present.
  b. Poor for return to normal function if:
    i. Decreased anal tone
    ii. Decreased perineal sensation
    iii. Fecal incontinence
    iv. Urinary incontinence

BIBLIOGRAPHY

Slatter DH. *Textbook of Small Animal Surgery*. 3rd edition. Elsevier Science, Philadelphia, PA, 2003. Chapters 19, 127, 130, 134–137, 139–142, 146, 149, 150, 158.

Piermattei DL, Flo GL. *Handbook of Small Animal Orthopedics and Fracture Repair*. 3rd edition. WB Saunders, Philadelphia, PA, 1983.

Piermattei DL, Flo GL. *Handbook of Small Animal Orthopedics and Fracture Repair*. 4th edition. Elsevier Science, Philadelphia, PA, 2006.

BITE WOUND TRAUMA

David Holt

1. INTRODUCTION

a. Bite wounds occur frequently in dogs and cats and account for a substantial part of the small animal veterinarian's emergency caseload:

    i. The true incidence of dog and cat bites is unknown but dog bite wounds were responsible for 10% of canine admissions to an emergency service in one study (Kolata et al., 1974).

    ii. Bite wounds affecting the head, neck, or thorax can cause immediate, life-threatening injuries.

b. In many cases, bite wounds cause substantial tissue injury and infection, and cause systemic inflammation and sepsis.

c. This chapter will review the systemic and local effects of severe bite wounds and provide a plan for managing the bite wound patient that includes initial evaluation, stabilization, injury assessment, and definitive treatment.

2. SYSTEMIC EFFECTS OF BITE WOUNDS

a. Even small, single bite wounds can cause immediate morbidity or death if they affect an organ or body system vital for life.

b. Central nervous system:

    i. Bite wounds penetrating the cranial vault can cause coma or death.

    ii. Bite wounds affecting the cervical spinal cord can cause hypoventilation through injury to the nervous supply of the muscles of respiration, and tetraparesis/paralysis.

c. Respiratory system:

    i. Small perforations of the thoracic wall can cause a life-threatening open pneumothorax.

    ii. Crushing injuries to the larynx or trachea can cause respiratory obstruction.

d. Cardiovascular system:

    i. Lacerations of major vessels can cause severe hemorrhage.

    ii. Detailed management of neurologic, respiratory, and cardiovascular emergencies is covered in other chapters of this book (see Chapter 2: Triage and Primary Survey, Chapter 3: Shock in the Trauma Patient, Chapter 6: Trauma-Associated Thoracic Injury, Chapter 7: Traumatic Brain Injury).

e. Systemic inflammation:

    i. Systemic inflammation is often seen in animals with multiple, severe bite wounds.

    ii. Initiating factors:

        (a) Severe tissue trauma, with or without infection and/or devitalized, necrotic tissue results in activation and interaction of inflammatory, immunological, coagulation, and fibrinolytic cascades.

        (b) Inflammation is normally a protective physiological response but is usually tightly controlled by compensatory anti-inflammatory mechanisms.

(c) Systemic inflammation occurs as a result of excessive activation of the inflammatory mechanisms, loss of local and systemic compensatory anti-inflammatory mechanisms or a combination of the two.

iii. The systemic inflammatory response syndrome ("SIRS") is represented in a patient when two or more of the following conditions are present: Tachypnea, tachycardia, hyperthermia, and leukocytosis or leukopenia. "Sepsis" is defined as SIRS with a documented infection and often occurs in animals with bite wounds. This can progress to "severe sepsis" when a septic animal develops hemodynamic compromise or organ dysfunction (see Chapter 3: Shock in the Trauma Patient).

f. *Local* inflammation serves several important roles in normal wound healing:

i. Vasoconstriction, activation of platelets, and the intrinsic and extrinsic clotting cascades facilitate clot formation that minimizes blood loss in the wound area.

ii. Cytokines (proteins acting as intercellular signals) and growth factors are generated by injured cells, activated platelets, and the coagulation and complement pathways and stimulate local vasodilation; enzyme, antibody, and complement protein leakage into the wound; neutrophil and monocyte migration into the wound; and wound debridement and repair.

iii. The same cells and cytokines responsible for the normal protective inflammatory response to wounding can result in systemic inflammation and sepsis. The local inflammation becomes systemic (SIRS) when the inciting insult is overwhelming or local regulatory control of inflammation is lost.

iv. Large hematomas, remaining necrotic tissue, and bacteria will prevent migration of fibroblasts and capillaries into the wound. Infected, devitalized tissue delays wound healing and serves as stimulus for systemic inflammation. Wound repair only occurs once the wound is debrided and cleaned. This allows for fibroblasts and capillaries to migrate into the wound and form granulation tissue. The epithelium then migrates from the wound edges.

v. Clinical relevance:

(a) Wound healing will not progress past the "Inflammatory" phase until dead or infected tissue is removed.

(b) Wounds containing devitalized or infected tissue can serve as an ongoing stimulus for SIRS/sepsis.

(c) Treatment of SIRS/sepsis is unlikely to be successful until the inciting cause (treatment of the wound) of the systemic inflammation is removed.

(d) Once the animal is stabilized, wounds should be debrided to remove dead or infected tissue and lavaged using a balanced electrolyte solution under pressure to cleanse the wound. As the majority of bite wounds are contaminated, broad-spectrum, bacteriocidal antibiotics should be administered parenterally (see below).

3. LOCAL TISSUE INJURY

a. Compressive and tensile forces are involved in the majority of dog and cat bite wounds:

i. Tensile forces result in avulsion of tissues from underlying structures:

(a) Skin is often avulsed from the subcutaneous tissues.

(b) Subcutaneous tissues are avulsed from muscle.

(c) Muscles are avulsed from underlying bones:

(i) Avulsion of muscles often results in hernias and muscle devitalization.

ii. Compressive forces can result in either puncture wounds, crushing injury, or both, depending on the shape of the teeth:

(a) Compression by premolar and molar teeth of dogs causes crushing injuries of varying severity including fractures of skull, limbs, or the chest wall.

(b) Crushing causes swelling, ischemia, and necrosis:

(i) In experimental crush injury, tissue blood flow and resistance to infection decrease in proportion to the amount of energy absorbed by the wound.

b. Initial appearance of many bite wounds is deceptive ("the tip of the iceberg") and commonly the majority of tissue damage occurs below the skin such as limb fractures or body cavity penetration. Laceration, avulsion, and devitalization of muscle and subcutaneous fat create large areas of dead space. Inoculation of the devitalized area and dead space with bacteria optimizes the chances for infection to take hold.

 c. Clinical relevance:

  i. All open bite wounds and the vast majority of closed bite wounds should be considered *contaminated*, meaning that they contain bacteria, devitalized tissue, and sometimes foreign material. Untreated, bacteria will rapidly proliferate and invade the tissues, resulting in an *infected* wound.

4. INITIAL MANAGEMENT OF THE BITE WOUND PATIENT

 a. Initial management of an animal with bite wounds should proceed in a planned, orderly manner. The initial examination should focus on the major body systems and stabilization of immediate life threatening problems (see Chapter 1: Global Approach to the Trauma Patient):

  i. Rapid local hemorrhage control:

   (a) Bite wounds will occasionally lacerate a single large blood vessel and the animal will present with ongoing hemorrhage.

   (b) Rapid control of distal extremity bleeding can be achieved by placing a blood pressure cuff on the limb proximal to the hemorrhaging vessel and inflating it to a pressure just greater than systemic blood pressure (until hemorrhage is slowed or stopped).

   (c) Rapid control of proximal limb hemorrhage (i.e., femoral artery) can be achieved by direct pressure until stabilized by surgical ligation.

 b. Complete patient stabilization may not always be possible because of infection and necrotic tissue in the bite wounds. In these animals, delaying surgery in the hope of clinical improvement is usually of little benefit. The author prefers an aggressive period of stabilization (usually 2–4 hours) followed by anesthesia and surgery for exploration of wounds, management of specific injuries, debridement of necrotic tissue, lavage, and establishment of drainage.

 c. After stabilizing immediate life-threatening problems, a more thorough physical examination focusing on all body systems should be performed. All wounds should be covered at this time if possible to prevent further wound colonization with hospital bacteria that may have substantial antibiotic resistance. Broad-spectrum, bacteriocidal antibiotics are administered intravenously, pending culture and sensitivity results from tissue samples taken at surgery (see below). Further evaluation of the wound(s) should ideally be performed under aseptic conditions and should include the following:

  i. Assessing the extent of the injuries.

  ii. Minimizing the bacterial population in the wound through aggressive wound debridement and lavage.

  iii. Repairing fractures and defects in the thoracic and abdominal walls.

  iv. Deciding between immediate and delayed wound closure.

5. INJURY ASSESSMENT

 a. In an unpublished survey of 263 animals with bite wounds presented to an urban veterinary emergency room during a one-year period, the most common wound sites were: 1. The limbs; 2. The head and neck; 3. Regions over the thoracic and abdominal cavities; and 4. The perineal region (Parent C. Unpublished bite wound survey, University of Pennsylvania, School of Veterinary Medicine, 1993). There are specific evaluation and management concerns with wounds in each of these locations:

 b. *Limb wounds*:

  i. Viability of the leg can be assessed clinically by the temperature and color of the leg. Additionally, perfusion can be assessed by Doppler once the animal is adequately resuscitated.

   (a) Measurement of toe web temperature and selective angiography have been described but are not applicable to routine clinical practice.

  ii. Perform thorough orthopedic and neurologic examination. (Neurologic examination should be delayed until after resuscitation, as animals in shock are often poorly responsive to noxious stimuli.) Starting distally on each limb the bones are individually assessed for fractures and joints manipulated carefully for instability or luxation. Spinal reflexes, withdrawal, and pain sensation are assessed in each limb.

 c. *Head and neck wounds*:

  i. Bite wounds to the neck may result in cervical spinal fracture, luxation, or traumatic disc prolapse. Cervical spinal injury should be assumed and proper precautions should be taken to limit movement of the neck until complete assessment is completed If spinal injuries are suspected (i.e., quadraparesis) or documented the neck should not be manipulated and instead it should be stabilized (see Chapter 9: Traumatic Spinal Injury).

ii. Thorough evaluation for CNS and upper airway trauma should be performed.

iii. Thorough palpation of the skull, mandible, and cervical vertebrae should be performed:

(a) All areas of the skull should be palpated. The mouth should be evaluated for tooth fractures, avulsions, integrity of the hard palate, and lacerations or hematomas of the tongue (see Chapters 16: Trauma-Associated Musculoskeletal Injury to the Head and 17: Trauma-Associated Soft Tissue Injury to the Head and Neck). The mouth is opened, and closed to assess for function, pain and crepitus. The neck should be very carefully palpated and manipulated to assess for pain or crepitus. Immediately stop manipulation if crepitus, resistance or pain is noted.

(b) Subcutaneous emphysema may indicate skull sinus fracture, laryngeal, tracheal, or esophageal perforation.

(c) Rarely, bites to the neck can damage the caudal laryngeal nerves resulting in laryngeal paralysis resulting in inspiratory dyspnea, and stridor.

d. *Thoracic and abdominal wounds*:

i. Both radiography and blunt probing of thoracic or abdominal wounds to determine body cavity penetration are *unreliable* diagnostic tests:

(a) In many cases, there is no pneumothorax, pleural effusion, pneumoperitoneum, or peritoneal effusion visible radiographically, yet wounds obviously are identified that enter the affected body cavity at surgical exploration.

ii. The lateral and especially caudal abdomen is carefully palpated to rule out traumatic herniation of intra-abdominal contents (see Chapter 13: Trauma-Associated Body Wall and Torso Injury).

iii. The best method of assessment of these wounds is thorough surgical exploration.

e. *Perineal wounds*:

Perineal wounds should be carefully evaluated for rectal or urethral penetration. Placement of a urinary catheter may aid in the identification of the urethra during wound exploration. Wounds in this region are often severely contaminated with bacteria from the perineal skin. They should be treated as surgical emergencies and explored as soon as the animal is stabilized. Retrograde urethrocystography may be indicated to definitively rule out urethral trauma.

6. WOUND EXPLORATION, DEBRIDEMENT AND LAVAGE

a. Wound preparation:

i. Prior to clipping a sterile, water-soluble gel (K-Y Jelly, Johnson & Johnson) should be placed in the wounds to prevent further contamination.

ii. An extremely large area should be clipped around the wounds and prepared for aseptic surgery as tissue damage often extends far beyond the visible wound.

iii. Use of surgical scrub solutions in the wound itself controversial as bacteriocidal concentrations of both chlorhexidine diacetate (0.05%) and povidone-iodine (1%) are lethal to fibroblasts in vitro:

(a) The benefits of removing dirt, debris and killing bacteria should be weighed against the risk of damaging healthy tissue and impairing wound healing.

(b) Scrubbing the wound itself should probably be limited to wounds with gross contamination. All of the scrub solution in the wound should be flushed immediately with balanced electrolyte solution.

b. Debridement:

i. Debridement is best performed with sharp dissection. Vital structures (nerves, tendons) should be preserved wherever possible.

ii. In some cases, the surgeon must recognize that preservation of a limb is not possible and be prepared to perform an amputation.

iii. Bite wounds penetrating abdominal or thoracic cavity require special consideration and necessitate thorough exploration of affected body cavity. The surgeon should initially explore and debride the wound itself, but be prepared for a separate approach into the affected body cavity if necessary. In many cases, the thorax can be explored via lateral thoracotomy created by following and debriding bite wounds on the lateral thorax. In such cases the anesthetist should be prepared to provide manual or mechanically assisted positive pressure ventilation once the pleural space is entered. Bite wounds penetrating the abdominal cavity often necessitate a complete exploratory laparotomy via a ventral midline approach.

> (a) The lungs, liver, spleen, digestive, and urogenital tracts should be carefully examined for perforating or crushing injuries.

iv. Debridement of all necrotic and infected tissue is vital. Any remaining necrotic fat or muscle enhances bacterial growth and could contribute to inhibition of healing and bacterial infection due to low oxygen tension within devitalized tissue, which can impair bacterial killing by white blood cells.

v. Begin superficially and progress deeper into the wound.

vi. Tissue at each layer should be carefully assessed for viability before resection.

vii. All fat of questionable viability should be removed.

viii. Muscle viability can be determined by assessing bleeding at surgery.

c. Lavage:

i. Wounds should be copiously lavaged during exploration. The effectiveness of lavage is proportional to the volume of solution used.

ii. Lavage fluid must be delivered under pressure to be effective:

> (a) Use a 35-mL syringe and a 19-gauge needle to cleanse a wound of particulate matter, soil, and bacteria (see Figure 18.27, Chapter 18: Trauma-Associated Musculoskeletal Injury to the Appendicular Skeleton).
>
> (b) Higher lavage pressures force bacteria deeper into a wound and open deeper tissue planes.
>
> (c) Lactated Ringer's solution or phosphate buffered saline has been shown to be less damaging to fibroblasts in vitro than normal (0.9%) saline.

7. FRACTURES

i. Small avascular bone fragments should be removed during exploration. Larger bone fragments should be cultured and be retained as they may be useful for reconstruction.

ii. The opinions are divided over immediate fracture repair and this decision depends on the fracture type and extent of surrounding soft tissue injuries.

iii. Options include the following:

> (a) Immediate repair at the initial surgery.
>
> (b) Immobilization in splint, or padded bandage for 48 hours with the objective of having healthy soft tissues surrounding the fracture at the time of definitive repair (see Chapter 18: Trauma-Associated Musculoskeletal Injury to the Appendicular Skeleton).
>
> (c) Rigid immobilization is vital for bone healing in potentially infected fractures. Multidimensional external fixators or bone plates provide the necessary rigid fixation for definitive repair.
>
> (d) A large autogenous cancellous bone graft can be placed in and around the fracture after repair and lavage.

8. BODY WALL DEFECTS

a. Defects created in the thoracic and abdominal wall by debridement of necrotic tissue require reconstruction. Healthy tissue with an adequate blood supply is used for reconstruction if it is available.

b. Options for *thoracic wall reconstruction*: (*Note*: referral to clinicians that are experienced in thoracic wall reconstruction would be appropriate):

i. Advancing the diaphragm: only applicable to caudal defects.

ii. Latisimus dorsi muscle flap.

iii. External abdominal oblique, rectus abdominis muscle flaps.

iv. Multiple rib fractures with insufficient muscle for reconstruction of the chest wall:

> (a) Stabilize ribs by passing heavy gauge sutures around pairs of adjacent ribs.
>
> (b) Place a chest tube.
>
> (c) Close skin over the defect.
>
> (d) Alternatively:
>
> > (i) Resection of the damaged ribs can be performed followed by placement of a polypropylene mesh into the defect. The mesh should be sutured intrapleurally to the remaining muscles surrounding the defect:

1. The mesh should be covered with an omental pedicle flap mobilized through a separate flank incision.

c. Abdominal defects:

i. The cranial sartorius muscle flap can be used to reconstruct caudal abdominal wall defects.

ii. Polypropylene mesh/omentum can be used for large abdominal wall defect repairs.

9. WOUND REPAIR

a. The aim of debridement and lavage is to convert a contaminated wound containing devitalized tissue into one clean enough to be sutured closed. The previously held concept of a "golden period", that is a time from wounding to surgery within which surgical treatment allows all wounds to be closed (6–12 hours), has largely been abandoned. Although this 6–12 hour period after wounding is considered to be the time necessary for bacterial multiplication and invasion of the wound, the situation in many wounds, especially bite wounds, cannot be simplified to a judgment based on time alone.

b. The surgeon must evaluate a wound for the amount of local tissue trauma that might compromise the animal's defenses, the degree of contamination, the type and number of bacteria inoculated into the wound, and the adequacy of the wound's blood supply before deciding on open or closed wound management. Closure should be delayed if any doubt exists concerning the viability of tissue or amount of infection remaining in the wound.

c. Primary closure:

i. Strict adherence to basic surgical principles is essential.

ii. Only healthy tissues should be present after debridement and lavage.

iii. Hemostasis must be excellent, as blood clots provide a superior medium for bacterial growth.

iv. Tissue layers should be gently apposed to minimize dead space.

v. Wounds should be tension free.

vi. If dead space is present:

(**a**) Use one or more gravity-dependent, Penrose or closed suction drains (Figure 20.1).

(**b**) Drains should exit through separate stab incisions in the sterile field, rather than

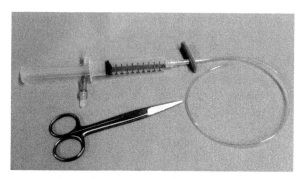

FIGURE 20.1 Closed suction drain. Extension set tubing is cut to length, the distal end fenestrated and placed in the wound. The tubing is connected to a syringe. Once the wound is closed, fluid and air are evacuated from any remaining dead space. The plunger of the syringe is then drawn back and stabilized with a needle to maintain subatmospheric pressure in the syringe. The system is clamped and the syringe emptied periodically.

the bite wound, and should be covered by a sterile dressing postoperatively.

d. Delayed primary closure:

i. This is often the best option for many bite wounds.

ii. The wound is left open after the initial debridement and covered with a sterile, permeable dressing, such as Vaseline-impregnated gauze (Adaptic, Johnson & Johnson Medical Ltd. Skipton, U.K.) followed by placement of a thick absorbent layer of padding, a conforming bandage, and an elastic, adhesive bandage layer.

iii. Application of a debriding bandage, such as a wet-to-dry bandage, or a topical debriding agent (e.g., Granulex-V, Beecham Inc., Bristol, TN) may be considered in wounds still grossly contaminated after initial debridement. A layer of moist sterile gauze is used as the contact layer. This is surrounded by absorbent cotton and a tertiary bandage layer. As the moist gauze dries, it adheres to the necrotic tissue, which is removed when the bandage is changed. A debriding bandage should not be used:

1. As a substitute for adequate initial debridement.

2. Instead of a second debriding surgery.

3. Once a healthy bed of granulation tissue has formed.

iv. Initial daily bandage changes and wound assessment should be performed.

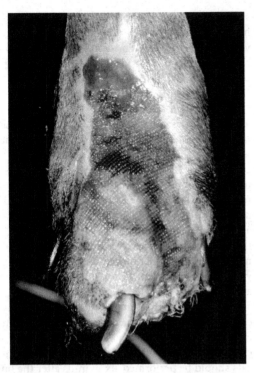

FIGURE 20.2 Healthy bed of granulation tissue 10 days after debridement and lavage of an injury involving the metacarpus and digits.

v. Definitive wound closure should be performed when all contamination debris and devitalized tissue are removed. This usually occurs 3–5 days after the initial surgery.

vi. In some areas such as the distal limbs, extensive skin loss necessitates the use of a skin graft or flap for definitive repair. A healthy bed of granulation tissue should be allowed to develop before a free skin graft is performed (Figure 20.2).

10. USE OF ANTIBIOTICS IN ANIMALS WITH BITE WOUNDS

a. The use of antibiotics in dogs and cats with bite wounds is poorly understood. There are few objective studies documenting the bacteria contaminating bite wounds in dogs and cats, and no studies documenting either risk factors for bite wound infection, indications for antibiotic treatment in bite wounds, or the bacteria causing true wound infections.

b. In human bite wounds, the use of antibiotics to prevent infection is controversial. Some authors favor antibiotic use in all cases, while others recommend antibiotics for wounds known to be at high risk of infection. There is one meta-analysis of randomized trials of antibiotics to prevent infection in humans with dog bite wounds. This study (Cummings, 1994) found the risk of infection in the control (nonantibiotic treated population) was 16%; the relative risk for infection in the patients given oral antibiotics was 0.56 (95% confidence interval, 0.38–0.82). In essence, these data imply that if 100 human patients with bite wounds were given oral antibiotics, 84 would not become infected regardless of treatment, 9 will become infected in spite of the treatment, and in 7 the antibiotics will prevent infection.

c. Risk factors for infection in humans:
   i. Full thickness puncture.
   ii. Hand or lower extremity wounds.
   iii. Wounds requiring surgical debridement or involving joints, tendons, ligaments, or bones.
   iv. Patients with compromised immune function.
   v. Patients with prosthetic implants.

d. Risk factor analysis for infection has not been performed for bite wounds in dogs and cats.

e. Culture studies in dogs:
   i. Zimbabwe (87 dogs, aerobic cultures only) (Kelly et al., 1992):
      (a) *Staphylococcus intermedius* (23%): 30% resistant to multiple drugs.
      (b) *Escherichia coli* (18%): Multiple drug resistance common.
      (c) Nonlactose fermenting coliforms (14%).
   ii. University of Pennsylvania (37 dogs; cultures taken before and during surgery) (Griffin and Holt, 2001):
      (a) *S. intermedius* was the most common bacteria cultured.
      (b) *Enterococcus* was cultured more frequently than E. coli (11 vs 10 isolates in 37 cases).
      (c) Wide range of other aerobic and *anaerobic* bacteria were also cultured.
      (d) Antibiotic sensitivities were variable.
      (e) Neither the bacterial isolates nor the likely antibiotic sensitivity could be predicted with any accuracy prior to the results of culture and sensitivity testing.

(f) No one antibiotic could be relied upon to kill all bacteria in all wounds.

f. Clinical recommendations:

i. Antibiotic treatment is justified in clinically infected wounds and probably warranted in fresh wounds that have full thickness punctures or lacerations with surrounding crush injury, cellulitis or avulsion, and in animals with decreased immune resistance due to diabetes mellitus, hyperadrenocorticism or sepsis.

ii. Antibiotics should not be used as a substitute for appropriate wound management.

iii. Given the uncertain flora and antimicrobial sensitivity in individual animals, cultures obtained at the time of surgical debridement is mandatory.

iv. Wounds with suspected postoperative infections should be re-cultured.

v. In animals requiring parenteral medication, either a penicillin combined with an aminoglycocide or a second-generation cephalosporin combined with a fluroquinolone will provide broad-spectrum coverage. However, the latter combinations will not kill the majority of Enterococcus species, which are often sensitive only to Ampicillin, Clavamox, Timentin, or Vancomycin.

vi. Editors note: If empiric oral antibiotic therapy must be chosen for dogs and cats with bite wounds, the four most commonly cultured bacteria from bite wounds have been shown to sensitive to amoxicillin-clavulonic acid (14 mg/kg PO q12 hours).

11. POSTOPERATIVE MANAGEMENT

a. The bite wound patient is monitored carefully and daily initially if it is severe. Tissues that appeared healthy on initial inspection can progress to necrosis in spite of appropriate debridement and antibiotic therapy.

b. Respiratory function should be assessed using clinical parameters (respiratory rate and effort) and blood gas measurement or pulse oximetry if the chest was damaged by the bite.

c. Cardiovascular status and perfusion are evaluated frequently in animals with severe bite wounds. These animals are at risk for sepsis in spite of early, aggressive medical management and wound debridement. Any deterioration in the animal's condition should raise suspicion of ongoing tissue necrosis in the wound. The wound(s) are inspected, and if there is any doubt about tissue viability, re-explored. The wound is again aggressively lavaged and debrided to healthy, bleeding tissue.

12. INFECTIOUS DISEASES

a. Bite wounds can transmit several viral diseases including rabies in both dogs and cats, and feline leukemia virus (FeLV) and feline immunodeficiency virus (FIV) in cats. The American Veterinary Medical Association approved guidelines for rabies control recommend that unvaccinated animals bitten by a mammal or bat that is not available for testing be euthanatized immediately. If the owner is not prepared to euthanatize the animal, it should be quarantined for 6 months and vaccinated 1 month prior to release. Animals that are vaccinated should be revaccinated immediately, kept under the owner's control, and observed carefully for 45 days. The chance of infection with either FeLV or FIV from a bite from an infected cat is difficult to predict. Serologic testing of bitten cats should be performed six months after the bite wound was sustained.

BIBLIOGRAPHY

Abello PA, Buchman TG, Bulkley GB. Shock and multiple organ failure. In: Armstrong D, ed. *Free Radicals in Diagnostic Medicine.* Plenum Press, New York, 1994; 253.

Beal AL, Cerra FB. Multiple organ failure syndrome in the 1990s. *JAMA* 1994; 271, 226.

Bright RM. Reconstruction of thoracic wall defects using Marlex mesh. *J Am Anim Hosp Assoc* 1981; 17: 415.

Bright RM. Repair of thoracic wall defects in the dog with an omental pedicle flap. *J Am Anim Hosp Assoc* 1982; 18: 277.

Buffa EA, Lubbe AM, Verstraete FJM, et al. The effects of wound lavage solutions on canine fibroblasts: an in vitro study. *Vet Surg* 1997; 26: 460.

Callaham M. Medical Emergency Management: dog bite wounds. *JAMA* 1980; 244: 2327.

Cardany CR, Rodeheaver G, Thacker J, et al. The crush injury: a high risk wound. *JACEP* 1976; 5: 965.

Cowell AK, Penwick RC. Dog bite wounds: a study of 93 cases. *Compend Contin Educ Pract Vet* 1989; 11: 313.

Cummings P. Antibiotics to prevent infection in patients with bite wounds: a meta-analysis of randomized trials. *Annals Emerg Med* 1994; 23: 535.

Davidson EB. Managing bite wounds in dogs and cats. Part I. *Compend Contin Educ Pract Vet* 1998; 20: 811.

Davies MG, Hagen P -O. Systemic inflammatory response syndrome. *Br J Surg* 1997; 84: 920.

de Holl D, Rodeheaver G, Edgerton MT. Potentiation of infection by suture closure of dead space. *Am J Surg* 1974; 127: 716.

Deitch EA. Multiple organ failure. Pathophysiology and potential future therapy. *Ann Surg* 1992; 216: 117.

Dire DJ. Emergency management of dog and cat bite wounds. *Emerg Med Clin North Am* 1992; 10: 719.

Donnelly SC, Robertson C. Mediators, mechanisms and mortality in major trauma. *Resuscitation* 1994; 28: 87.

Edlich RF, Rodeheaver GT, Morgan RF, et al. Principles of emergency wound management. *Ann Emerg Med* 1988; 17: 1284.

Galloway RE. Mammalian bites. *J Emerg Med* 1988; 6: 325.

Griffin GM, Holt DE. Dog-Bite wounds: bacteriology and treatment outcome in 37 cases. *J Am Anim Hosp Assoc* 2001; 37: 453–460.

Haury B, Rodeheaver G, Vensko J, et al. Debridement: an essential component of traumatic wound care. *Am J Surg* 1978; 135: 238.

Hohn DC, MacKay RD, Halliday B, et al. Effect of O_2 tension on microbicidal function of leucocytes in wounds and in vitro. *Surg Forum* 1976; 27: 18.

Johnston DE. Care of accidental wounds. *Vet Clin North Am Small Anim Pract* 1990; 20: 27.

Kelly PJ, Mason PR, Matthewman LA. Pathogens in dog bite wounds in dogs in Harare, Zimbabwe. *Vet Rec* 1992; 131: 464.

Kolata RJ, Kraut NH, Johnston DE, et al. Patterns of trauma in urban dogs and cats: A study of 1,000 cases. *J Am Vet Med Assoc* 1974; 164: 499.

Martin P. Wound healing - Aiming for perfect skin regeneration. *Science* 1997; 276: 75

Pavlettic M. *Atlas of Small Animal Reconstructive Surgery*. JB Lippincott Company, Philadelphia, PA, 1992; 309.

Peacock EE, Jr, van Winkle W, Jr. *Wound repair*. WB Saunders, Philadelphia, PS, 1976.

Rappolee DA, Mark D, Banda MJ, et al. Wound macrophages express TGF-α and other growth factors in vivo: analysis by mRNA phenotyping. *Science* 1988; 241: 708.

Ritter MA, Stringer EA. Intraoperative wound cultures: Their value and long-term effect on the patient. *Clin Ortho Relat Res* 1981; 155: 180.

St John RC, Dorinski PM. An overview of multiple organ dysfunction syndrome. *J Clin Lab Med* 124: 478, 1994

Sanchez IR, Nusbaum KE, Swaim SF, et al. Chlorhexadine diacetate and povidone-iodine cytotoxicity to canine embryonic fibroblasts and Staphylococcus aureus. *Vet Surg* 1988; 17: 182.

Shahar R, Shamir M, Johnston DE. A technique for management of bite wounds of the thoracic wall in small dogs. *Vet Surg* 1997; 26: 45.

Singer AJ, Clark RAF. Cutaneous wound healing. *New Eng J Med* 1999; 341: 738.

Singleton AO, Julian J. An experimental evaluation of methods used to prevent infection in wounds which have been contaminated with feces. *Ann Surg* 1960; 151: 912.

Stevenson TR, Thacker JG, Rodeheaver GT, et al. Cleansing the traumatic wound by high pressure syringe irrigation. *JACEP* 1976; 5: 17.

Talan DA, Citron DM, Abrahamian FM, et al. Bacteriologic analysis of infected dog and cat bites. *New Eng J Med* 1999; 340: 85.

Trott A. Mechanisms of surface soft tissue trauma. *Ann Emerg Med* 1988; 17: 1279.

Underman AE. Bite wounds inflicted by dogs and cats. *Vet Clin North Am Small Anim Pract* 1987; 17: 195.

Waldron Dr, Trevor P. Management of superficial skin wounds. In: Slatter D, ed. *Textbook of Small Animal Surgery*. 2nd edition. WB Saunders, Philadelphia, PA, 1993; 269.

TRAUMA-ASSOCIATED AURAL INJURY

William T. Culp and Philipp D. Mayhew

1. INTRODUCTION

a. Patients with aural trauma often have simultaneous head trauma, and signs such as altered mental status, seizures, and cardiovascular compromise induced by swelling of the brain require immediate intervention (see Chapter 7: Traumatic Brain Injury).

b. The long-term complications encountered with aural trauma can be significant and proper management of injury is a necessity.

c. Aural trauma is generally not considered immediately life-threatening and is addressed once patient stability has been achieved.

2. CLINICALLY IMPORTANT ANATOMY AND PHYSIOLOGY

a. The ear has several important functions, specifically in the control of balance and hearing. The anatomical and physiological functions of each of the components contributing to these functions should be thoroughly understood if appropriate management of these injuries is to be achieved:

  i. The ear is divided into three anatomical divisions: the external ear, middle ear, and inner ear.

  ii. The external ear:

    1. Pinna:

      a. Variable shape depending on the breed

      b. Formed by auricular cartilage

    2. Vertical canal:

      a. Funnel shaped

      b. Formed by auricular cartilage

    3. Horizontal canal:

      a. Communicates with short osseous external canal that projects from petrous temporal bone.

      b. Formed by annular cartilage and small proximal portion of auricular cartilage.

    4. The external ear functions to receive air vibrations and direct the vibrations toward the middle ear.

    5. The arterial blood supply to the external ear is derived from branches of the external carotid artery and venous blood drains into the maxillary vein:

      a. Arterial blood supply is evenly distributed across the pinna and consists of three arteries: lateral auricular artery, intermediate auricular artery, and medial auricular artery. The caudal auricular artery provides the blood supply to the ear canal.

      b. Venous drainage primarily occurs from two branches of the maxillary vein found on the lateral and medial margins of the pinna.

  iii. Middle ear:

    1. The tympanic membrane marks the division between the middle and external ear.

2. The middle ear primarily consists of the tympanic cavity, which is housed in an out-pouching of the temporal bone. The middle ear communicates with the nasopharynx via the auditory tube.

3. When sound waves strike the tympanic membrane, the vibration creates a ripple effect that is transmitted, via the auditory ossicles within the middle ear (malleus, incus, and stapes), to the inner ear.

4. Unlike dogs, the feline tympanic cavity consists of two compartments, a larger ventromedial and a smaller craniolateral compartment, which are separated by a bony septum.

   iv. Inner ear:

     1. Housed within the petrous temporal bone.

     2. Consists of the vestibule and semicircular ducts, which are involved with equilibrium, and the cochlea, which contributes to hearing function.

  b. Neural structures associated with the ear:

   i. Cranial nerve VII (facial):

     1. Leaves the petrosal bone via the stylomastoid foramen.

     2. Courses just ventral to the horizontal canal near the external acoustic meatus.

   ii. Cranial nerve VIII (vestibulocochlear):

     1. Communicates with the tympanic cavity within the middle ear.

     2. Damage to this nerve causes peripheral vestibular signs.

   iii. Axons from postganglionic sympathetic neurons:

     1. Course close to the wall of the middle ear in dogs and cats.

     2. More exposed in cats, and thus more sensitive to traumatic damage.

     3. Damage to these fibers can result in Horner's syndrome.

3. ETIOLOGY

a. While studies describing trauma specific to the ear are lacking, causes of injury may include motor vehicular accidents, nonaccidental physical injuries, bite wounds, rough play with other dogs, severe head shaking, and surgical trauma.

b. Many dogs that present with aural trauma will have sustained concurrent head or neck injuries

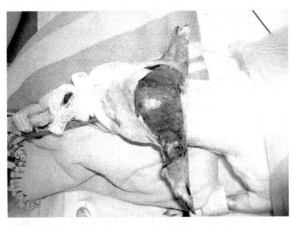

FIGURE 21.1 An anesthetized dog that has experienced blunt trauma to the head and ear. This patient was experiencing significant side effects associated with his head trauma. Once stabilized, the wound was debrided and closed and a left pinna amputation was performed due to devascularization.

(Figure 21.1):

   i. Soft tissue injuries to the head have been detected in 35% of cases of trauma-induced injury (Kolata, 1975).

   ii. Eleven percent of gunshot wounds are reported to be localized to the head (Fullington, 1997).

   iii. Of injuries induced nonaccidentally, 19% are reported to affect the head (Munro, 2001).

4. DIAGNOSTICS

  a. Physical examination:

   i. Perform thorough examination of both concave and convex surfaces of the pinna.

   ii. Palpation of the ear canal should be performed. Ear canal separation can be detected by palpating a loss of continuity of the ear canal between the horizontal and vertical canal. As you are palpating the ear canal in a dog or cat with an ear canal separation, a division between the vertical and horizontal ear canal can be felt. Additionally, the ear canal may be more mobile than usual.

  b. Otoscopy:

   i. Otoscopy can be used to diagnose tympanic membrane rupture.

   ii. An abrupt ending to the vertical canal and inability to visualize the horizontal canal suggests a traumatic ear canal separation.

c. Radiography:

i. Fractures of the petrous temporal bone or bulla can be noted on radiographs and may suggest the presence of middle and/or inner ear damage.

ii. Radiographs can demonstrate signs that are consistent with middle ear disease secondary to abscessation that may occur from traumatic ear canal separation or bite wounds. Radiographic findings suggestive of middle ear disease include increased soft tissue opacity within the bulla as well as thickening of the wall of the tympanic bulla.

d. Computed tomography (CT):

i. CT provides better visualization of the middle ear structures than radiographs because of greater image contrast and the ability to evaluate the middle ear in cross-section.

ii. CT is superior to MRI for diagnosing bony changes.

e. Magnetic resonance imaging (MRI):

i. MRI is capable of detecting disease earlier than can radiographs or CT.

ii. MRI can visualize the inner ear including the semicircular canals, vestibule and cochlea.

5. TRAUMATIC AURAL LESIONS

a. Pinna trauma:

i. Pinna lesions can affect the skin alone, the skin and underlying cartilage, or may involve full thickness lacerations through both skin surfaces and cartilage.

ii. Indications for surgery to the pinna include severe lacerations or perforations and avulsions.

iii. As with any cutaneous wound, attention should focus on debridement of any necrotic tissue and copious lavage with a sterile isotonic solution:

1. Minor lacerations of the skin may be left open to heal by second intention.

2. If the laceration results in a two- or three-sided flap, then surgery is recommended (Figure 21.2):

a. Skin laceration only: Skin edges should be apposed using a 3–0 or 4–0 monofilament suture in a simple interrupted pattern.

b. For wounds penetrating through the pinna, both the cartilage and skin on the convex surface should be aligned

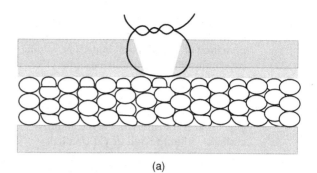

(a)

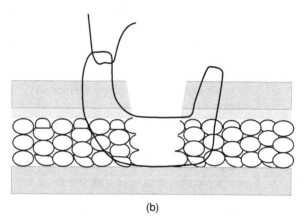

(b)

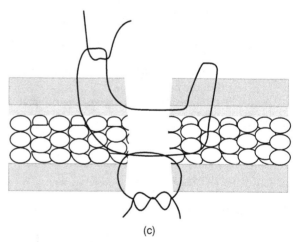

(c)

FIGURE 21.2 Proper suture placement for repair of lacerations that involve one skin layer (a), one skin layer and cartilage (b), and both skin layers and cartilage (c).

together with a vertical mattress pattern using a 3–0 or 4–0 monofilament suture (incorporate the cartilage on the deeper bite and appose the skin on the more superficial bite). The skin on the other side can be apposed with simple interrupted sutures (Figure 21.2).

3. Wounds that are located on the border of the pinna will require surgical correction, as wound contraction and epithelialization in this area will often result in defects that are not cosmetically acceptable to pet owners.

4. Partial pinna amputation:

   a. Necrotic pinna tissue (both skin and cartilage) should be removed leaving healthy tissue to suture together.

   b. The exposed skin edges are sutured together using a 3–0 or 4–0 monofilament suture in a simple continuous pattern.

5. More extensive injuries may require full pinna amputation or a skin flap:

   a. Skin flaps used in the treatment of pinna injuries generally come from the head or neck (e.g., caudal auricular axial pattern flap).

   b. Extensive injuries may require staged procedures over several weeks.

b. Aural hematomas:

   i. The pathogenesis of aural hematomas has not been fully elucidated. A direct causal relationship between trauma and aural hematomas has been questioned; however, many still believe that severe head shaking and other forms of pinna trauma precipitate the development of aural hematomas (Kagan, 1983; Dubielzig, 1984; Kuwahara, 1986):

      1. Fracture of the cartilage has been linked with hematoma formation (Dubielzig, 1984).

      2. Others have suggested an immune-mediated pathogenesis for aural hematomas based upon positive ANA titers and positive Coombs' tests (Kuwahara, 1986). Other authors have not corroborated these findings (Joyce, 1997).

   ii. Treatment:

      1. Nonsurgical options:

         a. Identify and treat the source of head shaking or ear scratching.

         b. Needle aspiration of the hematoma can be attempted, but this is generally ineffective long term and is associated with a high recurrence rate.

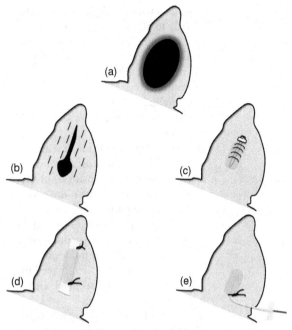

FIGURE 21.3 Treatment Options for Aural Hematomas (a). Cavity obliteration (b), Teat cannula (c), Penrose drain (d), Active drainage with a butterfly catheter (e).

         c. Systemic corticosteroids have been administered with variable success.

      2. Cavity obliteration (Figure 21.3):

         a. An incision is made over the full length of the hematoma on the concave surface of the pinna:

            i. A linear incision can be used for small hematomas.

            ii. Curved incisions are preferred in animals with large hematomas to reduce the degree of ear deformation resulting from contraction.

         b. The cartilaginous cavity is explored, and the fibrin clumps are removed.

         c. The cavity is flushed with sterile saline, and obliterated by proper suture placement (Figure 21.3):

            i. Place 3–0 to 4–0 monofilament nonabsorbable sutures about 1 cm from each other, oriented along the long axis of the ear (parallel to the incision).

            ii. Place full-thickness sutures in the area of the cavity and tie on the convex surface of the ear. Do not tie tightly to allow for swelling.

iii. The incision is left open and a wide gap should be left at the dependent aspect of the hematoma to encourage drainage.

3. Passive drainage (Figure 21.3):

   a. Teat cannula (Dr. Larson's™, Spring Valley, WI):

   i. A stab incision is made with a scalpel blade at the most dependent section (neutral ear position) of the aural hematoma cavity on the concave surface of the pinna.

   ii. The cavity is flushed thoroughly with sterile saline and encouraged to drain via manual manipulation.

   iii. A teat cannula is then placed into the stab incision and secured with 3–0 nylon to the skin.

   iv. The ear is massaged gently on a daily basis, and the cannula is left in place for 3–4 weeks.

   b. Penrose drain (Bard, Covington, GA):

   i. Two stab incisions are made with a scalpel blade—one at the proximal aspect of the hematoma and one at the distal aspect of the hematoma.

   ii. The contents of the hematoma are removed, and the cavity is flushed thoroughly with sterile saline.

   iii. A $\frac{1}{4}$ inch Penrose drain is placed into one incision and out the other and secured to the skin with 3–0 nylon.

   iv. These drains are generally kept in place for 2–3 weeks.

   v. Complications such as recurrence of the hematoma or seroma formation are associated with early drain removal.

4. Active drainage (Figure 21.3):

   a. The hub from a butterfly catheter (Abbott Laboratories, Chicago, IL) is removed and the tubing is placed into a tiny incision made at the most distal aspect of the hematoma. The needle of the butterfly catheter is then inserted into a blood collection tube that will generate negative pressure and result in drainage.

   b. The blood collection tube should be changed several times daily (Figure 21.3).

5. Other techniques that have been attempted for resolving aural hematomas include a sutureless technique involving an elliptical incision over the hematoma, a continuous suture around an elliptical incision made over the hematoma, placement of cyanoacrylate adhesive into the hematoma cavity, laser-created incisions, biopsy punch holes made over the hematoma, and intralesional injection of corticosteroids.

   iii. Regardless of the technique employed, recurrence is a common complication and multiple procedures may be required. No single technique has been shown to be superior and to result in fewer recurrences than any other.

   iv. If a surgical treatment (cavity obliteration, passive drainage, active drainage) is pursued, the ear should be pressure-wrapped postoperatively (Figure 21.4):

   1. Place absorbent bandages over the site of the hematoma, and wrap the entire head with a padded bandage for 10 days.

   2. The bandage should be changed every 3 days unless it becomes wet or dirty and then should be changed immediately.

c. Ear canal separations and abscessation:

   i. Trauma may lead to ear canal separations that can develop para-aural abscessation.

   ii. Separation occurs between the vertical and horizontal ear canals.

   iii. Signs of para-aural abscessation include the development of draining tracts ventral to the horizontal ear canal and para-aural swelling; however, reports of these cases have shown that the disease can remain undiscovered for as long as several months after the traumatic episode.

   iv. Diagnostics may include palpation, otoscopic examination, radiographs, and CT (see above).

   v. In the literature, all cases have been addressed surgically, and the procedures utilized most commonly included total ear canal ablation and a concurrent lateral bulla osteotomy. Other procedures that have been attempted include ventral bulla osteotomy and creating a hole in the horizontal canal (Boothe, 1992; McCarthy, 1995).

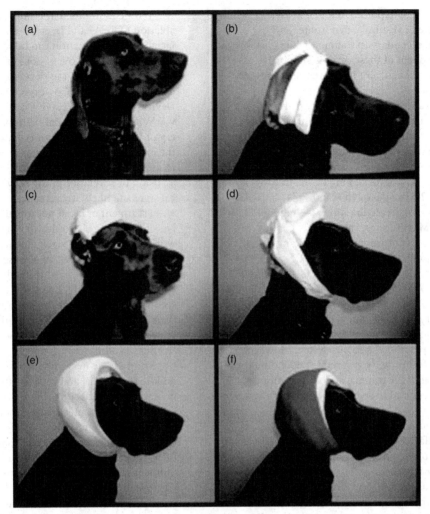

FIGURE 21.4 Placement of a pressure-wrap that would be used after surgical treatment of an aural hematoma in a large-breed dog (a). Tape is placed on the margins of the ear, and the ear is rotated to the dorsal aspect of the head in a comfortable position (b). Gauze sponges are placed on the top of the head in contact with the convex surface of the ear and on the incision that was made over the aural hematoma (c). The tape attached to the ear margins is wrapped around the neck to secure the gauze sponges in place (d). Cast padding is wrapped around the gauze sponges/ear and the neck (e). A final outer layer is used to keep the pressure-wrap tightly adhered to the ear (f).

vi. The prognosis with surgery in these cases is favorable.

d. Peripheral vestibular disease:

  i. Direct neuronal damage from fractures to the petrous temporal bone or tympanic bulla can result in vestibular signs. In addition, abscessation secondary to ear canal separations or bite wounds may result in inner ear disease and subsequent signs of peripheral vestibular disorder may be noted.

  ii. Clinical signs such as ataxia, head tilt, turning in tight circles, and/or horizontal or rotatory nystagmus may be noted with trauma-induced peripheral vestibular disease. Signs of peripheral vestibular disease should be differentiated from signs of central vestibular disease. Central vestibular disease may be a more likely differential when vertical nystagmus, proprioceptive and postural reaction deficits, and deficits in cranial nerves V, VII, IX–XII are present.

iii. One study reported that of 83 cases of peripheral vestibular syndrome, 7 (8%) occurred secondary to trauma (Schunk, 1983).

iv. Treatment of these cases is supportive as long as no concurrent injury requiring surgery is present:

    1. Nausea can be treated with antihistamines or alpha-2 receptor antagonists. Cats tend to have a better response to alpha-2 receptor antagonists than antihistamines.

        a. Meclizine: 25 mg PO q24h (dogs), 12.5 mg PO q24h (cats).

        b. Diphenhydramine: 2–4 mg/kg PO, IM q8h (dogs, cats).

        c. Chlorpromazine: 0.5 mg/kg IM, SC q6-8h (dogs, cats).

        d. Maropitant: 1 mg/kg IM, 2 mg/kg PO q24h (dogs).

    2. Keep pet in a padded area to prevent injury from falls due to ataxia.

v. Prognosis is good if dysfunction affects only the peripheral nervous system; however, the time for recovery is variable depending on the extent of the trauma, and several months may be required to see improvement of clinical signs.

e. Facial neuropathy:

i. The facial nerve innervates the superficial muscles of the head and face, including the auricular muscles and the caudal aspect of the digastricus muscle. The facial nerve also supplies the parasympathetic preganglionic neurons to the sublingual and mandibular salivary glands, nasal and lacrimal glands and sensation to the concave portion of the external ear.

ii. Signs associated with facial neuropathy include ptyalism, lack of movement of the ear, lip (droop) and eyelid (ptosis), loss of blink, and/or keratoconjunctivitis sicca (KCS).

iii. In a large retrospective study of animals with facial neuropathy, 14% of dog cases and 44% of cat cases were thought to occur secondary to surgical or nonsurgical trauma. Of the cases of nonidiopathic facial neuropathy, 55% and 58% of the cases of facial neuropathy were secondary to trauma in dogs and cats, respectively. Twenty-five percent of dogs and 44% of cats with facial neuropathy developed concurrent signs of vestibular disease (Kern, 1987).

iv. With conditions that require total ear canal ablation (TECA) and lateral bulla osteotomy, facial nerve dysfunction can be seen postoperatively. Twelve to 36% of dogs and 56–78% of cats have been shown to develop facial nerve dysfunction after TECA surgery (White, 1990; Devitt, 1997; Bacon, 2003; Doyle, 2004).

v. With traumatic facial neuropathy, recovery of facial nerve function is dependent on the extent of injury. Weeks to months may be required to see any improvement in signs. If avulsion or severance of the nerve occurs, clinical signs are likely irreversible.

vi. Treatment of facial neuropathy is supportive and consists of monitoring the patient for worsening of clinical signs at which point further diagnostics may be necessary. If KCS occurs, apply an artificial tear solution topically 4–6 times daily. Because KCS occurs secondary to trauma in this scenario rather than an immune-mediated condition, the use of cyclosporine will be of no benefit.

f. Horner's syndrome:

i. Sympathetic nerve fibers pass through the middle ear of dogs and cats and thus are susceptible to trauma affecting this area.

ii. Signs consistent with Horner's syndrome such as miosis, enophthalmos, protrusion of the third eyelid, and ptosis can be seen.

iii. Other reported causes of Horner's syndrome include intracranial lesions, otitis, cervical trauma or myelopathy, brachial plexus injuries, thoracic trauma, and thoracic masses. In many older dogs with Horner's syndrome, the condition may be idiopathic.

iv. Traumatic uveitis can often have many of the same signs as Horner's syndrome and these processes should be differentiated. Important differentiating features seen with traumatic uveitis include blepharospasm, photophobia, the presence of aqueous flare in the anterior chamber, and low intraocular pressures (see Chapter 15: Trauma-Associated Ocular Injury).

v. In one study, blunt vehicular trauma was the most common cause of Horner's syndrome in dogs and one of the two most common causes in cats. That study did not comment on the specific sympathetic nerve fibers that were damaged, however, and some of the patients had Horner's syndrome related to brachial plexus injury (Kern, 1989).

vi. Horner's syndrome can be seen after TECA surgery. This has been rarely documented in dogs; however, due to increased exposure of the sympathetic nerve fibers, 42% of cats can develop Horner's syndrome postoperatively (Bacon, 2003).

vii. As with facial neuropathy, treatment for trauma-induced Horner's syndrome consists of monitoring the patient for worsening of clinical signs.

g. Hearing loss:

i. The method generally employed to definitively judge hearing ability in companion animals is the brainstem auditory-evoked response (BAER):

    1. Simply stated, the BAER test measures the recordings of activity in the vestibulo-cochlear nerve and the auditory portion of the brainstem in response to sensory stimuli.

    2. The hearing threshold can be determined by use of the BAER technique, and hearing loss can be noted after trauma that affects this pathway.

ii. With tympanic membrane perforation, some hearing loss may occur:

    1. The tympanic membrane may heal and hearing ability may return to normal.

    2. In humans, it has been shown that damage to the ossicles of the middle ear results in more significant hearing loss than when only the tympanic membrane is perforated.

BIBLIOGRAPHY

Bacon NJ, Gilbert RL, Bostock DE, *et al.* Total ear canal ablation in the cat: indications, morbidity and long-term survival. *J Small Anim Pract* 2003; 44: 430–434.

Boothe HW, Hobson HP. Traumatic separation of auricular and annular cartilages in three dogs (abstract). *Vet Surg* 1992; 384.

Devitt CM, Seim HB, Willer R, *et al.* Passive drainage versus primary closure after total ear canal ablation-lateral bulla osteotomy in dogs: 59 dogs (1985–1995). *Vet Surg* 1997; 26: 210–216.

Doyle RS, Skelly C, Bellenger CR. Surgical management of 43 cases of chronic otitis externa in the dog. *Irish Vet J* 2004; 57: 22–30.

Dubielzig RR, Wilson JW, Seireg AA. Pathogenesis of canine aural hematomas. *J Am Vet Med Assoc* 1984; 185: 873–875.

Dvir E, Kirberger, Terblanche AG. Magnetic resonance imaging of otitis media in a dog. *Vet Radiol Ultrasound* 2000; 41: 46–49.

Dye TL, Teague D, Ostwald, *et al.* Evaluation of a technique using the carbon dioxide laser for the treatment of aural hematomas. *J Am Anim Hosp Assoc* 2002; 38: 385–390.

Fullington RJ, Otto CM. Characteristics and management of gunshot wounds in dogs and cats: 84 cases (1986–1995). *J Am Vet Med Assoc* 1997; 210: 658–662.

Garosi LS, Lamb CR, Targett MP. MRI findings in a dog with otitis media and suspected otitis interna. *Vet Rec* 2000; 146: 501–502.

Getty R, Foust, HL, Presley ET, *et al.* Macroscopic anatomy of the ear of the dog. *Am J Vet Res* 1956; 17: 364–375.

Hoskinson JJ. Imaging techniques in the diagnosis of middle ear disease. *Semi Vet Med Surg (Small Anim)* 1993; 8: 10–16.

Joyce JA. Treatment of canine aural haematoma using an indwelling drain and corticosteroids. *J Small Anim Pract* 1994; 35: 341–344.

Joyce JA, Day MJ. Immunopathogenesis of canine aural hematoma. *J Small Anim Pract* 1997; 38: 152–158.

Kagan KG. Treatment of canine aural hematoma with an indwelling drain. *J Am Vet Med Assoc* 1983; 183: 972–974.

Kern TJ, Erb HN. Facial neuropathy in dogs and cats: 95 cases (1975–1985). *J Am Vet Med Assoc* 1987; 191: 1604–1609.

Kern TJ, Aromando MC, Erb HN. Horner's syndrome in dogs and cats: 100 cases (1975–1985). *J Am Vet Med Assoc* 1989; 195: 369–373.

Kolata RJ, Kraut NH, Johnston DE. Patterns of trauma in urban dogs and cats: a study of 1,000 cases. *J Am Vet Med Assoc* 1974; 165: 499–502.

Kolata RJ, Johnston DE. Motor vehicle accidents in urban dogs: a study of 600 cases. *J Am Vet Med Assoc* 1975; 167: 938–941.

Kuwahara J. Canine and feline aural hematoma: clinical, experimental and clinicopathologic observations. *Am J Vet Res* 1986; 47: 2300–2308.

Lanz OI, Wood BC. Surgery of the ear and pinna. *Vet Clin North Am Small* 2004; 34: 567–599.

Leftwich MW. Cyanoacrylate adhesive for aural hematoma. *Vet Med* 1981; 76: 1155.

Love NE, Kramer RW, Spodnick GJ. Radiographic and computed tomographic evaluation of otitis media in the dog. *Vet Radiol Ultrasound* 1995; 36: 375–379.

McCarthy PE, McCarthy RJ. Surgery of the ear. *Vet Clin North Am Small* 1994; 24: 953–969.

McCarthy PE, Hosgood G, Pechman RD. Traumatic ear canal separations and para-aural abscessation in three dogs. *J Am Anim Hosp Assoc* 1995; 31: 419–424.

Munro HMC, Thrusfield MV. 'Battered pets': non-accidental physical injuries found in dogs and cats. *J Small Anim Pract* 2001; 42: 279–290.

Remedios AM, Fowler JD, Pharr JW. A comparison of radiographic versus surgical diagnosis of otitis media. *J Am Anim Hosp Assoc* 1991; 27: 183–188.

Rose WR. Pinna trauma. *Vet Med* 1978; 73: 164–167.

Schunk LK. Disorders of the vestibular system. *Vet Clin North Am Small* 1988; 18: 641–665.

Schunk KL, Averill DR. Peripheral vestibular syndrome in the dog: a review of 83 cases. *J Am Vet Med Assoc* 1983; 182: 1354–1357.

Steiss JE, Boosinger TR, Wright JC, *et al.* Healing of experimentally perforated tympanic membranes demonstrated by electrodiagnostic testing and histopathology. *J Am Anim Hosp Assoc* 1992; 28: 307–310.

Sturges BK, Dickinson PJ, Kortz GD, *et al.* Clinical signs, magnetic resonance imaging features, and outcome after surgical and medical treatment of otogenic intracranial infection in 11 cats and 4 dogs. *J Vet Intern Med* 2006; 20: 648–656.

Swaim SF, Bradley DM. Evaluation of closed-suction drainage for treating auricular hematomas. *J Am Anim Hosp Assoc* 1996; 32: 36–43.

Weber HO. A technique for surgical treatment of aural hematoma in dogs and cats. *Vet Med* 1979; 74: 1271.

White RAS, Pomeroy CJ. Total ear canal ablation and lateral bulla osteotomy (TECA/LBO) in the dog: indications, complications and long-term results in 100 procedures (abstract). *Vet Surg* 1990; 1981.

Wilson JW. Treatment of auricular hematoma, using a teat tube. *J Am Vet Med Assoc* 1983; 182: 1081–1083.

Wilson WJ, Mills PC. Brainstem auditory-evoked response in dogs. *Am J Vet Res* 2005; 66: 2177–2187.

INDEX

Note: Bold and italic page number refer to figures and tables.

Manual of Trauma Management in the Dog and Cat, First Edition. Edited by Kenneth J. Drobatz, Matthew W. Beal and Rebecca S. Syring.
© 2011 John Wiley & Sons, Inc. Published 2011 by John Wiley & Sons, Inc.

Printed in the United States
By Bookmasters